THE
SKULL

VOLUME

3

THE
SKULL

VOLUME
3

Functional and Evolutionary Mechanisms

EDITED BY

JAMES HANKEN AND BRIAN K. HALL

THE UNIVERSITY OF CHICAGO PRESS

Chicago and London

James Hanken is associate professor in the Department of Environmental, Population, and Organismic Biology at the University of Colorado, Boulder.
Brian K. Hall is Izaak Walton Killam Research Professor and professor of biology at Dalhousie University.

The University of Chicago Press, Chicago 60637
The University of Chicago Press, Ltd., London
© 1993 by The University of Chicago
All rights reserved. Published 1993
Printed in the United States of America

02 01 00 99 98 97 96 95 94 93   5 4 3 2 1

ISBN (cloth): 0-226-31571-1
ISBN (paper): 0-226-31573-8

Library of Congress Cataloging-in-Publication Data

The Skull / edited by James Hanken and Brian K. Hall.
          p.   cm.
      Includes bibliographical references and index.
      Contents: v. 1. Development—v. 2. Patterns of structural and systematic diversity—v. 3. Functional and evolutionary mechanisms.
      1. Skull Anatomy.   2. Skull—Evolution.   3. Anatomy, Comparative.
I. Hanken. James.   II. Hall, Brian Keith, 1941–.
      [DNLM: 1. Skull—anatomy & histology.   2. Skull—growth & development.   3. Skull physiology.   WE   705   S6291
QL822.S58   1993
596'.04'71—dc20
DNLM/DLC
for Library of Congress   92-49119
                                                                                      CIP

CONTENTS

VOLUME 3

Functional and Evolutionary Mechanisms

VOLUME 1

Development

VOLUME 2

Patterns of Structural and Systematic Diversity

PREFACE

JAMES HANKEN AND BRIAN K. HALL

This is the third in the series of three volumes on the vertebrate skull. It builds on the foundation laid by the preceding two volumes (*Development*, and *Patterns of Structural and Systematic Diversity*) in keeping with the general aims for the series overall: (a) to organize and present the results of recent studies of skull development and structure in such a way as to be of interest to specialists as well as to vertebrate morphologists generally; (b) to evaluate the implications of these results for fundamental questions in vertebrate structure and evolution; (c) to examine current studies of the functional bases and constraints of skull form; (d) to use the vertebrate skull to illustrate evolutionary patterns and processes and to test hypotheses to account for them; and (e) to promote further interest and research in these and related issues.

The present volume deals with the vertebrate skull both in the context of its function and in relation to the ecological and evolutionary mechanisms that underlie cranial diversity. These are two of the most active and exciting areas of investigation in cranial biology at the present time. The ten chapters comprise four related themes. Chapter 1 (Hanken and Hall) links this volume with the first two by discussing the role of developmental factors in mediating cranial diversification, and by emphasizing the need to integrate developmental and populational approaches in the study of cranial evolution. Chapters 2–6 address specific and prominent skull functions, namely feeding (Sanderson and Wassersug, Lauder and Shaffer, and Smith), locomotion (Wake), and hearing and sound transmission (Lombard and Hetherington). Three chapters are devoted to feeding because of the tremendous structural and functional diversity of the trophic apparatus in vertebrates, which exerts a predominant influence on skull design, and the fundamentally different problems posed by feeding in water versus on land. Chapters 7 (Weishampel) and 8 (Russell and Thomason) are concerned with the methodology for mechanical analysis of skull structure and function, as well as the practical limitations of these methods. They reveal how new engineering approaches have offered insights, and in some instances, solutions, into classical problems of skull design and evolution. The final two chapters address mechanisms of cranial evolution. Chapter 9 (Emerson and Bramble) emphasizes the importance of absolute size and size change for the evolution of cranial design and function, whereas chapter 10 (Liem) is primarily concerned with the interplay of ecology and morphology in cranial diversification. As in earlier volumes, chapters in this volume generally are intended to be synthetic overviews of a given topic, not exhaustive reviews. However, in chapter 2, on suspension feeding, and chapter 5, on locomotion, a more comprehensive treatment proved to be the only effective way to synthesize a widely scattered literature.

As an integrated whole, this volume provides an overview of a number of important and diverse functions of the vertebrate skull and relates these functions to patterns of cranial development and growth, as well as to ecological and evolutionary constraints, processes, and opportunities. In doing so, it offers a functional context for the treatments of skull development and diversity provided in the preceding two volumes. It is undeniably the most eclectic of the three volumes in this series. We would argue, however, that this is indicative of the field of functional and evolutionary morphology itself, where there is a wide range of research questions, analytical paradigms, and methodological approaches and techniques (Liem and Wake 1985). The volume does not cover all of these paradigms or approaches, or even all cranial functions, among other reasons because to do so would take several volumes in itself. More important, function and evolutionary mechanisms are arguably the most poorly understood of the three main areas of cranial biology covered in this series, and a truly comprehensive treatment is not possible at this time, however desirable. Rather, these chapters are intended to convey a sense of the range of topics, paradigms, and approaches that are being considered at present; in other words, what can or even should be done, and how. In this regard, many of the chapters focus on the authors' own work, as examples of the analysis of major problems. Consequently, the topics considered give an accurate assessment and representation of current interest and knowledge of skull function.

As in earlier volumes, we are pleased to thank the authors of the present volume for their excellent contributions.

REFERENCES

Liem, K. F., and D. B. Wake. 1985. Morphology: Current approaches and concepts. In *Functional Vertebrate Morphology,* M. Hildebrand, D. M. Bramble, K. F. Liem, and D. B. Wake, eds. Cambridge: Harvard University Press. pp. 366–377.

1

Mechanisms of Skull Diversity and Evolution

JAMES HANKEN AND BRIAN K. HALL

INTRODUCTION

THIS VOLUME ATTESTS TO the breadth of current interest and inquiry into the function and evolution of the vertebrate skull. One cannot come away from reading the following chapters without a great appreciation of the adaptive diversity of cranial form and function. They also reveal the need to consider the function and evolution of the skull in their proper context, whether this be the suite of nonskeletal cranial tissues with which the skull is functionally, anatomically, and developmentally integrated, or related aspects of behavior, physiology, and ecology.

We begin this broad, interdisciplinary approach with a brief consideration of the mechanisms for the evolution of cranial diversity. In particular, we concern ourselves with two aspects that we consider to be particularly important: the role of development, and particularly the embryonic neural crest from which much of the skull is derived; and the nature of intraspecific variability, and its role in morphological diversification. Both aspects are relatively poorly known in the context of cranial evolution, but we believe that a comprehensive understanding of the mechanisms of morphological diversification of the skull—indeed, of any structure—must incorporate them. In focusing on them here, we also hope to underscore the need for more work in each area.

SKULL DEVELOPMENT

The diversity of form displayed by the vertebrate skull is, on the one hand, great (compare the skull of the elephant with that of a shrew, a snake with that of a bird) and, on the other hand, limited—all vertebrate skulls are built upon the same basic plan. The fundamental structural similarity is a reflection of conservative developmental processes within and among vertebrate taxa. In this section, we deal with those fundamental developmental processes—the neural crest origin of much of the vertebrate skull, the epigenetic evocation of skull differentiation through tissue (epithelial-mesenchymal) and functional interactions, and the mechanisms for cranial patterning. It is these processes and their stability/modification during vertebrate phylogeny that provide the ontogenetic basis for both phylogenetic stability and for diversity of the vertebrate skull.

The Contribution of the Neural Crest to the Skull

The neural crest was first described by Wilhelm His in 1868 when he reported the existence of a specialized zone of cells between the neural and epidermal ectoderms at the boundary of the future neural tube (i.e., in the crests of the neural folds) in neurula-stage chick embryos. In the years since its discovery, our view of the neural crest and of neural crest cells has progressed from surprise, through mistrust, ridicule, heresy, ignorance, indifference, reawakening, reevaluation, reinvestigation, and orthodoxy, to the current enthronement of the neural crest as a quintessential vertebrate character (Hall 1988b; Gans 1993). As these authors indicate: "this embryonic tissue [the neural crest] (and the ectodermal neurogenic placodes) represents the common denominator for vertebrate synapomorphies" (Gans 1993 2:17); "The neural crest as part and parcel of a dorsal nerve cord and notochord is a quintessential vertebrate characteristic, or according to some *the* quintessential vertebrate characteristic" (Hall 1988b, 19–20).

The first challenge to orthodoxy, especially with regard to the origin and development of the skull, came from the studies of Kastschenko (1888) and Goronowitsch (1892, 1893a, b) who argued that some cranial mesenchyme in shark, fish, and bird embryos arose not from mesoderm, but from cells derived from the neural crest (de Beer 1947). Although unexpected, these studies did not occasion the controversy that followed Platt's (1893, 1897) assertion that the visceral arch cartilages of *Necturus* also arose from ectoderm, either neural crest or placodal head ectoderm. This heretical notion of an ectodermal origin of a skeletal (mesodermal) tissue, and its challenge to the firm grasp that the germ layer theory held on late-nineteenth-century biology and biologists, has been discussed elsewhere (Oppenheimer 1940; de Beer 1947; Hörstadius 1950; Hall 1988b).

Fortunately, prevailing orthodoxy did not discourage persistent and enquiring experimental embryologists from pursuing the problem of the origin of the head skeleton. Platt, on the basis of differences in yolk between ecto- and mesodermal cells, assigned the origin of the visceral arch cartilages to placodal ectoderm. A more comprehensive analysis of *Ambystoma jeffersonianum* by Landacre (1921) assigned the neural crest as the chondrogenic source; provided the first mapping of individual skeletal elements (the anterior aspects of the cranial base [trabeculae cranii] and visceral arch cartilages, except the second basibranchial, derived from the neural crest; the balance of the skull from mesoderm); and gave the first indication that the viscerocranial skeleton had a dual origin, arising in part from neural crest–derived and in part from mesodermally derived mesenchyme.

Descriptive studies being equivocal, Stone (1922, 1926, 1929), Raven (1931, 1936) and Harrison (1935a–c, 1938) extirpated neural crest from, and exchanged neural crests between, urodele and frog embryos. Using these techniques they mapped the migratory pathways of neural crest cells and confirmed the neural crest origins of viscerocranial cartilages. They further demonstrated that trunk neural crest cells could not substitute for extirpated cranial cells to prevent skeletal deficiencies—the now well-known dichotomy between the skeletogenic and odontogenic cranial neural crest and nonskeletogenic and nonodontogenic trunk neural crest (but see Smith and Hall [1990] for a reevaluation of this dichotomy).

Subsequent detailed analysis by Hörstadius and Sellman (1941, 1946), Chibon (1964, 1966, 1967, 1974) and Sadaghiani and Thiébaud (1987) have mapped the neural crest origin of the larval skulls and visceral arch skeletons of two urodeles (*Ambystoma mexicanum, Pleurodeles waltl*) and one anuran (*Xenopus laevis*). This neural crest contribution to amphibian skull development has now been extended to representatives of all classes of vertebrates (see Hall 1987b, 1988b for summaries). The major (in some cases the only) studies for each taxon are as follows:

Cyclostomes (lampreys): Damas (1944, 1951); Johnels (1948); Newth (1950, 1951, 1956); Langille and Hall (1986, 1988b, 1989b).

Teleosts: Matsumoto et al. (1983); Langille and Hall (1987, 1988a)

Reptiles: Toerien (1965a, b) (For the neural crest origin of cranial mesenchyme in turtles and alligators see Meier and Packard [1984] and Ferguson [1984, 1985].)

Birds: Johnston (1966), Le Lièvre (1971a, b, 1974, 1976, 1978); Le Lièvre and Le Douarin 1974, 1975); Noden (1978a, 1984); Johnston et al. (1979)

Mammals: Johnston and Hazelton (1972); Johnston et al. (1981); Tan and Morriss-Kay (1986); Morriss-Kay and Tan (1987); Smits-van Prooije et al. (1987, 1988) (For references on the neural crest origin of cranial mesenchyme in mammals see Hall [1988b, 62–72].)

Rather than provide an exhaustive list of elements of the skull and visceral skeleton derived from the neural crest (for which the papers and reviews listed above and Langille and Hall's chapter in volume 1 may be consulted), we utilize the scheme shown in figure 1.1, which depicts the regionalization (rostro-caudal extent) of the neural crest that forms the chondrocranial and visceral arch skeletons in a variety of vertebrates. It is very clear that regionalization of the skeletogenic neural crest is a highly

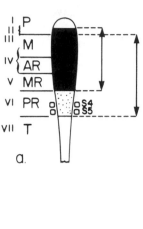

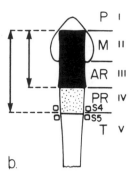

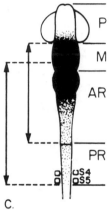

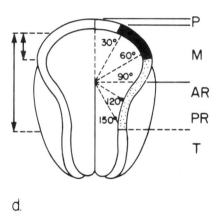

Fig. 1.1. Constancy of regionalization of the skeletogenic neural crest in (a)
Petromyzon marinus (a lamprey), (b) *Oryzias latipes* (the Japanese medaka, a teleost
fish), (c) *Gallus domesticus* (the common fowl), and (d) *Ambystoma mexicanum* and
Pleurodeles waltl (two urodele amphibians). Chondrocranial neural crest is shown in
black, viscerocranial neural crest is stippled; both are demarked by double-headed
arrows. The skeletogenic cranial neural crest extends from the anterior mesencephalon
(mid-prosencephalon in *P. marinus*) caudad to the level of somites 4 or 5 (S5, S5).
Other abbreviations: AR, anterior rhombencephalon; M, mesencephalon; MR, mid-
rhombencephalon; P, prosencephalon; PR, posterior rhombencephalon; T, trunk
neural crest. Roman numerals I–VII in (a) and I–V in (b) refer to boundaries of
regions excised to generate fate maps. The angles from the midline in (d) represent
sectors of neural crest excised from *P. waltl* by Chibon (1966, 1967), projected onto
the fate map for *A. mexicanum*. Reproduced from Hall (1988b) with permission of
the publisher.

TABLE 1.1   Regionalization of the skeletogenic neural crest in the lamprey, *Petromyzon marinus*, in relation to the rostro-caudal regions I to VII shown in figure 1.

	I	II	III	Regions IV	V	VI	VII
Trabeculae	√	√	√	√	√		
Branchial arches							
1–3			√√	√√	√√	√	
4 & 5			√	√√	√√	√√	
6 & 7				√	√√	√√	

Note: Single checks indicate only a minor contribution from this region.

conserved vertebrate feature; skeletogenic neural crest extends in all taxa from the anterior mesencephalon caudad to the level of somite 5. Although chondrocranial neural crest lies rostral to viscerocranial crest, the two regions overlap substantially. Regionalization is also evident *within* the chondrocranial and viscerocranial neural crest; more anterior elements arise from rostral, and more posterior elements from caudal, neural crest (table 1.1). (We have, however, minimal knowledge of how the neural crest itself is specified—see Hall [1988b] and Thomson [1988] for some discussion).

We take this rostro-caudal regionalization of the neural crest, the source of much of the cranial skeleton, to be a fundamental, ancient feature (synapomorphy) of the vertebrates (Langille and Hall 1989a). This dictates how we currently evaluate developmental mechanisms underlying diversity and evolution of the vertebrate skull.

Tissue Interactions in Skull Development

The skull arises epigenetically, largely through cell and tissue (epithelial-mesenchymal) interactions and through the action of adjacent nonskeletal tissues. It was in the pioneering study by Hörstadius and Sellman (1946) mapping the skeletogenic neural crest of *Ambystoma mexicanum* that evidence for induction of cranial cartilage by epithelia was obtained, viz. neural crest–derived visceral arch cartilage by pharyngeal endoderm and mesodermally derived otic capsule cartilage by otic vesicle epithelium. Such interactions have chiefly been studied in anuran amphibians (Holtfreter 1968; Cusimano-Carollo 1963, 1969, 1972; Cusimano et al. 1962), in urodeles [Wagner 1949; Okada 1955; Rollhaüser-ter-Horst 1977; Cassin and Capuron 1979; Corsin 1975; Drews et al. 1972; Epperlein and Lehmann 1975; Minuth and Grunz 1980; Graveson and Armstrong 1987), and in birds (Schowing 1968; Tyler and Hall 1977; Hall and Tremaine 1979; Bee and Thorogood 1980; Thorogood 1981; Thorogood and Smith 1984) (see Hall 1987b, 1988a for reviews). As known in greatest detail for the embryonic chick, every cartilage and bone in the developing skull

TABLE 1.2   Epithelia involved in the epithelial-mesenchymal interactions required for differentiation of the components of the viscerocranial and chondrocranial skeletons of the embryonic chick

Skeletal component	Epithelium
angular	mandibular arch epithelium
basisphenoid	rhombencephalon, notochord
dentary	mandibular arch epithelium
frontal	prosencephalon, mesencephalon, cranial ectoderm
maxilla	maxillary arch epithelium
Meckel's cartilage	dorsal cranial ectoderm
occipital	rhombencephalon
otic capsular cartilage	otic vesicle epithelium
palatine	palatal epithelium
parasphenoid	notochord
parietal	mesencephalon, rhombencephalon
pterygoid	palatal epithelium
scleral cartilage	pigmented retinal epithelium
scleral ossicles	scleral epithelial papillae
squamosal	mesencephalon
surangular	mandibular arch epithelium

Note: See Hall (1987b) for information on the timing of these interactions and for the primary literature.

depends for its differentiation on one or more epithelial-mesenchymal interactions (table 1.2). Discussion of the mechanism of these interactions, which is outside the scope of this paper, may be found in Hall (1987a, 1988a, 1989).

The timing of these epithelial-mesenchymal interactions is not constant throughout the vertebrates for, on the one hand, neural crest cells at different stages in their migration, and on the other hand, different epithelia, are involved in the interactions. That this is so for different skeletal elements in the same embryo is not surprising (table 1.2). For example, the dentary and the frontal arise from different neural crest cell populations which are differentially localized along the neural axis, migrate along different paths, and settle at different sites. Inevitably, these populations encounter different epithelial environments—cranial ectoderm, pharyngeal endoderm, and mandibular arch epithelium encountered by dentary mesenchyme; cranial ectoderm and mesencephalic neural ectoderm encountered by frontal mesenchyme.

However, divergence in time, space, and components involved in epithelial-mesenchymal interactions is also seen when development of the same skeletal element is compared across taxa, the best-documented examples being those interactions involved in the differentiation of Meckel's cartilage in urodele and anuran amphibians, birds, and mammals (Hall 1984, 1987b). Here we have, in representatives of each of these groups, a homologous structure arising from neural crest cells from the same rostro-caudal region of the neural crest, which follow similar migration pathways and encounter similar epithelia, but where the epithelium required for chondroblast differentiation varies from group to group. The active epithelium is cranial ectoderm adjacent to the neural tube in the embryonic chick, pharyngeal endoderm in anuran and urodele amphibians, and mandibular arch epithelium in the fetal mouse (fig. 1.2). What has altered or shifted during the evolution of amphibians, birds, and mammals apparently is not the neural crest component of the epithelial-mesenchymal interaction, but rather the epithelium providing the signal to which the neural crest–derived cells respond. Changes in the epithelia that evoke chondrogenic differentiation must relate to aspects of skull development other than basic structure, for basic chondrocranial form, including that of Meckel's cartilage, is largely conserved throughout the vertebrates.

Why should development of Meckel's cartilage in avian embryos require that the chondroblasts be specified earlier than in mammals or amphibians? Does the answer lie (a) in the amount of *in ovo* growth of Meckel's cartilage required to produce an elongated beak capable of func-

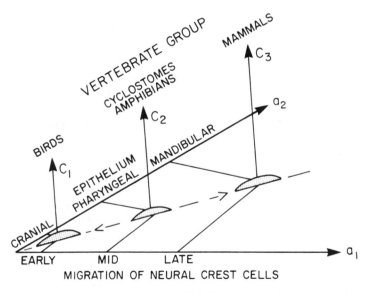

Fig. 1.2. Variation in the timing of the epithelial-mesenchymal interaction that initiates differentiation of Meckel's cartilage in amphibians, birds, and mammals, in terms of both the time during neural crest cell migration when the interaction occurs (a_1) and the epithelium involved in the interaction (a_2). If the amphibian condition is taken as primitive for extant tetrapods, then the interaction has been moved earlier in development during the evolution of birds (C_1) and later in development during the evolution of mammals (C_3). Modified from Hall (1984).

tioning immediately after hatching (Meckel's cartilage "controls" mandibular growth; Diewert 1982), extension of the time between epithelial-mesenchymal interactions and differentiation allowing more cells to be specified as chondroblasts, (b) in the fact that Meckel's cartilage persists unossified in many birds (except for the retroarticular process) but is transformed into ligaments or translated into ear ossicles in mammals, or (c) in some other aspect of avian mandibular development?

A parallel evolutionary change to that just described for Meckel's cartilage has been revealed by experiments transplanting facial ectoderm of anuran and urodelan embryos. The inability of anuran embryos to form a balancer and of urodele embryos to form an adhesive organ results from evolutionary changes in the epithelial rather than the mesenchymal component of the interactions. Thus, urodele epithelium can elicit development of a balancer from anuran mesenchyme and anuran epithelium can elicit development of an adhesive organ from urodelan mesenchyme (Spemann 1938, 350–366).

As epithelial-mesenchymal interactions determine the number of mesenchymal cells that will be able to differentiate into a particular cell type (chondroblasts) to make a particular skeletal element (Meckel's cartilage) at a particular site (the mandibular arch; Hall 1988a), the timing, duration, and/or strength of the interaction influences when the skeletal element arises in ontogeny and the extent of its subsequent growth. Variations in timing, duration, and strength of these interactions provide mechanisms for evolutionary change through heterochrony (Hall 1984; Smith and Hall 1990). Epithelial-mesenchymal interactions, however, are not isolated, single events. A cascade of inductive interactions has been demonstrated in the frog *Discoglossus pictus,* and in the urodele *Pleurodeles waltl,* such that, during jaw development, specification of chondroblasts is required before osteoblasts can arise, which in turn must be specified before teeth can form (see summary in Hall 1987b, 1988b). We do not know the cascades in other vertebrates (and indeed have only brief glimpses of the amphibian cascade) but it is clear that alteration in timing of the first step, specification of chondroblasts, could have a ripple effect on the subsequent development of other tissues. Alterations in the timing of even one epithelial-mesenchymal interaction involved in development of even a single skull element, must, on the one hand, be assessed in the context of such "epigenetic cascades," and on the other hand, provide a developmental mechanism for generating diversity during skull development (Hall 1988b; Smith and Hall 1990).

Patterning of the Skull

What are the consequences for patterning of the skull by epigenetic evocation of mesodermal and neural crest cells?

The knowledge that (a) key vertebrate characteristics are a consequence of the evolution of the neural crest and ectodermal placodes (because these characters either develop directly from, or under the influence of, neural crest cells in the epigenetic cascades noted earlier) and that (b) the cranial mesenchyme, much of the skull, and the viscerocranial skeleton are formed exclusively from neural crest cells, leads to the obvious corollary that (c) the vertebrate head is a new structure, a neomorph (Gans and Northcutt 1983; Northcutt and Gans 1983; Gans 1993). Thus, the classic notion, the origins of which lie in Goethe's famous 1790 inspiration while gazing at a sheep's skull in a Venetian cemetery, that the head and skull represent the anterior continuation of a segmented neuronal, muscular, and vertebral pattern seen in the trunk, is no longer tenable. In fact, the sequence is quite the reverse, for, as emphasized by Gans (1993) and Smith and Hall (1990), a postotic skull, and indeed, a trunk skeleton consisting of ossified vertebrae, arose only with the evolution of the jawed vertebrates. For discussions of our changing views on head segmentation see Huxley (1898), Russell (1916), de Beer (1937), Hall and Hanken (1985), and Gans (1993).

Cranial segmentation is confined to the neuromeres and myogenic somitomeres (Jacobson 1987). There is no evidence for segmentation of the cranial, nor indeed of the trunk neural crest, although as indicated in figure 1.1, cranial neural crest is regionalized on the basis of the arches to which mesenchyme migrates and of the neuro- and vicerocranial skeletal elements that arise from these regions: the neural crest is patterned but not segmented.

The recent mapping of homeobox genes in the mouse head indicates that *En-1* is distributed throughout the rostro-caudal extent of the neural tube, *En-2* is confined to mesencephalic and rostral metencephalic neural tube, and *Hox 1.5* and *2.1* do not extend more rostrally than the pre- and postotic myelencephalon respectively (Holland 1988; Holland and Hogan 1988). Homeobox gene distribution is regionalized and segmented, and this regionalization extends to the neural crest. No regionalization of the cranial mesoderm, however, has been found.

Does regionalization of the neural crest reflect a restricted morphogenetic capability with respect to ability to form specific components of the skull? Perhaps the situation is like that of the developing nervous system during neurulation, in which cells along the entire length of the neural axis undergo an equivalent cytodifferentiation into neurons, but where those neurons, because of inductions related to their position along the neural axis, organize themselves into distinct regions of the nervous system: fore-, mid-, hindbrain and spinal cord. If neural crest cells share this property with neuronal cells, then neural crest cells along the rostro-caudal extent of the cranial neural crest may possess a shared capability of cytodifferentiation into chondroblasts (which they do) but a restricted capability for the chondrocranial elements that they could form. Alternatively, morphogenetic specificity may be resident within these cells before they leave the neural tube, as the evidence of Wagner (1949), Hörstadius (1950), and Noden (1978a, 1984) suggests (see Hörstadius [1950] and Thorogood [1993] for discussions of these alternatives).

Thorogood et al. (1986) and Thorogood (1988, 1993) have demonstrated a spatial and temporal heterogeneity in the distribution of type II collagen along the neuroepithelium that corresponds to the sites of chondrocranial capsule formation and have argued that neural crest cells encountering this type II collagen during migration will receive the primary signal in specification of chondrocranial patterning, i.e., that irrespective of level along the cranial neural axis, neural cells that become trapped in particular sites should be able to produce a chondrocranial element appropriate to that site. As Thorogood puts it: "The (neuro) epithelium simply specifies, to a responsive mesenchyme where and when cartilage should form. Viewed in this way, differential lineage composition of 'homologous' skeletal elements, in terms of ectomesenchymal or mesodermal contributions, becomes largely irrelevant" (Thorogood 1988, 152).

This interpretation assumes no site-specificity in the epithelial-mesenchymal interactions that initiate or promote chondrogenesis, an issue that is currently unresolved (Hall 1986, 1988c, 1991). In fact, much of the facial ectoderm, at least in the avian embryo, arises from the most rostral region of the prosencephalic neural folds (Couly and Le Douarin 1987, 1988), a site consistent with the possibility that facial ectoderm may itself be regionalized during primary embryonic induction of the neural ectoderm.

Thus, there appears to be a hierarchy of epigenetic processes explaining both stability of basic skull form and diversity upon that basic theme. The localization of type II collagen provides a means of trapping cells that are migrating from the regionalized neural crest, thereby ensuring stability of basic chondrocranial form across the vertebrates. A diversity of subsequent tissue interactions, and their modification through heterochrony, permits variation on that basic structural scheme.

INTRASPECIFIC VARIATION

The Relevance of Intraspecific Variation

As emphasized in the previous section, knowledge of development offers valuable insights into the organismal mechanisms that may in some instances constrain, and in other instances facilitate, morphological diversification. Yet, an understanding of how cranial morphology evolves requires more than simply identifying embryonic tissues and eludicating developmental processes, or even using this information to delineate the potential range of organic form. Developmental events must also be linked to interspecific differences. In other words, it is also necessary to resolve how structural variation at the level of developmental processes translates into morphological variation among taxa. We consider this to be one of the most important challenges facing future investigators of the vertebrate skull. Valuable information may come from studies of the nature, extent, and causes of intraspecific variation in natural populations.

Remarkably little, however, is known about naturally occurring intraspecific variation in the cranium. This is especially surprising in view of the enormous literature dealing with, on the one hand, mechanisms of skull development and growth (see volume 1, this series), and, on the other, patterns of cranial diversity among taxa (volume 2). Moreover, much of the data that exist have been amassed in the context of taxonomic investigations where the primary interest has been to define the limits of variability for the purposes of delimiting taxa; there have been few studies of variation per se, including its nature, range, developmental/genetic basis, or ecological/evolutionary causes.

Perhaps the variation that is of most interest and relevance in the context of mechanisms of cranial diversity involves so-called discontinuous variants (Falconer 1981); that is, variation not simply involving mensural variables but characterized by discrete and often large-scale differences between variants, and which is largely independent of sex, age, and adult body size. Several examples of discontinuous, intraspecific variation involving cranial characters are listed in table 1.3. This list is neither comprehensive nor necessarily representative of the range or nature of variation within particular groups or among vertebrates generally. It is simply intended to convey some idea of the potentially enormous variability that exists in nature. Most of the examples, documented only in the last 10–20 years, differ widely with respect to both the magnitude of morphological differences involved and their ecological and evolutionary significance, but they can be readily divided among three distinct classes of variation—gross malformations, epigenetic polymorphisms, and trophic polymorphisms.

Classes of Intraspecific Variation

Type 1: Gross Malformations. This class of variation includes teratologies, deformities, and other gross malformations that typically lie outside a species' developmental "norm of reaction" (Schmalhausen 1949) (table 1.3). An excellent example is cleft palate, a common congenital malformation in humans that is also found in other vertebrates, including many squamates (Bellairs and Boyd 1957; Bellairs 1965). Such variants are of considerable biomedical importance when occurring in humans, and they

TABLE 1.3 Intraspecific variation involving discontinuous characters in the skull

Variant type/taxon	Variable character	Reference
Type 1: Gross malformations		
Caretta caretta (R)[1]	partial cyclopia, monorhinia	Bellairs 1983
Natrix maura (R)	cyclopia	in den Bosch and Musters 1987
Eunectes murinus, Natrix natrix, Vipera berus, Lacerta spp. (R)	cleft palate	Bellairs 1965; Bellairs and Boyd 1957
Type 2: Epigenetic polymorphisms		
Amia calva (F)	parietal bones paired or fused; number of postorbital, infraorbital, and extrascapular bones; frequent asymmetry	Jain 1985
Osteolepis macrolepidatus (F)	numbers of parietal shields and intertemporal bones	Graham-Smith 1978
Salvelinus alpinus (F)	number of foramina; bone fusion	Medvedeva and Savvaitova 1981
Bolitoglossa occidentalis (A)	prefrontal bone present or absent	Alberch 1983
Notophthalmus viridescens (A)	branchial cartilages present or absent; atavisic epibranchials	Reilly 1987; Reilly and Lauder 1988
Rhyacotriton olympicus (A)	nasal bone present or absent	Wake 1980
Taricha granulosa (A)	branchial cartilages present or absent	Reilly 1987
Thorius spp. (A)	nasal, prefrontal, and septomaxilla bones present or absent; asymmetry	Hanken 1984
Geochelone radiata (R)	parietal foramen present or absent	Crumly 1982
Phrynosoma solare (R)	epipterygoid bone present or absent	Axtell 1986
Megapodius freycinet, Chamaepetes goudotii, Crax pauxi, C. rubra, Penelope purpurascens, Tympanuchus phasianellus, Callipepla californicus, Acryllium vulturinum, Guttera plumifera, G. pucherani, Numida meleagris, Opisthocomus hoazin, Corythaixoides leucogaster, Crinifer piscator, Tauraco erythrolophus, T. hartlaubi, T. schalowi, Guira guira, Centropus goliath (B)	number and pattern of scleral ossicles	de Queiroz and Good 1988

Species (group)[1]	Trait	References
Erethizon dorsatum (M)	number of interparietal (wormian) and squamosal bones; squamosal foramen present or absent; masticatory and buccinator foramina separate or joined	Sutton 1972
Homo sapiens (M)	number of foramina, bone fusions, etc. (29 variants); number of interparietal bones	Berry and Berry 1967; Berry 1968; Pal 1987; Pal et al. 1984
Mus musculus (M)	number of foramina, bone fusions, etc. (24 variants)	Berry 1968; Berry and Searle 1963
Sciurus carolinensis, Cavia porcellus, Lemmus lemmus, Microtus agrestis, Peromyscus maniculatus, Micromys minutus, Rattus spp. (M)	number of foramina, bone fusions, etc. (10–22 variants per species)	Berry and Searle 1963
Type 3: Trophic polymorphisms		
Cichlasoma managuense (F) *Cichlasoma minckleyi, C. citrinellum, C. haitiensis* (F)	skull dimorphism: obtusorostral vs. acutorostral[2]; skull and tooth dimorphism: papilliform vs. molariform	Meyer 1987; Sage and Selander 1975; Liem and Kaufman 1984; Kornfield et al. 1982; Meyer 1989, 1990a,b, 1991
Ilyodon spp. (F)	skull dimorphism: tapered vs. blunt	Turner and Grosse 1980; Grudzien and Turner 1984a,b
Poeciliopsis sp. (F)	dentary polymorphism	Vrijenhoek 1978; Levinton 1988; Roberts 1974
Saccodon spp. (F)	jaw and tooth polymorphism: 3–4 morphs per species	Collins and Cheek 1983; Powers 1907; Pierce et al. 1983; Rose and Armentrout 1976;
Ambystoma tigrinum (A)	larval skull dimorphism: cannibal vs. typical	Lannoo and Bachman 1984
Scaphiopus spp. (A)	skull dimorphism: cannibal vs. typical (includes keratinized mouth parts)	Orton 1954; Bragg 1965; Bragg and Bragg 1959; Pomeroy 1981
Chondrohierax uncinatus (B)	bill size dimorphism: large vs. small	Smith and Temple 1982
Pyrenestes spp. (B)	bill size dimorphism: large vs. small	Smith 1987, 1990a, b, c
Peromyscus maniculatus (M)	mandible dimorphism: woodland vs. grassland	Holbrook 1982

[1] Abbreviations denote major group, as follows: A, amphibian; B, bird; F, jawed fish; M, mammal; R, reptile.
[2] Variation between morphs is not discontinuous. Instead, morphs denote extreme endpoints of a morphological continuum.

often provide useful models for examining basic processes underlying skull development generally. However, the often considerable morphological changes involved typically confer a tremendous decrease in fitness and have no obvious present or even potential adaptive value. Thus, variants of this type are of doubtful prospective significance and are unlikely vehicles of subsequent evolutionary change.

Type 2: Epigenetic Polymorphisms. The second class of discontinuous variation involves typically subtle variability of one or a few characters per individual in which the range of character states lies within, and in fact may define, the norm of reaction for the species or higher group involved (table 1.3). This variation is the result of a complex interplay between genome and environment, both of which exert a strong influence in determining the structure(s) involved. Instances of such variation have been termed "epigenetic polymorphisms" (Berry and Searle 1963), in recognition of the predominant role of developmental processes in mediating the interaction between genome and environment and in establishing the discontinuous nature of the variation. Although the mode of inheritance has been documented in relatively few instances, discontinuous variation that is characteristic of epigenetic polymorphisms is generally believed to reflect a developmental threshold acting on a continuously variable genetic liability (Berry 1968; Falconer 1981; fig. 1.3). Examples include the variable presence or absence of particular bones (e.g., nasal in the Olympic salamander, *Rhyacotriton olympicus;* Wake 1980; fig. 1.4), occasional fusion of typically paired elements (e.g., parietals in the bowfin, *Amia calva;* Jain 1985; fig. 1.5), and variation in the absolute number of bones or foramina (e.g., the accessory maxillary foramen in the house mouse, *Mus musculus;* Berry and Searle 1963).

Variability of this kind is important in several respects. First is the very obvious fact that it demonstrates the capacity, and possibly even the propensity, for natural populations to sustain sometimes substantial intraspecific variation in discontinuous characters. In certain instances, alternate character states are as different as those that distinguish species or even higher taxa. This variation represents a pool of discrete, alternate phenotypes that may provide the basis for subsequent evolutionary change and morphological diversification. Moreover, because the initial appearance of variant phenotypes may typically be regarded as incidental to subtle changes in either the genome or the environment and unrelated to current adaptation (equals "exaptation" of Gould and Vrba [1982]), the problem of explaining the initial evolution of novel morphologies, especially in the context of natural selection, is minimized. At the same time, should a novel variant prove to be selectively advantageous, all the ingredients are on hand for a transition, via genetic assimilation, from the chance occurrence

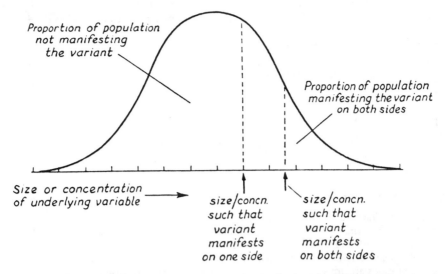

Fig. 1.3. Model for the developmental-genetic basis of epigenetic polymorphisms involving paired characters. The normal curve depicts the frequency distribution of a continuously varying genetic liability which, combined with two developmental thresholds, yields three variant classes in the population—absent, present on one side (i.e., asymmetry), present on both sides. (Reproduced with permission from Berry [1968].)

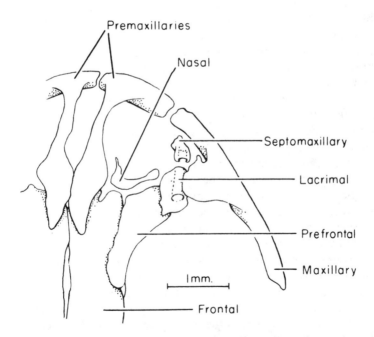

Figure 1.4. Nasal bone in the snout of the Olympic salamander, *Rhyacotriton olympicus* (dorsal view, right side). Of 16 specimens sampled from a single population, 8 had the bone on both sides, 7 had it on one side only, and 1 lacked it entirely. (Reproduced with permission from Wake [1980].)

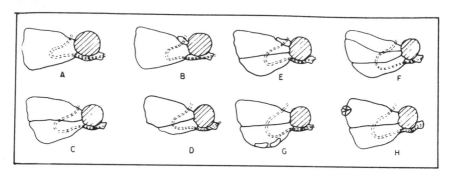

Figure 1.5. Variation in the number, size, and shape of postorbital bones in the skull of the bowfin, *Amia calva*. The modal number of postorbitals per side is 2 (n = 77 specimens), with a range from 1 to 3 or more and frequent asymmetry. Hatched circle denotes the orbit, dashed lines indicate the course of the lateral line sensory canal; all configurations are drawn as right sides. (Reproduced with permission from Jain [1985].)

of the variant in one or a few individuals to its incorporation as a characteristic feature of the entire population (Berry and Searle 1963).

Second, variants of this type may provide insight into the developmental mechanisms of evolutionary change in particular groups. For example, variable presence/absence of individual bones is frequently observed in paedomorphic taxa, i.e., those that fail to complete the ancestral cranial ontogenetic sequence during their own ontogeny. In such instances, the variable element typically is one that forms late in the ancestral ontogeny; its variable occurrence in descendant species reflects variability among individuals or even larger segments of the population (e.g., geographic regions; Wake 1980) in the degree to which they complete the ancestral ontogeny. In cases where a variant occurs at extremely low frequency, it is often interpreted as the atavistic "reappearance" of an ancestral feature (e.g., Alberch 1983). In most instances, however, there is insufficient information with which to eliminate the alternative interpretation that the variant has been continuously maintained in the population from the time of the ancestor, albeit at low frequency. Another example of the important role of epigenetic processes in evolution may be Bock's (1959, 1960) study of the evolution of secondary jaw articulations in birds, an important structural innovation which has evolved repeatedly in living taxa. Initial evolutionary steps likely involve the epigenetic development of an articulation between the mandible and the skull base, which are brought into incidental contact as a result of modifications that primarily affect other musculoskeletal components of the feeding apparatus. However, while the morphology of secondary articulations varies widely among taxa, polymorphisms involving variable development of these articulations within a species have not been reported.

Third, these variants may be useful in establishing homologies between anatomical features in ancestors and descendants. An excellent example is provided by Reilly and Lauder (1988), who used the presence of "atavistic" epibranchial cartilages in red-spotted newts (*Notophthalmus viridescens*) to resolve a long-standing debate concerning the homologies of branchial arch segments in urodeles with respect to bony fishes.

Type 3: Trophic Polymorphisms. The third class of variation involves the coexistence within a given population of two or more discrete cranial phenotypes, or morphs, that are distinguished from one another by coordinated changes involving a large number of individual characters. A second, fundamental characteristic of these variants is that the alternate morphs either represent an adaptive response to some environmental variable, or in some other way enhance the immediate fitness of the individual and/or species. In this way, this type of variation is readily distinguished from the gross malformations (type 1; see above) which, while frequently comprising a large number of characters, are maladaptive except under the most exceptional circumstances. Most of the polymorphisms of this type that have been reported involve structures pertaining to feeding; hence, they are termed trophic polymorphisms (table 1.3). Examples include the papilliform/molariform morphs of the Mexican cichlid fish *Cichlasoma minckleyi* (Liem and Kaufman 1984; Sage and Selander 1975; see also the review of trophic polymorphisms in cichlids by Meyer [1991]) and the large- and small-billed morphs in several species of African finches in the genus *Pyrenestes* (Smith 1987, 1990b).

Because of the magnitude of the morphological difference between constituent morphs and their frequently obvious relation to adaptation, these polymorphisms provide among the strongest evidence of the evolutionary significance of intraspecific variation in cranial features. At the same time, a great deal of fundamental information concerning their basic biology is unavailable for any trophic polymorphism so far described— information that must be obtained before their full significance for the evolution of morphological diversity can be assessed. Two questions are especially important:

(1) Is intraspecific trophic polymorphism an incipient stage in the evolution of interspecific morphological diversity? Qualitative and quantitative differences between trophic morphs may be remarkably large (fig. 1.6, 1.7). Some morphs are as different from one another as are related species or even genera (e.g., *Pyrenestes*; Smith 1987, 1990b); indeed, many were

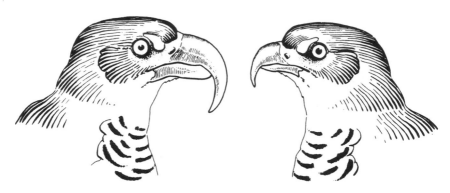

Fig. 1.6. Large- and small-billed morphs of the hook-billed kite (*Chondrohierax uncinatus*), a snail-eating raptor endemic to the New World tropics. Bill size is bimodally distributed in many parts of the species' range; variation is independent of sex and age. The distribution of bill sizes in regional populations is well correlated with the sizes of terrestrial snails, on which the birds feed almost exclusively. While these morphs likely are conspecific, previous studies have not been able to exclude the possibility that each morph represents a distinct species. (Reproduced with permission from Smith and Temple [1982].)

originally described as such (e.g., *Ilyodon:* Grudzien and Turner 1984a, b; Turner and Grosse, 1980; *Saccodon:* Roberts 1974; *Cichlasoma:* Sage and Selander 1975). It is therefore not surprising that trophic polymorphism has often been offered as a transitional stage, which need only be followed by segregation of the constituent morphs via speciation, in the evolution of interspecific morphological differentiation (e.g., Liem and Kaufman 1984; Meyer 1991; Orton 1954). This scenario is obviously tempting, for it circumvents many of the real problems that plague more traditional models for the evolution of large-scale, discontinuous differences among taxa, such as the difficulty in identifying the impetus for evolutionary transitions through putative intermediate stages that are seemingly maladaptive (Gould and Vrba 1982). It also avoids disputed features, such as random morphological change at speciation and species selection, that are central to certain hierarchical models of morphological evolution, such as punctuated equilibrium (Gould 1982; Gould and Eldredge 1977; Levinton 1988). Nevertheless, convincing, unequivocal evidence in favor of this model for the evolution of interspecific morphological diversity, which at the same time excludes alternative models, is lacking. Moreover, the seeming rarity of such discrete polymorphisms in many major taxa, including some, such as birds (Smith and Temple 1982), in which patterns of interspecific and intraspecific variation in the cranium are relatively well documented, suggests that trophic polymorphism is not a predominant "route" to interspecific diversification in cranial morphology in vertebrates generally.

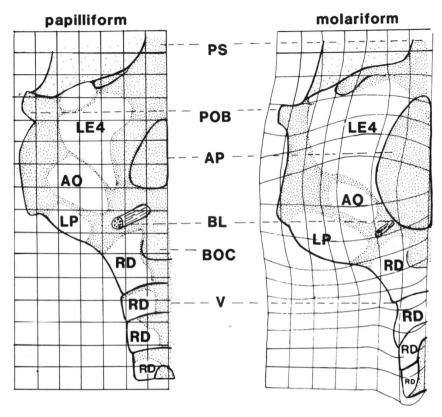

Fig. 1.7. Otic region of the neurocranium and anterior vertebrae of the two trophic morphs of the cichlid fish *Cichlasoma minckleyi*; ventral view, right side only. Unshaded areas depict origins of major muscles. Deformed Cartesian coordinates (standardized to the papilliform morph) graphically depict some of the morphological differences, and possible evolutionary transformation, between the morphs. Standard length for both specimens = 7.4 cm. Abbreviations: AO, adductor operculi; AP, pharyngeal apophysis of the parasphenoid; BL, Baudelot's ligament; BOC, basioccipital; LE4, fourth levator externus; LP, levator posterior; POB, postorbital process; PS, parasphenoid; RD, retractor dorsalis; V, vertebra. (Reproduced with permission from Liem and Kaufman [1984].).

Perhaps the most plausible example yet offered of trophic polymorphism as a vehicle for speciation is the Central American cichlid fish, *Cichlasoma citrinellum* (Meyer 1989, 1990a, b, 1991). In these fishes, two morphs (papilliform and molariform), which are distinguished by several features of cranial morphology and body form, are specialized for eating different prey types. Moreover, each morph is significantly correlated with a distinctive coloration, which is a primary cue for assortative mating. Thus, all the ingredients are at hand for morphological, ecological, and genetic isolation of the two morphs, which might eventually culminate in speciation. Indeed, Meyer (1990a, b, 1991) has offered this scenario as a mechanism for the explosive adaptive radiation of cichlid fishes in freshwater lakes of Africa and Central America.

An obvious alternative to the above view is that trophic polymorphism represents an evolutionary stable end point that bears no necessary relation to subsequent divergence culminating in speciation. According to this view, each polymorphism represents an adaptive "strategy" that enhances survival of the species by increasing the efficiency of trophic resource utilization and/or broadening the resource base (Kornfield et al. 1982; Liem and Kaufman 1984; Smith 1990c; Vrijenhoek 1978). While this may satisfy some of the preconditions for and enhance the likelihood of speciation (Maynard Smith 1966; McKaye et al. 1982), this would not be an inevitable outcome. Indeed, it has been argued that phenotypic plasticity, which underlies the development of variant morphs in many instances of trophic polymorphism, "may be a form of inertia against speciation" (Meyer 1987, 1366).

Both of these models are plausible; moreover, they are not mutually exclusive. A fundamental challenge to future studies is to establish which one predominates in nature and why. Predominance of the view of trophic polymorphism as an incipient stage of interspecific divergence would inevitably lead to investigation of how frequently morphological diversification among taxa involves polymorphisms of this type, viz., an initial phase in which alternate, discrete phenotypes are maintained within the same population. Predominance of the view of trophic polymorphism as a relatively stable end point within species would not diminish its role as a mechanism of morphological diversification per se, although its importance as a vehicle for interspecific divergence obviously would be lessened. Finally, it remains to be established what intrinsic factors (e.g., anatomical, genetic, developmental) and extrinsic factors (e.g., predator-prey relations, community structure, and dynamics) promote the appearance of trophic polymorphisms, and why they may be more common in some groups than in others.

(2) **What are the developmental and genetic bases of trophic polymorphisms?** The question of the developmental and genetic bases of a trophic polymorphism almost invariably follows its initial description. In general, morphological traits are under polygenic control (Falconer 1981; Levinton 1988), and it is reasonable to expect that this generalization applies to the characteristics of trophic morphs; see, for example, Atchley's (1993) discussion of the genetics of mandibular variation in mammals. Yet, the actual genetic basis of intrapopulation differences in cranial morphology, and especially the way genome and environment interact to mediate cranial de-

velopment, is poorly known for virtually every known instance of trophic polymorphism. Moreover, the answers that have been obtained to date are so variable that it is difficult to generalize. Nevertheless, two features are apparent. First, species that display trophic polymorphisms obviously possess genetic liability for the development of particular morphs; without this liability, the morphs could not form, regardless of the nature of the environmental stimuli. Second, many instances of trophic polymorphism involve a predominant role for the environment in making the developmental choice among alternate patterns of cranial ontogeny and, ultimately, cranial morphology (e.g., *Ilyodon;* Grudzien and Turner 1984a). Even such instances of environmentally controlled developmental polymorphisms, however, may be caused by different underlying genetic mechanisms; for example, a single shared genotype and a highly variable genotype could each be expressed as a series of discrete morphs given the right combination of environmental stimuli and developmental thresholds (Collins and Cheek 1983).

The environmental factor that perhaps most commonly promotes the development of alternate trophic morphs is food. Holbrook (1982), for example, implicated likely dietary differences between field mice (*Peromyscus*) inhabiting woodland or grassland habitats as the primary explanation for the distinctive mandibular morphotype characteristic of mice from each area. Interestingly, despite its predominantly environmental cause, the dimorphism is apparently quite stable, being present both in prehistoric and contemporary populations at three widely separated localities in the southwestern United States. Meyer (1987) documented that differences in food (and possibly feeding mode) underlie the considerable differences in jaw and snout structure between "acuto-rostral" and "obtuso-rostral" morphs in the cichlid fish, *Cichlasoma managuense.* These morphs represent the extremes of a continuum of morphological variation in this species, yet Meyer was able to evoke the differences by raising laboratory lines on different diets during the first eight months after the onset of feeding; moreover, the obtuso-rostral morph transformed to acuto-rostral following a change of diet (fig. 1.8). Finally, Pomeroy (1981) was able to produce tadpoles with hypertrophied jaw musculature characteristic of the naturally occurring carnivorous morph in the North American spadefoot toad, *Scaphiopus multiplicatus,* by varying diet in the laboratory. He also documented a "modest genetic effect" (p. 106) contributing to the appearance of the carnivorous morph in carefully controlled laboratory experiments.

Other environmental factors besides diet may also mediate trophic polymorphisms. In a controlled laboratory study of the tiger salamander (*Ambystoma tigrinum*), for example, high population density promoted the appearance of the distinctive larval cannibal morph independent of food

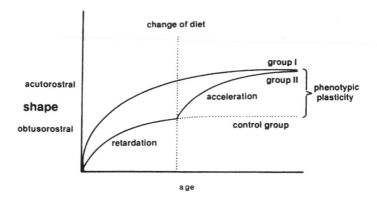

Fig. 1.8. Effects of diet and possibly feeding mode on cranial development in the cichlid fish *Cichlasoma managuense*. During ontogeny, the cranial morphology of group I, fed brine shrimp, changes from obtusorostral to acutorostral. Group II, fed flake food and worms, retains the obtusorostral morphology until 8.5 months of age (vertical dotted line), when a change of diet to shrimp promotes development of the acutorostral morph. (Reproduced with permission from Meyer [1987].)

level, which had no effect (Collins and Cheek 1983). Unlike diet or food processing, however, which likely mediate cranial development through changes in the mechanical environment of the musculoskeletal trophic apparatus, the specific way in which high density affects cranial morphogenesis is not known. Moreover, because the experimental design used in this study varied only food level, but not type, it is not known whether prey type or feeding mode may also promote the appearance of the cannibal morph.

Evidence suggesting that environmental stimuli may not be a primary cause of the development of all trophic polymorphisms, however, comes from another study of the cichlid fish *Cichlasoma minckleyi* (Sage and Selander 1975). When samples of broods were reared in aquaria on a soft diet, the fishes developed into both papilliform and molariform morphs. The latter is regarded as specialized to feed on a diet of hard food such as snails, but this food obviously is not required to evoke development of this morph. A predominantly genetic basis has also been claimed in other studies (e.g., Bragg 1965, Bragg and Bragg 1959; Smith 1987, 1990a), but the evidence is mostly preliminary, indirect, or circumstantial and does not exclude the possibility of a strong environmental component (see, however, Pomeroy 1981).

A final, intriguing aspect of the development basis of trophic polymorphisms that is only beginning to be explored is the possibility that variant morphs result from only slight perturbations to the normal developmental program characteristic of the species. Perhaps the best example to date is Meyer's (1987) study of the cichlid fish *Cichlasoma managuense* discussed earlier in which the variant obtuso-rostral morph, which can be evoked and sustained indefinitely by a particular diet, is an early and transient ontogenetic stage of fishes that typically develop into the acuto-rostral morph (fig. 1.8). Moreover, transformation from the "paedomorphic" obtuso-rostral morph to the acuto-rostral morph is readily achieved by a simple change in diet. A similar example is seen in *C. citrinellum*, in which all fish begin life as papilliform morphs; molariform morphs develop only following subsequent allometric growth as well as qualitative morphological changes (Meyer 1990b).

A second example comes from the so-called cannibal morph in North American spadefoot toads, *Scaphiopus*. The cannibals, or carnivorous tadpoles, differ from typical, omnivorous larvae in several cranial and postcranial features, including hypertrophied jaw musculature, fewer labial teeth and oral papillae, shorter intestine, and decreased melanization (Bragg and Bragg 1959; Orton 1954; Pomeroy 1981). All of these features typically accompany both natural and thyroid-hormone-induced metamorphosis in anurans (Etkin 1968; Fox 1984; Hanken and Hall 1988; Hanken and Summers 1988), including *Scaphiopus* (Pomeroy 1981). Thus, the carnivorous tadpole may represent a case of accelerated development, in which the appearance of certain postmetamorphic features has been accelerated into the larval period. This model, however, cannot explain such cannibal traits as the enlarged horny beak; the moderate-sized beak of omnivorous tadpoles does not enlarge at metamorphosis, but instead is shed.

These examples are important in at least two respects. First, they reveal that the initial evolution of trophic polymorphisms may be a relatively simple matter, that is, it need not require any fundamental or large-scale repatterning of the ontogenetic program of cranial development or of the underlying genome (Liem and Kaufman 1984). Second, they illustrate how the "novel" cranial configurations frequently represented by variant morphs are nevertheless a function of and constrained by the typical pattern of cranial development in each species.

CONCLUSION

Developmental Rules for Skull Specification during Ontogeny

As a means of generalizing the available information on the development of the skull and of relating ontogenetic mechanisms to phylogenetic change, we have assembled the following set of development rules (sensu Oster et al. 1988) that appear, with current knowledge, either to apply to skull development in all vertebrates, or to be capable of extrapolation to other vertebrate taxa from those for which data is available.

1. A regionalized, skeletogenic neural crest extends from the anterior mesencephalon/mid-prosencephalon caudad to somite 5 at the neurula stage of all vertebrates, providing a fundamental pattern of future skull-forming cells.

2. Transformation of epithelial neural crest cells (the state in the neural tube) to mesenchymal (mesectodermal, ectomesenchymal) cells occurs at the outset of migration.

3. Skeletogenic cells migrate from the neural tube as predictable streams, but not along predictable pathways, to "make" the head.

4. Extracellular matrix-mediated mechanisms trap regionalized subpopulations of neural crest−derived cells against neuroepithelia at sites of future cartilage capsule formation (so far demonstrated in avian and mammalian embryos), establishing the fundamental structural pattern of the vertebrate chondrocranium.

5. Initiation of chondrogenesis/osteogenesis requires interactions between neural crest−derived mesenchymal cells and epithelia. The timing of these interactions, the particular epithelia involved, and perhaps also the state of determination of the mesenchymal cells at the time of the interaction varies from group to group, and provides a mechanism, through heterochrony, of generating diversity on the basic structural plan of the skull.

6. Condensation (aggregation) of mesenchyme follows and is caused by the epithelial-mesenchymal interaction. Condensation size is important in determining the size of individual skeletal elements.

7. Cell-type specific molecules and macromolecules are synthesized and deposited into extracellular matrices as the mesenchymal cells differentiate into chondroblasts or osteoblasts. Variation in synthesis of extracellular matrix regulates skeletal form and growth.

8. Final determination of skull form involves integrated and coordinated growth of cartilaginous and bony elements, both among themselves and with respect to adjacent nervous, sensory, circulatory, muscular, and other connective tissues.

These eight rules provide the minimum number of developmental processes required to specify both the stability and the diversity of skull form among vertebrates. They are, however, derived from broad comparisons among mostly individual representatives of distantly related taxa. A fundamental challenge to future studies of skull morphology and evolution is to document the specific ways in which these (and possibly other) processes have been modified to achieve structural diversity in particular lineages, and how they relate to other mechanisms of adaptive and nonadaptive change.

Intraspecific Variation

Comprehensive understanding of the way that changes in developmental processes and patterns are translated into morphological differences among taxa requires consideration of the middle ground of intraspecific variation. As a beginning, we have considered three classes of cranial variants commonly observed in natural populations. *Gross malformations* offer an excellent opportunity to examine the basic mechanisms of cranial development and genetics. They also reveal the capacity for seemingly slight perturbations of developmental processes to effect large-scale changes in adult morphology. Nevertheless, because of the exceptional decrease in fitness typically conferred by these changes, we attribute little significance to them as vehicles of significant evolutionary change.

Epigenetic polymorphisms are routinely observed when adequate sample sizes are considered and may prove to be ubiquitous in natural populations. They provide a simple and rational mechanism for the initial appearance of novel, discontinuous variants and for subsequent incorporation of these initially rare variants into the population at large. Moreover, this mechanism is fully consistent with accepted principles of developmental genetics. Thus, epigenetic polymorphisms represent a likely source of the raw material necessary for directional change or diversification which may result from a variety of processes, such as natural selection, drift, and population fragmentation. For these reasons, we consider epigenetic polymorphisms to be of primary importance in morphological diversification among taxa.

Trophic polymorphisms are, except for sexual dimorphism, perhaps the most dramatic illustrations of intraspecific variation in cranial morphology in nature; they exemplify the fact that large-scale morphological change need not be contingent on speciation. They usually are of obvious selective value to the species involved, and pose a number of challenging and important questions that lie at the interface of ecology, morphology, development, genetics, and behavior. Yet, trophic polymorphisms in general would appear to be rare; while they may prove to be more abundant than now recognized in some groups, viz., teleost fishes, it is unlikely that they will prove to be a common phenomenon overall. They clearly represent a mechanism for morphological diversification that is distinct from more traditional models that entail speciation and subsequent divergence among taxa. At present, however, it remains unresolved how frequently trophic polymorphisms culminate in speciation and interspecific morphological differentiation, as opposed to remaining stable instances of intraspecific variation. Finally, the paucity of examples of adaptive cranial polymorphisms involving functional character complexes unrelated to feeding suggests that discontinuous variation of this type may be a viable mechanism for morphological diversification only for trophic structures within the skull.

ACKNOWLEDGMENTS

Drs. Axel Meyer and Thomas Smith provided helpful comments on earlier drafts and provided copies of manuscripts in press. Research of B. K. Hall supported by Natural Sciences and Engineering Research Council of Canada grant A-5056.

REFERENCES

Alberch, P. 1983. Morphological variation in the neotropical salamander genus *Bolitoglossa*. Evolution 37: 906–919.

Atchley, W. R. 1993. Genetic aspects of variability in the mammalian mandible. In *The Skull*, vol. 1, *Development*, J. Hanken and B. K. Hall, eds. Chicago: University of Chicago Press, pp. 207–247.

Axtell, R. W. 1986. The epipterygoids in *Phrynosoma solare*, still present, but disappearing. Journal of Herpetology 20: 79–81.

Bee, J., and P. V. Thorogood. 1980. The role of tissue interactions in the skeletogenic differentiation of avian neural crest cells. Developmental Biology 78: 47–66.

Bellairs, A. d'A. 1965. Cleft palate, microphthalmia, and other malformations in embryos of lizards and snakes. Proceedings of the Zoological Society of London 144: 239–251.

———. 1983. Partial cyclopia and monorhinia in turtles. In *Advances in Herpetology and Evolutionary Biology*, A. G. J. Rhodin and K. Miyata, eds. Cambridge: Museum of Comparative Zoology, pp. 150–158.

Bellairs, A. d'A, and J. D. Boyd. 1957. Anomalous cleft palate in snake embryos. Proceedings of the Zoological Society of London 129: 525–539.

Berry, A. C., and R. J. Berry. 1967. Epigenetic variation in the human cranium. Journal of Anatomy 101: 361–379.

Berry, R. J. 1963. Epigenetic polymorphism in wild populations of *Mus musculus*. Genetical Research, Cambridge 4: 193–220.

———. 1968. The biology of non-metrical variation in mice and men. In *The Skeletal Biology of Earlier Human Populations*, D. R. Brothwell, ed. Oxford: Pergamon Press, pp. 103–133.

Berry, R. J., and A. G. Searle. 1963. Epigenetic polymorphism of the rodent skeleton. Proceedings of the Zoological Society of London 140: 577–615.

Bock, W. J. 1959. Preadaptation and multiple evolutionary pathways. Evolution 13: 194–211.

———. 1960. Secondary articulation of the avian mandible. Auk 77: 19–55.

Bragg, A. N. 1965. *Gnomes of the Night: The Spadefoot Toads*. Philadelphia: University of Pennsylvania Press.

Bragg, A. N., and W. N. Bragg. 1959. Variation in the mouth parts in tadpoles of

Scaphiopus (Spea) bombifrons Cope (Amphibia: Salientia). Southwestern Naturalist 3: 55–69.

Cassin, C., and A. Capuron. 1979. Buccal organogenesis in *Pleurodeles waltlii* Michah (urodele amphibian): Study by intrablastocelic transplantation and in vitro culture. Journal de biologie buccale 7: 61–76.

Chibon, P. 1964. Analyse par la méthode de marquage nucléaire à la thymidine tritiée des dérivés de la crête neurale céphalique chez l'urodèle *Pleurodeles waltlii*. Comptes rendus, Académie des Sciences 259: 3624–3627.

———. 1966. Analyse expérimentale de la régionalisation et des capacités morphologénétiques de la crête neurale chez l'amphibien urodèle *Pleurodeles waltlii* Michah. Mémories, Société de zoologie, France 36: 1–107.

———. 1967. Marquage nucléaire par la thymindine tritiée des dérivés de la crête neurale chez l'amphibien urodèle *Pleurodeles waltlii* Michah. Journal of Embryology and Experimental Morphology 18: 343–358.

———. 1974. Un système morphogénétique remarquable: La crête neurale des vertébrés. Année biologique 13: 459–480.

Collins, J. P., and J. E. Cheek. 1983. Effect of food and density on development of typical and cannibalistic salamander larvae in *Ambystoma tigrinum nebulosum*. American Zoologist 23: 77–84.

Corsin, J. 1975. Différenciation in vitro de cartilage à partir des crêtes neurales céphaliques chez *Pleurodeles waltlii* Michah. Journal of Embryology and Experimental Morphology 33: 335–342.

Couly, G. F., and N. M. Le Douarin. 1987. Mapping of the early neural primordium in quail-chick chimeras. II. The prosencephalic neural plate and neural folds: Implications for the genesis of cephalic human congenital abnormalities. Developmental Biology. 120: 198–214.

———. 1988. The fate map of the cephalic neural primordium at the presomitic to the 3-somite stage in the avian embryo. Development 103 (suppl.): 101–114.

Crumly, C. R. 1982. The "parietal" foramen in turtles. Journal of Herpetology 16: 317–320.

Cusimano, T., A. Fagone, and G. Reverberi. 1962. On the origin of the larval mouth in the Anurans. Acta embryologiea et morphologiea experimentalis 5: 82–103.

Cusimano-Carollo, T. 1963. Investigation on the ability of the neural folds to induce a mouth in the *Discoglossus pictus* embryo. Acta embryologiea et morphologiea experimentalis 6: 158–168.

———. 1969. Phenomena of induction by the transverse neural fold during the formation of the mouth in *Discoglossus pictus*. Acta embryologiae et morphologiae experimentalis 1: 97–110.

———. 1972. On the mechanism of the formation of the larval mouth in *Discoglossus pictus*. Acta embryologiea et morphologiae experimentalis 4: 289–332.

Damas, H. 1944. Recherches sur le développement de *Lampetra fluviatilis* L.: Contribution à l'étude de la céphalogénèse des vertébrés. Archives de biologie. Paris 55: 1–284.

———. 1951. Observations sur le développement des ganglions of crâniens chez *Lampetra fluviatilis* (L). Archives de biologie. Paris 62: 5–95.

de Beer, G. R. 1937. *The Development of the Vertebrate Skull*. Oxford: Clarendon Press. Reprinted with an introduction by B. K. Hall and J. Hanken, 1985, Chicago: University of Chicago Press.

————. 1947. The differentiation of neural crest cells into visceral cartilages and odontoblasts in *Amblystoma*, and a re-examination of the germ-layer theory. Proceedings of the Royal Society of London (B) 134: 377–398.

de Queiroz, K., and D. A. Good. 1988. The scleral ossicles of *Opisthocomus* and their phylogenetic significance. Auk 105: 29–35.

Diewert, V. M. 1982. Contribution of differential growth of cartilages to changes in craniofacial morphology. In *Factors and Mechanisms Influencing Bone Growth*, A. D. Dixon and B. G. Sarnat, eds. New York: Alan R. Liss, pp. 229–242.

Drews, U., U. Kocher-Becker, and U. Drews. 1972. The induction of visceral cartilage from cranial neural crest by pharyngeal endoderm in hanging drop cultures and the locomotory behaviour of the neural crest cells during cartilage differentiation. Wilhelm Roux Archiv' fur Entwicklungsmechanik 171: 17–37.

Epperlein, H. H., and R. Lehmann. 1975. The ectomesenchymal-endodermal interaction system (EEIS) of *Triturus alpestris* in tissue culture. 2. Observations of differentiation of visceral cartilage. Differentiation 4: 159–174.

Etkin, W. 1968. Hormonal control of amphibian metamorphosis. In *Metamorphosis: A Problem in Developmental Biology*, W. Etkin and L. I. Gilbert, eds. New York: Appleton-Century-Crofts, pp. 313–348.

Falconer, D. S. 1981. *Introduction to Quantitative Genetics*, 2d ed. London: Longman.

Ferguson, M. W. J. 1984. Craniofacial development in *Alligator mississippiensis*. Symposium of the Zoological Society of London 52: 223–274.

————. 1985. Reproductive biology and embryology of the crocodilians. In *Biology of the Reptilia*, vol. 14, *Development A*, C. Gans, F. Billett, and P. F. A. Maderson, eds. New York: John Wiley & Sons, pp. 329–492.

Fox, H. 1984. *Amphibian Morphogenesis*. Clifton, N.J.: Humana Press.

Gans, C. 1993. Evolutionary origin of the vertebrate skull. In *The Skull*, vol. 2, *Patterns of Structural and Systematic Diversity*, J. Hanken and B. K. Hall, eds. Chicago: University of Chicago Press, pp. 1–35.

Gans, C., and C. Northcutt. 1983. Neural crest and the origin of vertebrates: A new head. Science 220: 268–274.

Goronowitsch, N. 1892. Die axiale und die laterale Kopfmetamerie der Vögelembryonen. Die Rolle der sog. "Ganglienleisten" im Aufbaue der Nervenstämme. Anatomischer Anzeiger 7: 454–464.

————. 1893a. Untersuchungen über die Entwicklung der sogenannten "Gantlienleisten" im Kopfe der Vögelembryonen. Morphologische Jahrbuch 20: 187–259.

————. 1893b. Weiters über die ektodermal Entstehung von Skeletanlagen im Kopfe der Wirbeltiere. Morphologische Jahrbuch 20: 425–428.

Gould, S. J. 1982. The meaning of punctuated equilibrium and its role in validating a hierarchical approach to macroevolution. In *Perspectives on Evolution*, R. Milkman, ed. Sunderland: Sinauer Associates, pp. 83–104.

Gould, S. J., and N. Eldredge. 1977. Punctuated equilibria: The tempo and mode of evolution reconsidered. Paleobiology 3: 115–151.

Gould, S. J., and E. S. Vrba. 1982. Exaptation—A missing term in the science of form. Paleobiology 8: 4–15.

Graham-Smith, W. 1978. On the lateral lines and dermal bones in the parietal region of some Crossopterygian and Dipnoan fishes. Philosophical Transactions of the Royal Society of London 282B: 41–105.

Graveson, A. C., and J. B. Armstrong. 1987. Differentiation of cartilage from cranial neural crest in the axolotl (*Ambystoma mexicanum*). Differentiation 35: 16–20.

Grudzien, T. A., and B. J. Turner. 1984a. Direct evidence that the *Ilyodon* morphs are a single biological species. Evolution 38: 402–407.

Grudzien, T. A., and B. J. Turner. 1984b. Genic identity and geographic differentiation of trophically dichotomous *Ilyodon* (Teleostei: Goodeidae). Copeia: 102–107.

Hall, B. K. 1981. Specificity in the differentiation and morphogenesis of neural crest–derived scleral ossicles and of epithelial scleral papillae in the eye of the embryonic chick. Journal of Embryology and Experimental Morphology 66: 175–190.

———. 1984. Developmental processes underlying heterochrony as an evolutionary mechanism. Canadian Journal of Zoology, 62: 1–7.

———. 1986. Initiation of chondrogenesis from somitic, limb, and craniofacial mesenchyme: Search for a common mechanism. In *Somites in Developing Embryos*, R. Bellairs, D. A. Ede, and J. W. Lash, eds. Advanced Science Institute Series A: Life Sciences. New York: Plenum Publishing Corporation, pp. 247–259.

———. 1987a. Earliest evidence of cartilage and bone development in embryonic life. Clinical Orthopaedics and Related Research 225: 252–272.

———. 1987b. Tissue interactions in the development and evolution of the vertebrate head. In *Developmental and Evolutionary Aspects of the Neural Crest*, P. F. A. Maderson, ed. New York: John Wiley and Sons, pp. 215–259.

———. 1988a. The embryonic development of bone. American Scientist 76 (2): 174–178.

———. 1988b. *The Neural Crest*. Oxford: Oxford University Press.

———. 1988c. Patterning of connective tissues in the head: Discussion report. Development 103 (suppl.): 171–174.

———. 1989. Morphogenesis of the skeleton: Epithelial or mesenchymal control? In *Second International Symposium on Vertebrate Morphology*, H. Splechtna and H. Hilgers, eds. Fortschritte der Zoologie (Progress in Zoology) 35: 198–201. Stuttgart: Gustav Fisher Verlag.

———. 1991. Cellular interactions during cartilage and bone development. Journal of Craniofacial Genetics and Developmental Biology 11: 238–250.

Hall, B. K., and J. Hanken. 1985. Foreword to *The Development of the Vertebrate Skull*, by G. R. de Beer. Chicago: University of Chicago Press, pp. vii–xxviii.

Hall, B. K., and R. Tremaine. 1979. Ability of neural crest cells from the embryonic chick to differentiate into cartilage before their migration away from the neural tube. Anatomical Record 194: 469–476.

Hanken, J. 1984. Miniaturization and its effects on cranial morphology in plethodontid salamanders, genus *Thorius* (Amphibia: Plethodontidae). I. Osteological variation. Biological Journal of the Linnean Society 23: 55–75.

Hanken, J., and B. K. Hall. 1988. Skull development during anuran metamorphosis: II. Role of thyroid hormone in osteogenesis. Anatomy and Embryology 178: 219–227.

Hanken, J., and C. H. Summers. 1988. Skull development during anuran metamorphosis: III. Role of thyroid hormone in chondrogenesis. Journal of Experimental Zoology 246: 156–170.

Harrison, R. G. 1935a. Factors concerned in the development of the ear in *Amblystoma punctatum*. Anatomical Record 64 (suppl. 1): 38–39.

———. 1935b. Heteroplastic grafting in embryology. Harvey Lectures 29: 116–157.

———. 1935c. On the origin and development of the nervous system studied by the methods of experimental embryology. Croonian Lecture. Proceedings of the Royal Society of London (B) 118: 155–196.

———. 1938. Die Neuralleiste Erganzheft. Anatomischer Anzeiger 85: 3–30.

Holbrook, S. J. 1982. Ecological inferences from mandibular morphology of *Peromyscus maniculatus*. Journal of Mammalogy 63: 399–408.

Holland, P. W. H. 1988. Homeobox genes and the vertebrate head. Development 103 (suppl.): 17–24.

Holland, P. W. H., and B. L. M. Hogan. 1988. Expression of homeobox genes during mouse development: A review. Genes and Development 2: 773–782.

Holtfreter, J. 1968. Mesenchyme and epithelia in inductive and morphogenetic processes. In *Epithelial-Mesenchymal Interactions,* R. Fleischmajer and R. E. Billingham, eds. Baltimore: Williams & Wilkins, pp. 1–30.

Hörstadius, S. 1950. *The Neural Crest.* Oxford: Oxford University Press.

Hörstadius, S., and S. Sellman. 1941. Experimental studies on the determination of the chondrocranium in *Ambystoma mexicanum*. Arkiv för Zoologi, Uppsala 33A (13): 1–8.

———. 1946. Experimentelle untersuchungen über die Determination des Knorpeligen Kopfskelettes bei Urodelen. Nova acta Regiae societatis scientiarum Uppsaliensis, ser. 4 (13): 1–170.

Huxley, T. H. 1898. On the theory of the vertebrate skull. In *The Scientific Memoirs of T. H. Huxley,* vol. 1, M. Foster and E. Ray Lankester, eds., London: John Murray, pp. 538–606.

in den Bosch, H. A. J., and C. J. M. Musters. 1987. Scalation and skull morphology of a cyclopian *Natrix maura*. Journal of Herpetology 21: 107–114.

Jacobson, A. G. 1987. Determination and morphogenesis of axial structures: Mesoderm metamerism, shaping of the neural plate and tube, and segregation and functions of the neural crest. In *Developmental and Evolutionary Aspects of the Neural Crest,* P. F. A. Maderson, ed. New York: John Wiley and Sons, pp. 147–180.

Jain, S. L. 1985. Variability of dermal bones and other parameters in the skull of *Amia calva*. Zoological Journal of the Linnean Society 84: 385–395.

Johnels, A. G. 1948. On the development and morphology of the skeleton of the head of *Petromyzon*. Acta Zoologica, Stockholm 29: 139–279.

Johnston, M. C. 1966. A radioautographic study of the migration and fate of cranial neural crest cells in the chick embryo. Anatomical Record 156: 143–156.

Johnston, M. C., and R. D. Hazelton. 1972. Embryonic origins of facial structures related to oral sensory and motor function. In *Third Symposium on Oral Sensation and Perception: The Mouth of the Infant*, J. F. Bosma, ed. Springfield: C. C. Thomas, pp. 76–97.

Johnston, M. C., D. M. Noden, R. D. Hazelton, J. L. Coulombre, and A. J. Coulombre. 1979. Origins of avian ocular and periocular tissues. Experimental Eye Research 29: 27–45.

Johnston, M. C., K. W. L. Vig, and L. J. H. Ambrose. 1981. Neurocristopathy as a unifying concept: Clinical correlations. In *Neurofibromatosis: Genetics, Cell Biology, and Biochemistry*, J. J. Mulvihill and V. M. Riccardi, eds. New York: Raven Press, pp. 97–104.

Kastschenko, N. 1888. Zur Entwicklungsgeschichte der Selachier Embryos. Anatomischer Anzeiger 3: 445–467.

Kornfield, I., D. C. Smith, D. S. Gagnon, and J. N. Taylor. 1982. The cichlid fish of Cuatro Cienegas, Mexico: Direct evidence of conspecificity among distinct trophic morphs. Evolution 36: 658–664.

Landacre, F. L. 1921. The fate of the neural crest in the head of the Urodeles. Journal of Comparative Neurology 33: 1–43.

Langille, R. M., and B. K. Hall. 1986. Evidence of cranial neural crest cell contribution to the skeleton of the sea lamprey, *Petromyzon marinus*. In *New Discoveries and Technologies in Developmental Biology*, pt. B, H. C. Slavkin, ed. New York: Alan R. Liss, pp. 263–266.

———. 1987. Development of the head skeleton of the Japanese medaka, *Oryzias latipes* (Teleostei). Journal of Morphology 193: 135–158.

———. 1988a. Role of the neural crest in development of the cartilaginous cranial and visceral skeleton of the medaka, *Oryzias latipes* (Teleostei). Anatomy and Embryology 177: 297–305.

———. 1988b. Role of the neural crest in development of the trabeculae and branchial arches in the embryonic sea lamprey, *Petromyzon marinus* (L). Development 102: 301–310.

———. 1989a. Developmental processes, developmental sequences, and early vertebrate phylogeny. Biological Reviews 64: 73–91.

———. 1989b. Neural crest–derived branchial arches link lampreys and gnathostomes. In *Second International Symposium on Vertebrate Morphology*, H. Splechtna and H. Hilgers, eds. Fortschritte der Zoologie (Progress in Zoology) 35: 210–212. Stuttgart: Gustav Fisher Verlag.

Lannoo, M. J., and M. D. Bachmann. 1984. Aspects of cannibalistic morphs in a population of *Ambystoma t. tigrinum* larvae. American Midland Naturalist 112: 103–109.

Le Lièvre, C. 1971a. Recherches sur l'origine embryologique des arcs viscéraux chez l'embryon d'Oiseau par la méthode des greffes interspécifiques entre Caille et Poulet. Comptes rendus des séances, Société de Biologie 165: 395–400.

———. 1971b. Recherche sur l'origine embryologique du squelette viscéral chez l'embryon d'Oiseau. Comptes rendus, Association d'anatomie 152: 575–583.

———. 1974. Rôle des cellules mésectodermiques issues des crêtes neurales céphaliques dans la formation des arcs branchiaux et du squelette viscéral. Journal of Embryology and Experimental Morphology 31: 453–477.

———. 1976. Contribution des crêtes neurales à la genèse des structures céphaliques et cervicales chez les Oiseaux. Thèse d'état, Nantes, France.

———. 1978. Participation of neural crest derived cells in the genesis of the skull in birds. Journal of Embryology and Experimental Morphology 47: 17–37.

Le Lièvre, C., and N. M. Le Douarin. 1974. Origine ectodermique du derme de la face et du cou, montrée par des combinaisons interspécifiques chez l'embryon d'Oiseau. Comptes rendus des Séances, Académie de Science, Paris. 278: 517–520.

———. 1975. Mesenchymal derivations of the neural crest: Analysis of chimaeric quail and chick embryos. Journal of Embryology and Experimental Morphology 34: 125–54.

Levinton, J. 1988. *Genetics, Paleontology, and Macroevolution*. Cambridge: Cambridge University Press.

Liem, K. F., and L. S. Kaufman. 1984. Intraspecific macroevolution: Functional biology of the polymorphic cichlid species *Cichlasoma minckleyi*. In *Evolution of Fish Species Flocks*, A. A. Echelle and I. Kornfield, eds., Orono: University of Maine Press, pp. 203–215.

McKaye, K. R., T. Kocher, P. Reinthal, and I. Kornfield. 1982. A sympatric sibling species complex of *Petrotilapia* Trewavas from Lake Malawi analysed by enzyme electrophoresis (Pisces: Cichlidae). Zoological Journal of the Linnean Society 76: 91–96.

Matsumoto, J., T. J. Lynch, S. Grabowski, C. M. Richards, S. L. Lo, C. Clark, D. Kern, J. D. Taylor, and T. T. Tchen. 1983. Fish tumor pigment cells: Differentiation and comparison to their normal counterparts. American Zoologist 23: 569–580.

Maynard Smith, J. 1966. Sympatric speciation. American Naturalist 100: 637–650.

Medvedeva, K. D., and K. A. Savvaitova. 1981. Intrapopulation and geographic variability of the skull in charrs. In *Charrs: Salmonid Fishes of the Genus Salvelinus*, E. K. Balon, ed. The Hague: W. Junk Publishers, pp. 435–440.

Meier, S., and D. S. Packard, Jr. 1984. Morphogenesis of the cranial segments and distribution of neural crest in the embryo of the snapping turtle, *Chelydra serpentina*. Developmental Biology 102: 309–323.

Meyer, A. 1987. Phenotypic plasticity and heterochrony in *Cichlasoma managuense* (Pisces, Cichlidae) and their implications for speciation in cichlid fishes. Evolution 41: 1357–1369.

———. 1989. Cost of morphological specialization: Feeding performance of the two morphs in the tropically polymorphic cichlid fish, *Cichlasoma citrinellum*. Oecologia 80: 431–436.

———. 1990a. Ecological and evolutionary consequences of the trophic polymorphism in *Cichlasoma citrinellum* (Pisces: Cichlidae). Biological Journal of the Linnean Society 39: 279–299.

———. 1990b. Morphometrics and allometry in the trophically polymorphic cichlid fish *Cichlasoma citrinellum:* Alternative adaptations and ontogenetic changes in shape. Journal of Zoology, London 221: 237–260.

————. 1991. Trophic polymorphisms in cichlid fish: Do they represent intermediate steps during sympatric speciation and explain their rapid adaptive radiation? In *New Trends in Ichthyology,* J. H. Schroeder, ed. Berlin: Paul Parey. In press.

Minuth, M., and H. Grunz. 1980. The formation of mesodermal derivatives after induction with vegetalizing factor depends on secondary cell interactions. Cell Differentiation 9: 229–238.

Morriss-Kay, G. M., and S-S. Tan. 1987. Mapping cranial neural crest cell migration pathways in mammalian embryos. Trends in Genetics 3: 257–261.

Newth, D. R. 1950. Fate of the neural crest in lampreys. Nature 165: 284.

————. 1951. Experiments on the neural crest of the lamprey embryo. Journal of Experimental Biology 28: 247–260.

————. 1956. On the neural crest of the lamprey embryo. Journal of Embryology and Experimental Morphology 4: 358–375.

Noden, D. M. 1978a. The control of avian cephalic neural crest cytodifferentiation. I. Skeletal and connective tissues. Developmental Biology 67: 296–312.

————. 1978b. The control of avian cephalic neural crest cytodifferentiation. II. Neural tissues. Developmental Biology 67: 313–329.

————. 1984. The use of chimeras in analysis of craniofacial development. In *Chimeras in Developmental Biology,* N. M. Le Douarin and A. McLaren, eds., Orlando: Academic Press, pp. 241–280.

Northcutt, R. G., and C. Gans. 1983. The genesis of neural crest and epidermal placodes: A reinterpretation of vertebrate origins. Quarterly Review of Biology 58: 1–28.

Okada, E. W. 1955. Isolationsversuche zur Analyse der Knorpelbildung aus Neuralleistenzellen bei Urodelenkeim. Memoirs of the College of Science of Kyoto University, ser. B22: 23–28.

Oppenheimer, J. M. 1940. The non-specificity of the germ layers. Quarterly Review of Biology 15: 1–27.

Orton, G. R. 1954. Dimorphism in larval mouthparts in spadefoot toads of the *Scaphiopus hammondi* group. Copeia: 97–100.

Oster, G. F., N. Shubin, J. D. Murray, and P. Alberch. 1988. Evolution and morphogenetic rules: The shape of the vertebrate limb in ontogeny and phylogeny. Evolution 42: 862–884.

Pal, G. P. 1987. Anatomical note: Variations of the interparietal bone in man. Journal of Anatomy 152: 205–208.

Pal, G. P., B. P. Tamankar, R. V. Routal, and S. S. Bhagwat. 1984. The ossification of the membranous part of the squamous occipital bone in man. Journal of Anatomy 138: 259–266.

Pierce, B. A., J. B. Mitton, and F. L. Rose. 1983. Head shape and size in cannibal and noncannibal larvae of the tiger salamander from west Texas. Copeia: 1006–1012.

Platt, J. B. 1893. Ectodermic origin of the cartilages of the head. Anatomischer Anzeiger 8: 506–509.

———. 1897. The development of the cartilaginous skull and of the branchial and hypoglossal musculature in *Necturus*. Morphologisches Jahrbuch 25: 377–464.

Pomeroy, L. V. 1981. Characteristics and determinants of polymorphism in the larvae of the spadefoot toad, *Scaphiopus* spp. Ph.D. thesis, University of California, Riverside.

Powers, J. H. 1907. Morphological variation and its causes in *Ambystoma tigrinum*. Studies of the University of Nebraska 7: 197–274.

Raven, C. P. 1931. Zur Entwicklung der Ganglienleiste. I. Die Kinematik der Ganglienleisten Entwicklung bei den Urodelen. Wilhelm Roux' Archiv für Entwicklungsmechanik 125: 210–293.

———. 1936. Zur Entwicklung der Ganglienleiste. V. Über die Differenzierung des Rumpfganglienleistenmaterials. Wilhelm Roux' Archiv für Entwicklungsmechanik 134: 122–145.

Reilly, S. M. 1987. Ontogeny of the hyobranchial apparatus in the salamanders *Ambystoma talpoideum* (Ambystomatidae) and *Notopthalmus viridescens* (Salamandridae): The ecological morphology of two neotenic strategies. Journal of Morphology 191: 205–214.

Reilly, S. M., and G. V. Lauder. 1988. Atavisms and the homology of hyobranchial elements in lower vertebrates. Journal of Morphology 195: 237–245.

Roberts, T. R. 1974. Dental polymorphism and systematics in *Saccodon,* a neotropical genus of freshwater fishes (Parodontidae, Characoidei). Journal of Zoology, London 1973: 303–321.

Rollhäuser-ter-Horst, J. 1977. Artificial neural induction in amphibia. II. Host embryos. Anatomy and Embryology 151: 317–324.

Rose, F. L., and D. Armentrout. 1976. Adaptive strategies of *Ambystoma tigrinum* Green inhabiting the Llano Estacado of West Texas. Journal of Animal Ecology 45: 713–729.

Russell, E. S. 1916. *Form and Function: A Contribution to the History of Animal Morphology.* London: John Murray. Reprinted with an introduction by G. V. Lauder, 1982, Chicago: University of Chicago Press.

Sadaghiani, B., and C. H. Thiébaud. 1987. Neural crest development in the *Xenopus laevis* embryo, studied by interspecific transplantation and scanning electron microscopy. Developmental Biology 124: 91–110.

Sage, R. D., and R. K. Selander. 1975. Trophic radiation through polymorphism in cichlid fishes. Proceedings of the National Academy of Sciences, U.S. 72: 4669–4673.

Schmalhausen, I. I. 1949. *Factors of Evolution: The Theory of Stabilizing Selection,* I. Dordick, trans.; T. Dobzhansky, ed. Philadelphia: Blakiston Company. Paperback reprint, Chicago: University of Chicago Press, 1986.

Schowing, J. 1968. Influence inductrice de l'encéphale embryonaire sur le développement du crâne chez le Poulet. III. Mise en evidénce du rôle inducteur de l'encéphale dans l'ostgénèse du crâne embryonnaire du Poulet. Journal of Embryology and Experimental Embryology 19: 83–94.

Smith, M. M., and B. K. Hall. 1990. Developmental and evolutionary origins of vertebrate skeletogenic and ondotogenic tissues. Biological Reviews 65: 277–373.

Smith, T. B. 1987. Bill size polymorphism and intraspecific niche utilization in an African finch. Nature 329: 717–719.

———. 1990a. Natural selection on bill characters in the two bill morphs of the African finch *Pyrenestes ostrinus*. Evolution 44: 832–842.

———. 1990b. Patterns of morphological and geographic variation in trophic bill morphs of the African finch *Pyrenestes*. Biological Journal of the Linnean Society 41: 381–414.

———. 1990c. Resource use by two bill morphs of an African finch: Evidence for intraspecific competition. Ecology 71: 1246–1257.

Smith, T. B., and S. A. Temple. 1982. Feeding habits and bill polymorphism in hook-billed kites. Auk 99: 197–207.

Smits-van Prooije, A. E., C. Vermeij-Keers, J. A. Dubbledam, M. M. T. Mentink, and R. E. Poelmann. 1987. The formation of mesoderm and mesectoderm in presomite rat embryos cultured in vitro using WGA-Au as a marker. Anatomy and Embryology 176: 71–77.

———. 1988. The formation of mesoderm and mesectoderm in 5- to 41-somite embryos cultured in vitro, using WGA-A as a marker. Anatomy and Embryology 177: 245–256.

Spemann, H. 1938. *Embryonic Development and Induction*. New York: Yale University Press.

Stone, L. S. 1922. Experiments on the development of the cranial ganglia and the lateral line sense organs in *Amblystoma punctatum*. Journal of Experimental Zoology 35: 421–496.

———. 1926. Further experiments on the extirpation and transplantation of mesectoderm in *Amblystoma punctatum*. Journal of Experimental Zoology 44: 95–131.

———. 1929. Experiments showing the role of migrating neural crest (mesectoderm) in the formation of head skeleton and loose connective tissue in *Rana palustris*. Wilhelm Roux' Archiv für Entwicklungsmechanik 118: 40–77.

Sutton, J. F. 1972. Notes on skeletal variation, tooth replacement, and cranial suture closure of the porcupine (*Erethizon dorsatum*). Tulane Studies in Zoology and Botany 17: 56–62.

Tan, S.-S., and G. M. Morriss-Kay. 1986. Analysis of cranial neural crest cell migration and early fates in postimplantation rat chimaeras. Journal of Embryology and Experimental Morphology 98: 21–58.

Thomson, K. S. 1988. *Morphogenesis and Evolution*. New York: Oxford University Press.

Thorogood, P. V. 1981. Neural crest cells and skeletogenesis in vertebrate embryos. Histochemical Journal 13: 631–642.

———. 1988. The developmental specification of skull form. Development 102 (suppl.): 141–154.

———. 1993. Differentiation and morphogenesis of cranial skeletal tissues. In *The Skull*, vol. 1, *Development*, J. Hanken and B. K. Hall, eds. Chicago: University of Chicago Press, pp. 112–152.

Thorogood, P. V., J. Bee, and K. Von derMark. 1986. Transient expression of collagen type II at epithelio-mesenchymal during morphogenesis of the cartilaginous neurocranium. Developmental Biology 116: 497–509.

Thorogood, P. V., and Smith, L. 1984. Neural crest cells: The role of extracellular matrix in their differentiation and migration. In *Matrices and Cell Differentiation,* R. B. Kemp and J. R. Hinchliffe, eds., New York: Alan R. Liss, pp. 171–185.

Toerien, M. J. 1965a. An experimental approach to the development of the ear capsule in the turtle, *Chelydra serpentina.* Journal of Embryology and Experimental Morphology 13: 141–149.

———. 1965b. Experimental studies on the columella-capsular interrelationships in the turtle, *Chelydra serpentina.* Journal of Embryology and Experimental Morphology 14: 265–272.

Turner, B. J., and D. J. Grosse. 1980. Trophic differentiation in *Ilyodon,* a genus of stream-dwelling goodeid fishes: Speciation versus ecological polymorphism. Evolution 34: 259–270.

Tyler, M. S., and B. K. Hall. 1977. Epithelial influences on skeletogenesis in the mandible of the embryonic chick. Anatomical Record 188: 229–240.

Vrijenhoek, R. C. 1978. Coexistence of clones in a heterogeneous environment. Science 199: 549–552.

Wagner, G. 1949. Die Bedeutung der Neuralleiste für die Lopfgestaltung der Amphibienlarven: Untersuchungen an Chimaeren von Triton. Revue suisse de zoologie 56: 519–620.

Wake, D. B. 1980. Evidence of heterochronic evolution: A nasal bone in the Olympic salamander *Rhyacotriton olympicus.* Journal of Herpetology 14: 292–295.

2

Convergent and Alternative Designs for Vertebrate Suspension Feeding

S. Laurie Sanderson and Richard Wassersug

INTRODUCTION

SUSPENSION-FEEDING AQUATIC ANIMALS capture planktonic prey as water flows past the feeding apparatus. Vertebrate suspension feeders include species of fishes, tadpoles, whales, and birds and are of evolutionary, ecological, and economic importance. Ancestral vertebrates are thought to have been suspension feeders as larvae (Jollie 1982; Northcutt and Gans 1983) or as adults (Mallatt 1985). Suspension feeding appears to have evolved independently multiple times in teleost fishes and in elasmobranchs (Moss 1977, 1981; Cavender 1970). By consuming phytoplankton, zooplankton, and/or detritus, suspension feeders obtain their energy at a relatively low level in the trophic pyramid and may attain large standing stocks (e.g., herrings and sardines) or large body size (e.g., whales and whale sharks).

The morphology and physiology of a large number of invertebrate suspension-feeding species have been described (reviews in Wallace and Merritt 1980; Jørgensen 1966, 1975; Vanderploeg 1990; Wotton 1990). The physical mechanisms operating in trophic fluid transport systems and in biological filters have been examined through the application of theoretical fluid mechanics to invertebrate suspension feeding (Shimeta and Jumars 1991; LaBarbera 1990, 1984; Jørgensen 1983; Rubenstein and Koehl 1977). The hydrodynamics of feeding in aquatic vertebrates have only recently received attention (Sanderson et al. 1991; Lauder and Shaffer 1986; Muller and Osse 1984; Lauder 1980; Weihs 1980), and the mechanics of vertebrate suspension feeding remain an open field for research. Ecological information on vertebrate suspension feeding far exceeds our understanding of the functional morphology involved. For example, functional morphological studies are needed to establish the structure of the prey-capturing surfaces. But more important, the pattern and velocity of water flow within the oral and (in fishes) opercular cavities must be deter-

Order of authorship is alphabetical.

37

mined. Without these data, the physical mechanism(s) used by vertebrates during suspension feeding cannot be fully understood.

In this chapter, we (1) provide an extensive list of vertebrate species that are known to suspension feed, (2) summarize the mechanistic components of vertebrate suspension feeding, (3) examine morphological and ecological patterns relating to convergent and alternative designs for vertebrate suspension feeding, and (4) identify potential research topics in this area.

Definitions of Suspension Feeding

Suspension feeding, as we use the term, involves both microphagy and planktivory. Microphagy is the consumption of prey too small to be sensed and engulfed as individual particles (Jørgensen 1966). Thus, more than one prey item is typically engulfed during each feeding bout, and some degree of nonselectivity is implied. Planktivory is the separation of particles from ambient water only. We exclude from consideration those animals that "bottom feed" by separating food from surrounding inorganic material and other nonfood particles at the sediment-water interface or that "deposit feed" by directly consuming particulate matter on or in the bottom (e.g., Hlohowskyj et al. 1989; Robotham 1982; Jørgensen 1966). Our definition, however, does not exclude feeding on material from the bottom that is brought into suspension by the activity of the animal. In this situation, inorganic material and other nonfood particles are often swallowed with the food rather than separated from the food in the oral cavity.

Jørgensen (1966) considered suspension feeders to be "typically nonselective feeders, which clear the surrounding water of particles at rates that are independent of the concentration of the particles below certain levels and of their value as food, and which feed continuously when undisturbed" (Jørgensen 1966, 134). As our knowledge of suspension-feeding organisms has grown, it has become clear that this definition may apply to a limited number of sessile invertebrate suspension feeders, but suspension-feeding activity in many other species is constantly regulated in a dynamic fashion. Vertebrates that suspension feed generally (1) respond to a reduction in the concentration of particles below a certain level by ceasing to suspension feed, (2) adjust their suspension-feeding rates in response to characteristics of the particles, and (3) do not suspension feed continuously when undisturbed (see, e.g., Runge et al. 1987; Gibson and Ezzi 1985; Durbin and Durbin 1975; O'Connell and Zweifel 1972; Seale et al. 1982; Viertel 1990). Jørgensen (1983, 89) offered a less restrictive definition that applies equally well to vertebrate and invertebrate suspension feeders, namely "aquatic animals that have evolved special structures to process the surrounding water and to retain small suspended particles, including food particles such as phytoplankton." It is, of course, those "special structures" that are our primary concern here.

Mechanistic Components of Vertebrate Suspension Feeding

In this chapter, we examine three mechanistic components of vertebrate suspension feeding: transport of water into the mouth, transport of water past entrapment surfaces and out of the mouth, and separation of particles from the water. Two additional components are transport of captured food from the oropharyngeal feeding structures to the esophagus, and deglutition (Zweers et al. 1977). The least amount of information is available regarding these latter two processes and they are beyond the scope of this review (but see Zweers et al. 1977; Kooloos et al. 1989; Friedland 1985; Bertmar et al. 1969; Nelson 1967a).

Many invertebrate suspension feeders have entrapping surfaces located external to the mouth and rely on ambient currents to transport water to them (Vogel 1981). Consequently, authors analyzing invertebrate suspension feeding have not always included transport of water into the mouth as one of the stages in suspension feeding (e.g., Jørgensen 1983; LaBarbera 1984). For some vertebrates, notably those that lack gill slits, transport of water into the mouth is a process distinct from transport of water past the suspension-feeding structures, with the direction of flow differing between the two processes by as much as 180°.

TRANSPORT OF WATER INTO THE MOUTH

To fill the mouth with water, animals can use their own forward velocity, generate suction within the oral cavity, or use a combination of the two (Alexander 1967). We identify four categories of vertebrate suspension feeders, based on the methods used to transport water into the mouth (Sanderson and Wassersug 1990): (1) continuous ram feeders, (2) intermittent ram feeders, (3) continuous suction feeders, and (4) intermittent suction feeders (table 2.1). In the first two categories, extracranial body movements alone deliver water into the mouth. In the latter two, specializations of the jaws and pharyngeal structures produce pulses of negative pressure to suck in water.

Ecological Patterns

Continuous Ram Feeders. Ram feeders engulf a volume of water by swimming forward with an open mouth (figs. 2.1, 2.2). Continuous ram feeders allow water to escape posteriorly from the mouth as they swim, maintain-

TABLE 2.1 Characteristics of the four categories of vertebrate suspension feeders, with a listing of previous authors' terms

	Ram feeders		Suction Feeders	
	Continuous	Intermittent	Continuous	Intermittent
Other terms in the literature[1]:	Skimmers (Nemoto 1970) Tow-net filter feeders (Lazzaro 1987) Continuous (Krushinskaya 1986)	Swallowers (Nemoto 1970) Gulpers, gulping, engulfment (Matthews 1978; Pivorunas 1979) Pulse (Krushinskaya 1986)		Gulpers (Janssen 1976) Pump filter feeders (Drenner, O'Brien et al. 1982)
Some general characteristics:	Prey small, nonevasive Uses forward body velocity to overtake prey Forward body velocity causes water to exit Body size moderate to large	Prey larger, more mobile Uses forward body velocity to overtake prey Muscular contraction and elastic recoil force water to exit Body size large	Prey small, nonevasive No forward body movement, uses suction to engulf prey Muscular contraction forces water to exit Body size small to moderate	Prey small, nonevasive Limited forward velocity, uses suction to engulf prey Muscular contraction forces water to exit Body size moderate to large
Examples:	Whale shark, menhaden, anchovy, right whale	Rorqual whales	Ammocoete larvae, tadpoles, flamingos, mallard	Tilapia, gizzard shad, cisco, megamouth shark

[1]Citations do not necessarily indicate the first or only use of that term.

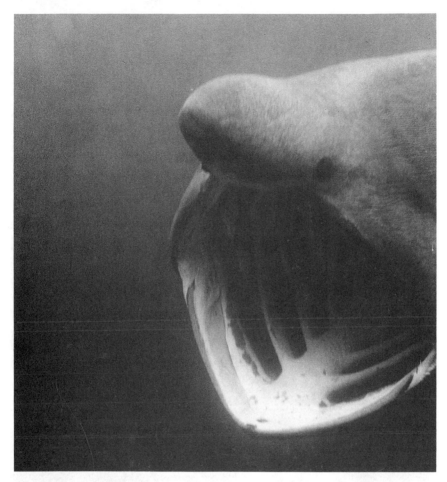

Fig. 2.1. Basking shark, *Cetorhinus maximus* (8 m total length), continuous ram feeding in Carmel Bay, California. The ventral portions of the gill arches are visible inside the mouth, which is about 1 m wide. (From Hallacher 1977)

ing an open mouth for sustained periods of time. The mouth may remain fully open for half a second to several minutes (Runge et al. 1987; Batty et al. 1986; Hallacher 1977; Colin 1976; O'Connell and Zweifel 1972). The mysticete whales that Nemoto (1970) referred to as "skimmers," the right and bowhead, are continuous ram feeders (table 2.2). The fishes described by Lazzaro (1987) as "tow-net filter feeders" are also included in this category.

Table 2.2 lists vertebrates that have been observed to feed in this manner or that are inferred to be continuous ram feeders on the basis of di-

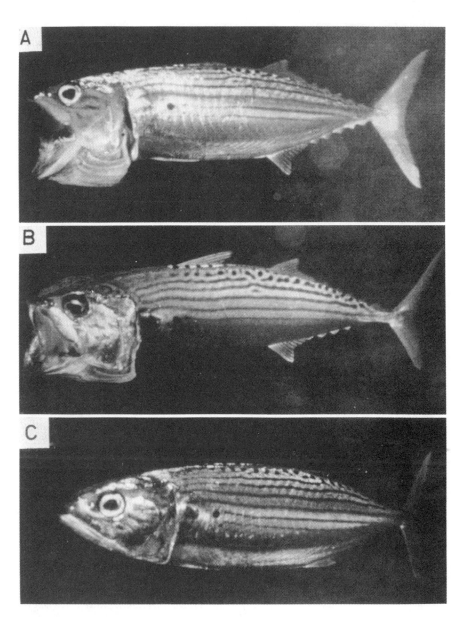

Fig. 2.2. Indian mackerel, *Rastrelliger kanagurta* (20–30 cm standard length), continuous ram feeding off Mbengga Island, Fiji (A, B) and swimming with mouth closed (C). (From Colin 1976)

gestive tract contents and the morphological features that are described below. Fishes that have a diet of phytoplankton, or that consume plankton species relatively nonselectively in the approximate proportions present in the environment, are suspension feeders by definition. Species listed in table 2.2 that have not been observed while feeding may be continuous ram feeders and/or intermittent suction feeders. With the possible exception of the basking shark, the fish species listed in table 2.2 are likely to be facultative suspension feeders. Most appear to be able to select individual food items from the water or off the bottom, in addition to continuous ram feeding (see references in table 2.2).

The whales that are continuous ram feeders consume smaller and less evasive prey relative to their intermittent ram-feeding relatives; i.e., they are microplanktophagous as opposed to macroplanktophagous, in the terminology of Tomilin (1967). The feeding structures inside their mouths present a high resistance to water flow and the resulting large pressure drag retards acceleration when the mouth is open. Continuous ram feeders are unable to capture large evasive prey that swim out of the open mouth's path (Tomilin 1967).

Intermittent Ram Feeders. Intermittent ram feeders use their forward velocity to force their mouths open widely (fig. 2.3) and fill their buccal cavity in a single pulse (Lambertsen 1983; Orton and Brodie 1987). As a feeding strategy, intermittent ram feeding is limited to the largest of all animals, the rorqual whales (table 2.3), swimming at a high (approximately 10^6) Reynolds number. No teleost fish or shark is known to feed in this manner.

In order for intermittent ram feeding to work, the inertial forces must be very high and the buccal floor compliant, otherwise the pressure head anterior to the animal would push water and food away. The rorqual whales direct their attacks on schools of fishes or local concentrations of krill. Complex herding behaviors may be used to further concentrate prey in front of the whales before they open their mouths (Hain et al. 1982; Watkins and Schevill 1979; Jurasz and Jurasz 1979).

Continuous Suction Feeders. An odd collection of animals comes under this heading: ammocoetes, tadpoles, certain ducks, and flamingos (table 2.4). What these organisms share is a dependence on an oscillating buccopharyngeal pump to generate feeding currents. Continuous suction feeders remain relatively stationary when feeding and thus, unlike most other suspension feeders, their locomotor capability is not directly linked to their feeding morphology. For continuous suction feeders with gill slits, the pharyngeal arches and associated musculature form the piston for the pump. For those that lack gill slits, the tongue and hyoid make up the pump.

TABLE 2.2 Continuous ram feeders

Family, species	Body length[1]	Prey[2]	Reference
Cetorhinidae			
Cetorhinus maximus[3] (basking shark)	> 6–10 m	Z	Hallacher 1977
Clupeidae[4]			
Alosa aestivalis (blueback herring)	7.2–29.0 cm FL	Z, D, B	Stone and Daborn 1987
Alosa pseudoharengus[3] (alewife)	5.0–33.8 cm FL	Z, P, D, B	Janssen 1976, 1978; Stone and Daborn 1987
Brevoortia tyrannus[3] (menhaden)	> 4 cm FL	Z, P, D, B (> 13–16 μm)	Durbin and Durbin 1975; Edgar and Hoff 1976; Friedland et al. 1989
Clupea harengus[3] (herring)	5–34 cm	Z, fish eggs, small fishes	Last 1989; Gibson and Ezzi 1990
Ethmalosa fimbriata (shad)	5.3–30.4 cm	Z, P, D, S	Blay and Eyeson 1982; Fagade and Olaniyan 1972
Gilchristella aestuarius (round-herring)		Z, P, B, S	White and Bruton 1983
Hilsa kelee (shad)	3–16 cm SL	Z, P	Blaber 1979
Sardinops caeruleus (Pacific sardine)	11.0–28.5 cm SL	Z, P	Hand and Berner 1959
Sardinops ocellatus (pilchard)	2–22 cm SL	Z, P	King and Macleod 1976
Sardinella longiceps (Indian oil sardine)	13.0–19.9 cm TL	Z, P	Bensam 1964
Engraulidae[5]			
Cetengraulis mysticetus[3] (anchoveta)	3–15 cm	Z, P, S	Bayliff 1963; Hobson 1963
Engraulis anchoita (Argentine anchovy)	0.3–9.0 cm	Z, P, B, S (> 100 μm)	Ciechomski 1967
Engraulis capensis[3] (Cape anchovy)	2–16 cm SL	Z, P, B, S (≈100 μm–2 cm)	King and Macleod 1976; James 1987; James and Findlay 1989
Engraulis encrasicholus maeoticus (Azov anchovy)	2.0–5.0 cm	Z, P, B	Mikhman and Tomanovich 1977
Engraulis mordax[3] (northern anchovy)	4.0–21.5 cm SL	Z, P, B, S (> 40 μm)	Leong and O'Connell 1969; Loukashkin 1970; Hunter and Dorr 1982

Mobulidae[6]			
Mobula hypostoma (devil ray)	< 1.3 m breadth	Z, S, small fishes	Radcliffe 1914; Coles 1916
Mobula thurstoni (devil ray)	0.6–2.3 m breadth	Z	MacGinitie 1947; Notarbartolo-di-Sciara 1988
Manta birostris (manta ray)		Z?, small fishes	Bigelow and Schroeder 1953
Polyodontidae			
Polyodon spathula[3] (paddlefish)	> 12 cm TL	fish (5–10 cm), Z, S	Fitz 1966; Michaletz et al. 1982; Rosen and Hales 1981; Weed 1925
Rhiniodontidae			
Rhiniodon typus[3] (whale shark)	14 m	Z, squid, small fishes	Gudger 1941b
Scombridae			
Rastrelliger kanagurta[3] (Indian mackerel)	5.5–30.0 cm TL	Z, P, fish eggs	Bhimachar and George 1952; Colin 1976; Rao and Rao 1957
Scomber japonicus[3] (Pacific mackerel)	20–25 cm SL	Z	O'Connell and Zweifel 1972
Scomber scombrus[3] (Atlantic mackerel)	adult	Z	Runge et al. 1987; Pepin et al. 1988
Balaenidae[7]			
Balaena mysticetus[3] (bowhead whale, Greenland right whale)	14–18 m TL	Z (3–4 mm copepods predominantly, euphausiacean krill), B (gammarid amphipods), S (pebbles)	Tomilin 1967; Nemoto 1970; Würsig et al. 1985; Reeves and Leatherwood 1985
Eubalaena glacialis[3] (right whale)	10–17 m TL	Z (3–4 mm copepods predominantly)	Tomilin 1967; Nemoto 1970

[1]TL = total length from tip of snout to end of caudal fin rays; SL = standard length from tip of snout to start of fork in caudal fin rays; breadth = breadth of body from wing tip to wing tip; FL = fork length from tip of snout to start of fork in caudal fin rays.

[2]Z = zooplankton; P = phytoplankton; D = detritus; B = benthic organisms; S = sediment.

[3]Direct observations of feeding made in field or laboratory. Species that have not been observed while feeding may be continuous ram feeders and/or intermittent suction feeders, but have been placed in this table on the basis of morphological features.

[4]Additional clupeid species reviewed in James 1988.

[5]Additional engraulid species reviewed in James 1988.

[6]Additional mobulid species discussed in Notarbartolo-di-Sciara 1988.

[7]On morphological grounds the pygmy right whale could be added to this list, but it is not included because its diet and behavior are so poorly known (Baker 1985).

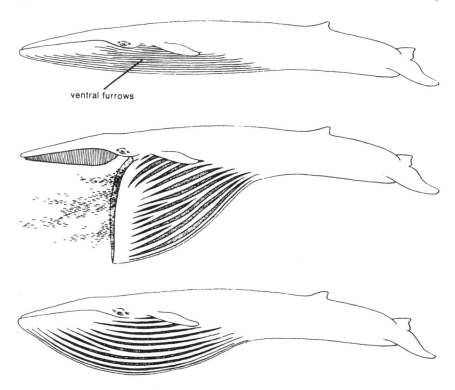

ventral furrows

Fig. 2.3. Intermittent ram feeders, the rorqual whales, use their forward motion to fill their buccal cavity during feeding. The ventral furrows and compliant tissue of the buccal floor facilitate this expansion (Orton and Brodie 1987). Observations of whales feeding in the wild (e.g., Watkins and Schevill 1979) indicate that, while on the surface at least, whales rarely swim in a straight path as they open their mouths. Pitching and rolling motions that bring the baleen on one side and the rostrum upward are common. These motions may facilitate the closing of the mouth and the draining of water through the baleen. (From Pivorunas 1979)

Continuous suction feeders, of course, do not feed *all* of the time, but when they are feeding the pump oscillates continuously at a rather high frequency to maintain the flow of water and food to surfaces on which food particles are captured. These vertebrates feed on very small particles compared to their own size. Certain tadpoles, for example, can grow to metamorphosis on single-celled phytoplankton and bacteria < 10 μm in diameter. Since continuous suction feeders are often either within (e.g., ammocoetes) or on (e.g., tadpoles, flamingos) the bottom when they feed, they can resuspend bottom material when feeding (Seale and Wassersug 1979; Chapman 1905) and, depending on the species, detritus may form an important part of their diet.

There appear to be two groups of continuous suction feeders. Mem-

TABLE 2.3   Intermittent ram feeders

Family, species	Body length	Prey[1]	Reference
Balaenopteridae			All data from Tomilin 1967; Nemoto 1970; Ridgway and Harrison 1985; or cited therein
Balaenoptera musculus (blue whale)	22–27 m	Euphausiacean krill (2–7 cm)	
Balaenoptera physalus (fin whale)	18–24 m	Euphausiacean krill (3–6 cm), large swarming copepods, schooling fishes, squid	
Balaenoptera edeni (Bryde's whale)	13–15 m	Pelagic fishes (e.g., pilchard, mackerel, herring), euphausiacean krill, copepods	
Balaenoptera borealis[2] (sei whale)	12–20 m	Copepods principally; also amphipods, euphausiacean krill and small schooling fishes (e.g., anchovies) occasionally	
Balaenoptera acutorostrata (minke whale)	6–10 m	Schooling fishes, euphausiacean krill	
Megaptera novaeangliae (humpback whale)	12–14 m	Euphausiacean krill, schooling fishes (e.g., mackerel, herring, capelin); benthic organisms occasionally	

[1] Prey are given in approximate order of preference from Nemoto (1970).
[2] Of all of the balaenopterid whales, the sei consistently feeds on the smallest prey and can capture some food by continuous ram feeding at the surface as well as intermittent ram feeding (Nemoto 1970; Mitchell 1974; Gaskin 1976; Krushinskaya 1986). It is included in this table rather than the previous one on taxonomic grounds.

bers of the first group, ammocoetes and tadpoles, are small benthic or midwater forms for which mucus entrapment and ciliary transport are essential components of their suspension-feeding mechanism. They all have gill slits with internal entrapment surfaces that are part of their gill system. For these organisms, feeding and respiration are tightly linked (Feder et al. 1984; Wassersug and Murphy 1987). The second group, containing suspension-feeding birds, is made up of air breathers that are restricted to feeding in either shallow water or at the water's surface. They

TABLE 2.4   Continuous suction feeders

Family, genera	Body length	Prey	Reference
Petromyzonidae, Geotriidae and Mordaciidae ammocoetes (lamprey larvae)	10–20 cm	Diatoms, desmids, protozoa, rotifers, detritus	Hardisty and Potter 1971; Mallatt 1981, 1982; Youson 1981
Anuran Larvae (tadpoles of most families and genera)	< 1-≈10 cm	Algae, detritus	Wassersug 1975; Seale and Beckvar 1980; Seale 1980 (plus other references cited therein)
Anatidae (Anatine ducks) many species in genera such as: *Anas* (mallard, shovelers), *Stictonetta* (freckled duck), *Malacorhynchus* (pinkeared)	35–80 cm	A variety of phyto- and zooplankton, such as *Daphnia*, calanoid copepods, and other microcrustaceans; seeds of terrestrial and aquatic herbs and grasses. Particles as small as 0.2 mm and as large as 4.4 mm depending on the species.	Douthwaite 1977; Crome 1985; Kooloos et al. 1989 (plus other references cited therein)
Phoenicopteridae (Flamingos)			
Phoenicopterus sp. (greater flamingos)	125–145 cm	Assorted small invertebrates, including gastropods (e.g., *Cerithium*), crustacea, insects (e.g., chironomid larvae), seeds, some algae. Preferred food between 1–10 mm.	Jenkin 1957; Hurlbert et al. 1986
Phoeniconaias minor (lesser flamingo)	80–90 cm	Primarily blue-green algae, diatoms, some small invertebrates. Preferred food between 0.02–0.1 mm.	Jenkin 1957
Phoenicoparrus sp. (Andean flamingos)	≈150 cm	Similar to *Phoeniconaias*	Jenkin 1957

lack gill slits and have lamellae at the margins of their jaws that form the filters. For them, entrapment surfaces are anatomically independent of respiratory surfaces.

All of the continuous suction feeders have a reduced oral gape with sensory structures at the margin to assess the size and texture of particles entering the mouth. They also all have ways of excluding particles above a certain size. Such adaptations are not necessary for continuous ram feeders because they feed in the open water where there is normally little abiotic material to clog their filters.

Intermittent Suction Feeders. Compared to continuous suction feeders, species in this category generate suction with aperiodic pulses. Teleost fishes are the only vertebrates clearly documented to feed in this manner (table 2.5), although the megamouth shark is thought to use this feeding mode (Compagno 1990). Drenner, O'Brien et al. (1982) referred to intermittent suction feeding in fishes as "pump filter feeding," but this term does not allow a distinction between continuous suction feeding and intermittent suction feeding.

The way water is transported into the mouth by intermittent suction feeders is similar to that used by the myriad of planktivorous fishes that visually locate, attack, and engulf individual prey items using suction (Drenner 1977). However, during suspension feeding, the predator does not usually alter its swimming speed or direction to focus attention on individual plankters (Johnson and Vinyard 1987; Gibson and Ezzi 1985; Drenner, O'Brien et al. 1982; Drenner 1977). In terms of the frequency, duration, and magnitude of mouth opening, intermittent suction feeding is intermediate between continuous ram feeding and suction feeding on individual prey.

Under various circumstances, fishes in this category may use a number of prey-capture techniques in addition to intermittent suction, including attacks on individual plankters and continuous ram feeding (e.g., Hoogenboezem et al. 1992; Batty et al. 1990; Gibson and Ezzi 1990; Ehlinger 1989; Drenner, Vinyard et al. 1982; Holanov and Tash 1978; Janssen 1976, 1978). The size of the predator, the size and density of the prey, and the ambient light level determine feeding behavior in such species (Crowder 1985). A predator with a gape that is large enough to engulf more than one prey at a time may use intermittent suction feeding when the prey are not dense enough or are too large to elicit continuous ram feeding (Gibson and Ezzi 1985; Janssen 1976). Janssen (1976) described three distinct feeding behaviors in the alewife that are dependent on the size of the fish. Small specimens are "particulate" feeders in that they visually select and engulf individual zooplankton, large fish are continuous ram feeders, and medium-sized fish use an intermittent suction-feeding technique that Janssen termed "gulping."

Morphological Patterns

Continuous Ram Feeders. *Head Size and Shape.* In continuous ram feeders, the head tends to be a very large portion of the body. Cranial dimen-

TABLE 2.5 Intermittent suction feeders

Family, species	Body length[1]	Prey[2]	Reference
Atherinidae			
Menidia audens[3] (Mississippi silverside)	5.6 cm SL	Z	Drenner and McComas 1980
Catostomidae			
Ictiobus cyprinellus (bigmouth buffalo)	24–83 cm TL	Z	Starostka and Applegate 1970
Cichlidae[4]			
Enterochromis nigripinnis	6.2–8.0 cm TL	P	Moriarty et al. 1973; Moriarty and Moriarty 1973
Oreochromis aureus[3] (blue tilapia)	7–25 cm SL (> 7 μm)	Z, P, D, B, S	Spataru and Zorn 1978; Drenner, Taylor et al. 1984; McDonald 1987; Vinyard et al. 1988
Oreochromis esculentus (tilapia)		P	Denny et al. 1978
Sarotherodon galilaeus[3] (Galilee Saint Peter's fish)	2.0–12.7 cm SL	Z, P (> 6–10 μm)	Drenner, Vinyard et al. 1982; Drenner, Hambright et al. 1987; Vinyard et al. 1988
Oreochromis mossambicus (tilapia)	16–36 cm TL	Z, P, D, B, S	Bowen 1982; Maitipe and De Silva 1985
Oreochromis niloticus[3] (tilapia)	15.7–22.1 cm TL	P, suspended bacteria	Moriarty et al. 1973; Moriarty and Moriarty 1973; Beveridge et al. 1989; Northcott et al. 1991
Clupeidae			
Alosa pseudoharengus[3] (alewife)	12–16 cm	Z	Janssen 1976, 1978
Clupea harengus[3] (herring)	15–16 cm TL	Z	Gibson and Ezzi 1985
Dorosoma cepedianum[3] (gizzard shad)	> 2.4 cm TL	Z, P, D, B (≥ 10 μm)	Bodola 1966; Cramer and Marzolf 1970; Drenner 1977; Drenner, Mummert et al. 1984; Drenner, O'Brien et al. 1982; Kutkuhn 1958; Pierce et al. 1981
Dorosoma petenense[3] (threadfin shad)	4–14 cm TL	Z, P, B	Holanov and Tash 1978; Miller 1967

Cyprinidae			
Abramis brama[3] (bream)	9.5–35.5 cm FL	Z	Lammens 1985
Carassius auratus (goldfish)	1.3–4.3 cm TL	P ($\geq$ 10 μm)	Iwata 1976
Cyprinus carpio[3] (carp)	8–38 cm SL	Z, P, D, B, S, suspended bacteria (> 250 μm)	Sibbing 1988; Beveridge et al. 1991
Hypophthalmichthys molitrix (silver carp)	6 gm–adult	Z, P, D, suspended bacteria (8–100 μm)	Kuznetsov 1977; Cremer and Smitherman 1980; Burke et al. 1986
Hypophthalmichthys nobilis (bighead carp)	adult	Z, P, D (17–3,000 μm)	Cremer and Smitherman 1980; Jennings 1988
Notemigonus crysoleucas[3] (golden shiner)	5.8–11.0 cm SL	Z (360–1,100 μm)	Ehlinger 1989; Hall and Ehlinger 1989
Orthodon microlepidotus[3] (blackfish)	5.1–30.8 cm SL	Z, P, D, B, S ($\geq$ 20 μm)	Byers and Vinyard 1990; Johnson and Vinyard 1987; Murphy 1950
Megachasmidae			
Megachasma pelagios (megamouth shark)	4.5 m	Z	Taylor et al. 1983; Compagno 1990
Mochokidae			
Brachysynodontis batensoda (scaleless catfish)	12.0–13.0 cm SL	Z, D ($\geq$ 80 μm)	Gras et al. 1981
Mugilidae			
Mugil cephalus[3] (striped mullet)	> 3 cm SL	P, D, B, S	Odum 1970
Osteoglossidae			
Heterotis niloticus (abuli)	40–60 cm SL	P	d'Aubenton 1955
Rhiniodontidae			
Rhiniodon typus[3] (whale shark)	14 m	small fishes	Gudger 1941b
Salmonidae			
Coregonus artedii[3] (cisco)	13–26 cm TL	Z	Engel 1976; Janssen 1978
Coregonus hoyi[3] (bloater)	9–26 cm TL	Z	Janssen 1978

[1] TL = total length from tip of snout to end of caudal fin rays; SL = standard length from tip of snout to start of caudal fin rays; FL = fork length from tip of snout to start of fork in caudal fin rays.

[2] Z = zooplankton; P = phytoplankton; D = detritus; B = benthic organisms; S = sediment.

[3] Direct observations of feeding made in field or laboratory. Species not observed feeding are thought to be intermittent suction feeders, rather than continuous ram feeders, on the basis of morphological features.

[4] Additional cichlid species reviewed in Reinthal 1990a, b; and Bowen 1982.

sions in these fishes and whales clearly relate to buccal volume (and opercular volume, in the case of the fishes) and to area of the filtering structures. In the basking shark and whale shark, the head length from the snout tip to the fifth gill slit is 25 to 28% of the total body length (Uchida 1983; Matthews and Parker 1950). The cranial cavities of these sharks are generally much larger than their brains (Matthews and Parker 1950; Denison 1937), and the increased skull size is used to support massive filtering structures. Head lengths of the mackerels *Scomber* and *Rastrelliger,* measured from the snout to the posterior margin of the opercle, are 20 to 26.5% of the standard length (Matsui 1967; Kishinouye 1923). In these teleosts, however, the large head size is due to the large opercular bones rather than the neurocranium (Allis 1903).

In balaenid whales, the head can be up to a third the total length of the animal (Matthews 1978). Such a large cranium results principally from rostral expansion, with specialized processes of the maxillae extending caudally to brace the palate to the braincase. The elongated rostrum supports the baleen plates. This cranial morphology is part of the telescoping of the cetacean skull discussed in detail in Miller (1923), Kellogg (1928), and Howell (1930). However, the rostrum of the paddlefish is an elongated protrusion that does not support the filtering apparatus (Gregory 1933; Imms 1904). In the whale shark, the width of the neurocranium greatly exceeds the length, and the rostrum is extremely reduced (fig. 2.4a).

The basking shark and mysticete whales in general have smaller brains than their non–suspension-feeding relatives (Denison 1937; Krushinskaya 1986; Worthy and Hickie 1986). The orbits and eyes are also reduced, and the eyes are directed laterally, as they are in most suspension-feeding vertebrates. In these species, vision is not an important factor in prey selection and capture. However, the anchovy *Engraulis* (fig. 2.4b) and the mackerels have large orbits, occupying as much as one half the length of the skull in the Atlantic mackerel. Anchovies and mackerels are rapid swimmers that are reported to switch from ram feeding to feeding on individual prey particles, depending on prey size, density, and location (Runge et al. 1987; O'Connell and Zweifel 1972; Loukashkin 1970; Hatanaka et al. 1957; Rao and Rao 1957).

Chapman (1944a) reported that the bones of the palatine and hyoid arches in the anchovy *Anchoa compressa* tend to be large and heavily ossified. He suggested that this strengthening was related to the feeding behavior of anchovies, in which the gill covers and associated structures flare at an angle of 30 to 45° from the vertical. The opercular bones themselves are thin and without strengthening ridges (Chapman 1944a). From their experiments on sunfish, Lauder and Lanyon (1980) determined that opercular bone strain results from the rapid reduction of pressure in the opercular cavity occurring during suction feeding. Two prominent orthogonal

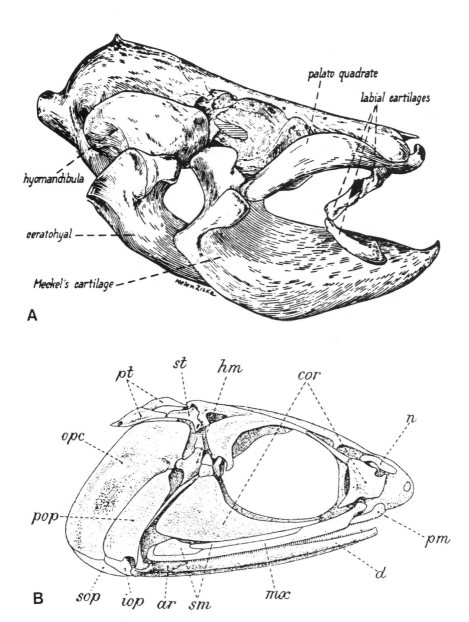

Fig. 2.4. A. Lateral view of skull in the whale shark, *Rhiniodon typus,* a continuous ram feeder and intermittent suction feeder. (From Denison 1937). B. Lateral view of skull in the anchovy, *Engraulis,* a continuous ram feeder. Abbreviations: ar, articular; cor, circumorbital bones; d, dentary; hm, hyomandibular, iop, interopercular; mx, maxilla; n, nasal; opc, opercular; pm, premaxilla; pop, preopercular; pt, post-temporal; sm, surmaxilla; sop, subopercular; st, supratemporal. (From Ridewood 1904)

bony struts on the medial opercular surface appear to resist the medial deformation caused by the generation of negative pressure. Lauder and Lanyon (1980) suggested that this thickening of the operculum is a functional correlate of an inertial suction strategy of prey capture. Consistent with this hypothesis, the anchovy feeds on plankton primarily by utilizing forward body velocity and has not evolved bony reinforcements on the operculum.

All mysticete whales have a large, anteriorly sloping occipital shield compared to odontocetes, although this feature is not as extreme in balaenids as it is in balaenopterids (Miller 1923; Howell 1930). The occipital expansion increases the area for the attachment of epaxial muscles, which may help to dorsiflex the head, but more probably contract isometrically to resist the downward torque on the head when the mouth is open. The problem of torque is partially reduced in balaenid whales because of the enormous arching of their skulls, which brings the open mouth in line with the long axis of the vertebral column. Furthermore, the balaenid whales have the shortest cervical region of any mammal (2.4% of body length in *Eubalaena;* Howell 1930). The cervical vertebrae are fused, greatly limiting any movement of the head on the body. Continuous ram-feeding fishes may have similar adaptations to stabilize the head on the body when the mouth is open. In the mackerel *Scomber,* anterior extensions of the epaxial muscles are located in two deep longitudinal grooves that begin near the lateral edge of the skull, posterior to the middle of the orbit, and widen posteriorly to occupy most of the dorsal surface of the skull (Allis 1903).

Oral Size and Shape. In continuous ram feeders, the mouth aperture is in a plane perpendicular to the direction of forward movement (e.g., mackerels, Matsui 1967; clupeids, Harder 1958). The independent evolution of continuous ram feeding in three families of elasmobranchs (Cetorhinidae, Mobulidae, and Rhiniodontidae) has, in each case, shifted the mouth from the ventral position found in other extant sharks back to its presumed ancestral position at the front of the snout (Moss 1981).

The oral orifice of continuous ram feeders tends to have a very large cross-sectional area. For a basking shark with a total length of approximately 7 m, the area of the open mouth was calculated by Matthews and Parker (1950) to be at least 0.5 m^2. At a swimming speed of about 3.7 km/hr while feeding (Matthews and Parker 1950), the volume of water filtered must be at least 1,850 m^3/hr.

In a whale shark 9.6 m long, the width of the slightly opened mouth was 1.1 m (Gudger 1941a). The tremendous transverse enlargement of the mouth in this species results from the laterally directed suspensorium (Denison 1937). The hyomandibula is a massive cartilage that projects almost directly laterad from the cranium. A groove and two flanges on the hyomandibula articulate with the otic region of the cranium. These flanges restrict antero-posterior movement of the hyomandibula, but dorso-ventral movement is free except for the dorsal limit of the opisthotic process of the cranium. The levator hyomandibuli is a large, powerful muscle (Denison 1937).

Balaenid whales have an anterior gap between their left and right baleen rows, through which water flows into the mouth when the jaws are depressed. Although the jaws do not open very far during ram feeding in the right whale, Nemoto (1970) still estimated a cross-sectional area of 8.9 m^2 for the oral orifice. The oral cavity in balaenids is largely filled with the muscular tongue (see for example figures in True 1904), which can deflect water laterally toward the baleen, but limits buccal volume. Still, because of the high arch of the skull, when the tongue is depressed the buccal volume can be enormous in these whales. Howell (1930) estimated that the buccal volume exceeds the combined volume of the thoracic and abdominal cavities. While this is probably high, there is no question that the buccal volume exceeds the volume of the rib cage.

Upper and Lower Jaws. Continuous ram feeders are characterized by dentition that is either reduced or absent (e.g., Taylor et al. 1983; Moss 1981; Monod 1961; Moona 1959; Chapman 1944b; Gudger 1935; Kishinouye 1923; Radcliffe 1914; Imms 1904; Kellogg 1928). Baleen whales have teeth only as fetuses. While other sharks in the order Lamniformes have fewer than 60 rows of teeth in each jaw, the basking shark has more than 200 rows of small teeth (Taylor et al. 1983). Each jaw of a large whale shark (> 9 m) may have 3,000 to 3,500 backwardly pointed teeth about one eighth of an inch long (Gudger 1941a). Within the teleost group Clupeomorpha, there is a repeated evolutionary trend toward loss of teeth (Nelson 1973).

The bones of the upper and lower jaws may be elongated and broadened (Moss 1981) but usually are not thickened or heavily ossified in continuous ram feeders (Whitehead 1985; Taylor et al. 1983; Moss 1981; Chapman 1944a; Kishinouye 1923). This is consistent with their function as regulators of water flow into the oral cavity rather than as active elements of prey capture.

The maxillae and intermaxillary elements of mysticete whales are relatively narrow. The rostrum of mysticetes is therefore narrow, particularly in the right and bowhead whales. The lower jaws, however, bow outward, allowing them to corral the baleen plates, which hang down from above, when the jaws are closed. In lateral view, the dentary of these balaenid whales is straight, thin, and lacks a coronoid process. There is little room for the attachment of adductor muscles and, as expected, adductor musculature is reduced compared to that of the odontoceti or even the Balaenopteridae. Because the rostrum arches upward in balaenid whales but the mandible does not, the sides of the mouth would remain open with baleen plates exposed even when the jaws were closed, except for the presence of a tall (approaching 2 m), tough, and resilient lower lip that rises from the lower jaw to cover the sides of the mouth (Slijper 1979; Matthews 1978).

The palatoquadrate cartilage of the whale shark is slender and atrophied compared to Meckel's cartilage, which is wide but extremely thin (White 1930). In a whale shark 9.6 m long, the palatoquadrate articulated with Meckel's cartilage at two points, at the knob that formed its proximal end and at a concave facet approximately 10 cm antero-mesiad. Although Denison (1937) suggested that this type of double articulation indicates that the mouth is kept open habitually, Moss (1972) reported a similar articulation in carcharhinid sharks that consume a variety of larger prey.

Intermittent Ram Feeders. The rorqual whales that constitute the intermittent ram feeders are characterized by longitudinal grooves in their gular region that can extend back to the umbilicus. The grooves allow the skin to expand when water is taken into the mouth (Tomilin 1967; Brodie 1977). That expansion can be astonishing (fig. 2.3): the lower jaw rotates back some 45° (P. Brodie, personal communication), and possibly as much as 90° (Gaskin 1976). According to one estimate, a blue whale can, in a matter of seconds, increase its volume by more than 600% (Storro-Patterson 1981). A more common and realistic estimate is that a full-grown blue whale engulfs 60 m³ or 60 metric tons of water, approximately 50% of its body volume (Orton and Brodie 1987; Pivorunas 1979; Sears 1983).

Essential for this process is the large size and high inertia of the swimming whale. Orton and Brodie (1987) modeled the pressure head on a fin whale as it opened its mouth. Using data from their stress/strain analysis of soft tissue in the throat region of fin whales, they concluded that "there is enough force generated by static pressure at a velocity less than 3.0 m/s to completely expand the buccal cavity." Thus, no buccopharyngeal pump is necessary and cranial specializations for intermittent ram feeding are largely of the soft tissue that must expand to contain the water.

The tongue of the adult blue whale has been described as weighing as much as an elephant, i.e., 2.5% of the whale's total weight (Slijper 1962). Whereas this value may have been inflated by the inclusion of sublingual tissue in the estimate (A. Pivorunas, personal communication), there is no question that mysticete tongues in general constitute a much larger proportion of total body mass than the tongues of non–suspension-feeding mammals. The balaenopterid tongue differs from that of balaenid whales in that it is made predominantly of spongy connective tissue, rather than muscle, and lies as a flaccid, immobile mass on the buccal floor (Lambertsen 1983). The tongue has a midline cleft and, under the impetus of the inflowing water, inverts completely into an intermuscular fascial cleft below it (the *cavum vertrale* of Schulte 1916), partially lining the water-filled buccal pouch (Pivorunas 1979).

A musculoskeletal feature associated with this first stage, the filling stage, of intermittent ram feeding is the large area for attachment of the semispinalis capitis on the occipital shield above the occiput. This muscle can contract in concert with the remainder of the erector spinae musculature, to resist forward pitch when the mouth opens. The horizontal fluke of the whale may be brought into play to further control forward pitch or even to extend the head and back. Side-to-side rolling motions and pitching over onto the back are common body motions observed during feeding in rorqual whales (e.g., Watkins and Schevill 1979; Storro-Patterson 1981; Sears 1983).

The jaws must close quickly around the mouthful of water to prevent prey from swimming out. This is accomplished by specializations of the mandibular joints and adductor musculature. Mysticete mandibles are not fused at the symphysis but form a loose, kinetic joint (Brodie 1977). The jaw symphysis resembles an intervertebral disc with a nucleus pulposus and anulus fibrosus (Lillie 1915). The articular heads of the mandibles are balls that fit into open sockets, rather than hinge joints. Thus the mandibles are free to rotate around their long axes as well as to swing up, down, left, and right. The right whale has a synovial temporomandibular joint, but in some, if not all, rorquals, that joint is replaced partially or fully by a fibrocartilage mass (Perrin 1870; Beauregard 1882; van Beneden 1882). As the jaw opens and the buccal floor stretches, the dorsal edge of each mandible rolls laterally (Lillie 1915; Pivorunas 1977). This has the effect of increasing the space between the rami by as much as three quarters of a meter in a 12 m humpback whale.

Two mechanisms assist in returning the jaw to its normal position. First, the fibrous tissue in the temporomandibular and intermandibular joints stores energy as elastic strain when the jaws are forced open by the oncoming water. Thus, in one sense, the jaws are spring-loaded and designed to snap shut automatically. Second, balaenopterid whales retain a coronoid process and have extensive temporal fossae for the attachment of large external adductor muscles of the mandible. The masseter and temporalis are not balanced by large internal adductors; rather the pterygoidei, and the pterygoid fossae from which they would originate, are greatly reduced (Carte and Macalister 1868; DeLage 1886; Schulte 1916). Therefore, a net torque is applied to the dentary along its long axis when the adductors contract. The result is not only that the jaws close but that the upper edge of the mandible rolls inward to press against the lateral margins of the baleen plates (Lillie 1915). This helps to buttress the baleen, keeping it from being pushed outward as the water flows out of the buccal cavity.

It is important that the lower jaws encircle the baleen plates as the mouth is closed, so that the baleen remains medial to the jaws despite the outward pressure of water extruded from the mouth. The rolling movements of the jaws just described may assist in this action. The fact that each lower jaw can roll somewhat independently inward and outward between the temporomandibular and the symphysis should help the mandibles clear the baleen during closure. Gross body movements, which alter the pressure of the water against the jaw (Brodie 1977) and swing the jaws from side to side, may also aid in repositioning the mandible.

Continuous Suction Feeders. *Ammocoetes.* Ammocoetes feed within burrows and are the most sessile of all vertebrate suspension feeders. Mallatt (1982) viewed them as specialized for pumping water at a slower rate than other suspension feeders but able to handle very concentrated suspensions. Forward-directed oral cirri surround the entrance of the mouth and act as a screen to prevent large particles from entering. In *Petromyzon marinus* the cirri exclude particles larger than 340 μm (Youson 1981).

Ammocoetes propel water into their mouths by rhythmic contractions of the pharyngeal wall and by oscillations of the velum, a pair of muscular flaps that lie between the oral orifice and the pharynx. Contraction of the pharynx is achieved by circular constrictors acting on a cartilaginous lattice, the branchial skeleton (Hardisty 1981). Elastic rebound in the branchial basket reduces intrapharyngeal pressure and draws water into the mouth (fig. 2.5). Mallatt (1981) considered the parabranchial chambers of ammocoetes to be similar to those of Chondrichthyes and felt that the ventilatory mechanism was fundamentally the same between fishes that use a dual ventilatory pump (the "force-suction pump" of Hughes 1960a, b) and ammocoetes. However, when lamprey larvae are undisturbed, the amplitude of pharyngeal contractions approaches zero (Rovainen and Schieber 1975). In that situation, velar movements continue as the sole pumping mechanism.

The velar flap on each side has an internal mucocartilage skeletal bar and protracting/retracting muscles. The medial edges of the velar flaps approximate as they move backward and separate as they move forward; thus they can fulfill both a piston and valvular function (Mallatt 1981). Flaps across the external branchiopores also act as branchial valves, opening and closing with each contraction of the branchial baskets (fig. 2.5). They act passively such that there is some reflux of water into the pharynx through the branchiopores as the pharynx begins to expand.

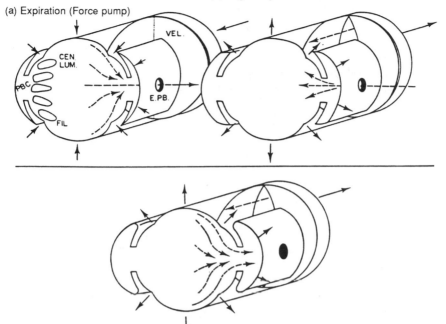

(a) Expiration (Force pump)

(b) Begin inspiration

(c) Inspiration (Suction pump)

Fig. 2.5. Model of water flow within the ventilating ammocoete pharynx. The pharynx is viewed from behind, anterior is to the right. Only one of seven pharyngeal segments is represented; central lumen and gill pouch are treated as a single unit. Water flow directions are indicated by dashed arrows, while movements of pharyngeal structures are indicated by solid arrows. Positions of the gill filaments are indicated in the left half of the top left diagram. During expiration (top left), the pharynx contracts and the velum moves posteriorly, forcing water over gill filaments and out the external branchiopore. At the onset of inspiration (top right), the velum moves forward and the pharynx begins to expand. Enlargement of the central lumen and parabranchial chambers draws some water in through the branchiopore under the still-closing branchial valve (black), and flow over the gills is medial. Later in inspiration (bottom center), the gill pores are entirely shut, and the expanding parabranchial chambers draw water laterally again across the filaments. Steps (a) and (c) comprise the force and suction pumps respectively of the classic piscine ventilatory mechanism (Hughes 1960a, b). Occasionally during ventilation, no pharyngeal movements occur. When that is the case, flow patterns of steps (a) and (b) do not differ from the above, but in step (c) no lateral flow across the gill occurs. CEN. LUM. = central lumen of pharynx, E.PB. = external branchiopore, FIL. = gill filament, PB.C. = parabranchial chamber, VEL. = velum. (From Mallatt 1981, courtesy of the Zoological Society of London)

Tadpoles. Tadpoles feed from a stationary position either midwater (e.g., most pipids and microhylids) or along the substrate (most other tadpoles). Facultative suspension-feeding tadpoles (Seale 1982) are benthic grazers that have external keratinized beaks and denticles, which they use to reduce detritus, macrophytes, and periphytic films to a size small enough to be brought into the mouth in suspension (Duellman and Trueb 1985; Altig and Johnston 1986). Obligate suspension feeders that live in midwater lack keratinized mouthparts. In both cases, the water transport system and particle entrapment mechanisms used are essentially the same (Seale and Wassersug 1979; Wassersug 1980).

The buccal pumping mechanism of anuran larvae has been investigated by a number of workers in recent decades. The most comprehensive studies are those of DeJongh (1968), Kenny (1969a), and Gradwell (1968, 1971, 1972a, b, 1975); older studies are cited therein. The essential feature of the pump is a medially expanded ceratohyal plate on each side that articulates laterally with the palatoquadrate. The ceratohyal plates serve as the piston for the buccal pump (fig. 2.6). Muscles that run from the lateral arm of the ceratohyal to the muscular process of the palatoquadrate, primarily the orbitohyoideus (Satel and Wassersug 1981; Wassersug and Pyburn 1987), cause the central portion of the ceratohyal to drop when they contract. A transverse sling of muscle below the ceratohyal that also attaches to the lateral arms of the ceratohyals, the interhyoideus, elevates the buccal floor when it contracts. Gradwell (1972b) has pointed out that the musculature of the ceratobranchials behind the ceratohyals may constrict and elevate the branchial baskets, thus acting as a secondary pump. It is not known, however, whether the slight movements of the branchial baskets observed when the tadpole buccal floor oscillates during normal feeding and breathing are passive or active.

Severtzov (1969) contrasted the horizontal expansion and ventral/dorsal movement of the tadpole ceratohyal with the fore-aft movement of the urodele larva's gill arches. An important aspect of the plane of movement of the tadpole buccal pump is the extreme elongation and horizontal orientation of the palatoquadrates, with which the ceratohyals articulate (Wassersug and Hoff 1982). This orientation of the jaw suspension distinguishes tadpoles from all other vertebrates, including adult frogs. In suspension-feeding tadpoles, this unusual design for the jaw suspension is associated with short Meckel's cartilages and a small oral orifice. At metamorphosis, the tadpole branchial skeleton completely rebuilds: the palatoquadrate shortens and takes up a more vertical orientation, Meckel's cartilage elongates, and the tadpole buccal pump disappears. With that, the anuran goes from being a small-mouthed microphagous tadpole to a big-mouthed macrophagous frog.

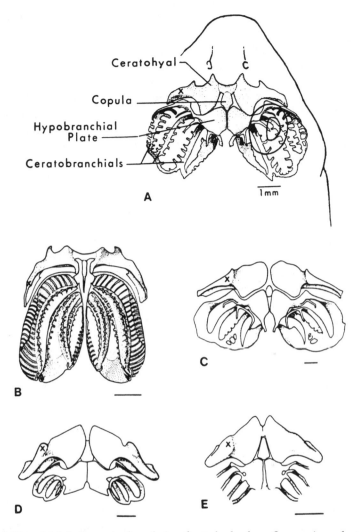

Fig. 2.6. Branchial skeletons in dorsal view for tadpoles from five species, selected to illustrate basic structures and diversity. Anterior is toward the top of the page. The "x" on each drawing indicates the point of articulation of the ceratohyal with the palatoquadrate bar on one side (not shown). The ceratobranchials form the branchial baskets and the gill filters arise from the ceratobranchials. All elements are cartilage. A. *Rana pipiens,* with major structures labeled. This larva is a dietary generalist, feeding on a coarse suspension of particles generated through the action of its keratinized beaks and denticles. B. *Gastrophryne carolinensis,* an obligate suspension feeder. C. *Heleophryne natalensis,* a benthic tadpole adapted to fast flowing water. This larva has a large suctorial mouth and grazes on periphyton. D. *Anotheca spinosa,* an arboreal, macrophagous, carnivorous larva. E. *Hyla microcephala,* a pond tadpole that ingests large filamentous plant fragments and zooplankton. (From Wassersug and Hoff 1979)

There is a spectrum of particle sizes on which tadpoles of different species preferentially feed, and these preferences can be correlated with differences in the buccal pump design among tadpoles (Wassersug and Hoff 1979). At one extreme, there are midwater, obligatorily microphagous larvae (fig. 2.6a, b). They tend to have a ceratohyal with a small medial surface area and short lateral lever arm (poor mechanical advantage). Wassersug and Hoff demonstrated that this was a design that achieved a large buccal volume by depressing a small buccal floor area a relatively long distance, i.e., "a small bore, long stroke" design. This design does not favor sucking in resistant prey, but by having a small buccal floor area these tadpoles have more cranial space left for gill filters. They have, indeed, the most extensive gill filters of any tadpoles. At the other extreme are the larvae of a few species that have evolved into obligatorily macrophagous forms (fig. 2.6c, d, e). These tadpoles have a longer lateral lever arm on their ceratohyal (high mechanical advantage) and a larger buccal floor area. They have a powerful buccal pump (associated with disproportionately large buccal floor depressor musculature; Satel and Wassersug 1981), but one that is not depressed very far, i.e., "a large bore, short stroke" design. They can pull into their mouths large and resistant prey, but space for their large buccal pump is at the expense of their gill filters. These tadpoles have little (e.g., *Anotheca*, Hylidae) or no (e.g., *Hymenochirus*, Pipidae) gill filters and the ceratobranchials—the skeletal elements that support the gill filters—are reduced in length and occasionally even in number (Wassersug et al. 1981).

There are several valves in tadpoles that control one-way flow. The mouth opens as the buccal floor is depressed and closes just before the buccal floor is elevated (e.g., DeJongh 1968; Kenny 1969a). The internal nares have simple, passive, valvular flaps that close as buccal pressure rises (Wassersug 1980; Wassersug and Heyer 1988). There is an elegant, internal valve mechanism built around a nonmuscular flap of tissue, called the ventral velum (not homologous with the velum in ammocoetes). The ventral velum of tadpoles extends caudally from the ceratohyal over the branchial baskets in most tadpoles (fig. 2.7). It has a cartilaginous skeleton made of spicules projecting rearward from the hypobranchial plate. Because the hypobranchial plate is overlapped rostrally by the ceratohyal, when the ceratohyal is depressed, the front of the hypobranchial plate is depressed also. The caudal part of the hypobranchial plate, however, moves upward because the plate rotates around a transverse axis (DeJongh 1968). This pushes the posterior free edge of the ventral velum against the buccal roof and seals the buccal cavity to the front from the pharyngeal cavity behind. As the buccal floor is elevated and buccal pressure rises, the ventral velum comes down and water is injected into the branchial baskets

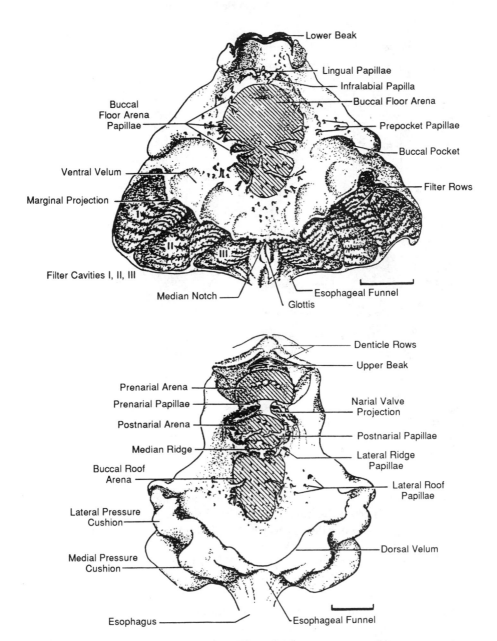

Fig. 2.7. The floor (above) and the roof (below) of a *Hyla femoralis* larva with major morphological features labeled. The complex surface features sense, sort, and direct particulate matter carried into the mouth of the tadpole in water currents. The scale line equals 1 mm. (From Wassersug 1980)

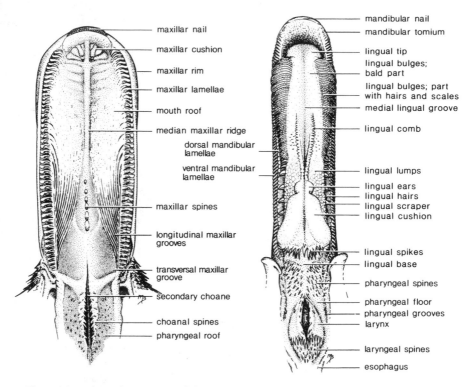

Fig. 2.8. Epidermal structures of the maxilla and pharynx of the mallard, *Anas platyrhynchos,* in a ventral view (left) and of the mandibula, tongue, and pharynx in a dorsal view (right). (Adapted by G. A. Zweers from Kooloos 1986 and Kooloos et al. 1989)

(Gradwell and Pasztor 1968). Another transverse flap, called the dorsal velum, descends from the buccal roof behind the ventral velum and helps to direct the jet of water down toward the gill filters and the mucus entrapment surfaces.

Tadpoles in the genus *Xenopus* (Pipidae) lack a valvular ventral velum. In those species, flaps on the body wall cover the opercular chamber and open and close with each stroke of the buccal pump; they serve as passive valves like the flaps over the branchiopores in ammocoetes.

Ducks and Flamingos. Suspension-feeding ducks (table 2.4) have relatively long and broad bills (Avilova 1978). The larger, upper bill in these birds bows upward in cross section to canopy completely the lower bill and the tongue when the mouth is closed. A row of keratinized lamellae lines the lateral margins of both beaks (fig. 2.8). When the mouth is slightly ajar, the lamellae on the upper jaw oppose the lamellae on the lower jaw and may act as sieves for straining particles from the water.

Unlike the comparatively amorphous tongue of suspension-feeding mammals, tongues of suspension-feeding birds are morphologically complex (see fig. 2.8 and figures in Crome 1985; Kooloos 1986; Kooloos et al. 1989). In anatines the tongue is broad, with two large, swollen areas that act as pistons to draw water into the mouth (Zweers et al. 1977; Kooloos and Zweers 1991). The more anterior area, the region of the lingual bulges, is pressed against the roof of the mouth as the tongue is drawn backward, but moves away from the roof when that portion of the tongue advances. Thus the bulges act as both a piston and a valve. The more posterior swelling, the lingual cushion, is bounded laterally by projections called lingual scrapers that ride past the lamellae. The cushion terminates posteriorly in a field of spikes. As the cushion oscillates back and forth, the scrapers remove food particles from the lamellae and draw ingested material posteriorly toward the esophagus. The spikes ultimately help to drive particles into the esophagus.

The tongue moves rapidly; in *Anas platyrhynchos* the tongue tip travels back and forth 11 mm in cycles that last 60–70 msec (Zweers et al. 1977). Cycle frequencies are only slightly lower in other species (Kooloos et al. 1989). The underlying musculoskeletal system that allows these complex lingual movements to take place so rapidly is described in detail in Zweers (1974).

With each cycle, the jaws open and close slightly (maximum and minimum gape during feeding in *A. platyrhynchos* equal 14 mm and 3 mm, respectively; Zweers et al. 1977). This is accomplished as much by elevation of the maxillae, which rotate through ≤ 13° with each cycle, as by depression of the mandible. The fast oscillations of the jaws help suck water into the mouth and give it momentum. Since these beak movements take place against the resistance of water and often mud, they require some force. Anatine ducks are characterized by a large retroarticular process on the mandible for the insertion of a large depressor muscle complex. The jaw adductors, specifically the vertically oriented pterygoid muscles, are equally large. Heavy jaw protractor muscles arise from a large lateral extension of the lacrymal bone. The lacrymo-mandibular and occipitomandibular ligaments, which help control jaw kinetics, are also very large, as are, of course, the surfaces from which they originate.

The jaw and tongue movements together bring water into the front of the mouth as a thin sheet. Water is then expelled from the mouth along the posterior 70% to 95% of the rim (Kooloos et al. 1989). It takes from 2 to 7 cycles for food particles to travel from outside the mouth, past the lingual bulges, and onto the collecting surfaces. It takes another 3 or 4 cycles for that ingested material to reach the esophagus.

One can contrast some of these features of ducks with those of the ultimate suspension-feeding birds, the flamingos. In flamingos, the tongue is a narrower, more cylindrical structure which lies in a bony trough formed within the deep lower jaws. Depending on the genus, the upper beak has either a deep or shallow median keel that descends toward the tongue and forms a cap over the lingual trough. Multiple rows of fine lamellae cover the interfacing regions of the upper and lower jaws (Jenkin 1957). The shape of the tongue and its tight confinement suggest that it functions as a simple piston, although the details of its movements have not been described. There are spines on the tongue posteriorly that may help to move food particles toward the esophagus, but the contact region for those spines with the lamellar fields on the beaks is far less than in the ducks.

In both flamingos and suspension-feeding ducks, the mouth opens and closes slightly with each tongue cycle. The mesokinetic skull of flamingos allows the upper jaw to be elevated when the lower one is depressed, but there are no quantitative data on how much rotation actually takes place for either jaw during a typical feeding cycle, as there is for ducks (Zweers et al. 1977; Kooloos 1986; Kooloos et al. 1989).

As in ducks, the feeding cycles are rapid; Jenkin (1957) reported four hyoidean/tongue cycles per second for *Phoenicopterus antiquorum,* whereas deJong and Zweers (1981) gave cycle lengths of 60 msec for the closely related *Phoenicopterus ruber.* According to Jenkin, in *Phoenicopterus* water is drawn in along the sides of the beaks and not just at the front. Lateral head movements are a common part of flamingo feeding and are thought to stir up water and bottom material, but may actually be part of the driving force propelling water through the beaks (deJong and Zweers 1981).

The small gape of all suspension-feeding birds helps exclude unwanted material from the mouth. Although it has not been rigorously documented, Jenkin (1957) inferred from the anatomy of the flamingo that the role of valves—crucial for assuring one-way flow—is achieved by the subtle movements of the jaws in relation to each other. By opening and closing the jaws, or possibly by lateral movements of the jaws, the spacing between lamellae can be greatly modified and the resistance to flow altered (Jenkin 1957). The jaw movements that are possible differ between ducks and flamingos. This is testified to by the quadrate-articular joint, which is a flat, open joint in the former and a ball and socket in the latter.

Both anatine and phoenicopterid birds share unusually long retroarticular processes for the attachment of jaw depressors. The beaks are narrower in flamingos than in ducks, so resistance from the surrounding water to jaw depression may be less; however, flamingos face the unique problem of having to depress their lower jaws against gravity since they feed with their heads upside down.

Similarities between anatine and phoenicopterid feeding structures vary with the species compared. According to Crome (1985), the freckled duck *Stictonetta naevosa* "has bill features more characteristic of flamingos," than other ducks. Based on the features just outlined it is too simplistic to say, as did Olson and Feduccia (1980b, ii), that "the structure of the feeding apparatus of flamingos is . . . entirely different from that of the Anseriformes" (see "Discussion").

Intermittent Suction Feeders. A large number of species in the cichlid genera *Oreochromis* and *Sarotherodon* are planktivorous (Bowen 1982; Philippart and Ruwet 1982). While only a few of these species have been observed to use intermittent suction feeding (Gophen et al. 1983; Drenner, Vinyard et al. 1982), the presence of phytoplankton in the diets of other species indicates that they use a mode of suspension feeding. These species demonstrate remarkable trophic plasticity, feeding opportunistically on phytoplankton, benthic algae, aquatic macrophytes, detritus, zooplankton, and periphyton (Bowen 1982; Philippart and Ruwet 1982). Since the mode of suspension feeding that we refer to as intermittent suction feeding is very similar to suction feeding on individual prey items, it is not surprising that intermittent suction feeders do not appear to possess unique morphological features related to the transport of water into the mouth. Like continuous ram feeders, however, intermittent suction feeders tend to have reduced dentition (e.g., *Coregonus:* Dorofeyeva et al. 1980; Vladykov 1970; Norden 1961; *Dorosoma cepedianum:* Miller 1960) and, in the case of suspension-feeding sharks, reduced heterodonty (Compagno 1990).

Although there have been no observations of feeding in megamouth sharks (*Megachasma pelagios,* Megachasmidae), this species can generate suction to draw water into its mouth during respiration (Lavenberg 1991), and the consensus is that it feeds using suction (Compagno 1990; Lavenberg 1991). Taylor et al. (1983) noted a number of morphological features that distinguish *Megachasma* from the basking and whale sharks. While the basking shark has slightly protrusile jaws, megamouth can protrude its jaws forward to expand the oral orifice well in front of the snout. Taylor et al. (1983) suggested that the hyomandibulae and the jaws move downward, anteriorly, and laterally during protrusion. Megamouth's stout jaws, which are much longer than its cranium, contrast with the slender, weak jaws of continuous ram feeders. The enlarged jaws increase the diameter of the oral orifice, and the thick hyaline cartilage provides support. Relative to these huge jaws, the adductor mandibulae muscles are, as expected of suspension feeders, small and weak (Taylor et al. 1983).

Compagno (1990) also discussed important differences between the morphology of the continuous ram-feeding basking shark and that of megamouth. The basking shark has: (a) a small, flat tongue, (b) gill rakers that do not substantially impede water flow through the gill openings, and (c) enormously enlarged gill openings that extend onto the dorsal and ventral surfaces of the head. Megamouth, in contrast, has: (a) a large, thick, and broad tongue enclosing a greatly enlarged basihyoid cartilage, so that the tongue almost fills the oral cavity when the jaws are closed, (b) papillose gill rakers in dense clusters that screen the internal gill openings, and (c) moderately large gill openings that do not extend onto the dorsal or ventral surfaces of the head. In addition, Compagno (1990) diagrammed how the hyoid of megamouth can reverse direction, to lie with the hyomandibulae and ceratohyals anteroventral to their normal position. This movement of the hyoid would cause the tongue, basihyobranchial skeleton, and pharynx to be depressed ventrally, increasing the volume of water in the mouth. Compagno (1990) also noted a cranial morphological feature of megamouth that allows the upper jaws to tuck in under the cranium. The orbital processes of the palatoquadrates fit into a deep, prominent pit in the basal plate on each side of the ventral surface of the cranium. These characteristics of megamouth, in combination with its weak body musculature and soft fins, indicate that megamouth is an intermittent suction feeder (Compagno 1990).

Iridescent tissue has been reported on the upper jaw and palate of megamouth (Compagno 1990), and Taylor et al. (1983) suggested that the skin of the lower jaw and tongue might be luminescent. Although Diamond (1985) speculated on the possible advantages of luminescent tissue in attracting prey, Lavenberg (1991) stated that there was no evidence of luminescence in a live specimen observed in captivity.

TRANSPORT OF WATER PAST THE FEEDING STRUCTURES AND OUT OF THE MOUTH

Water transported into the mouth must be moved past the feeding structures and must exit the mouth. The forward motion of continuous ram feeders directs water posteriorly through the gape and past the feeding structures. Water exits laterally from the corners of the mouth in continuous ram-feeding whales or from the gill slits in fishes. Contraction of the buccal floor directs water into and through the baleen plates in intermittent ram-feeding whales. All continuous and intermittent suction feeders possess valves to preclude reflux of unprocessed water and use their lingual, pharyngeal, or buccal pumps to force the water through feeding structures.

Continuous Ram Feeders. Swimming fishes in general use the reduced pressure behind the operculum or gill slits, induced by the Bernoulli effect, to draw water out the gill slits (Vogel 1988). Continuous ram-feeding whales possibly make use of this phenomenon also, but this is strictly conjecture since no data are available on water pressures around the heads of freely swimming and feeding whales. The large tongue in balaenid whales directs water toward the baleen fringe. When right and bowhead whales are skimming at the surface, the arch of their rostra means that a pressure head of water can build up within their mouths between the tongue and baleen. Gravity may then help drive water through the baleen plates posteriorly.

Intermittent Ram Feeders. Next to moving their tails up and down, the expelling of water from their mouths by rorqual whales is the most massive, single action taken by any organism that has ever lived. Yet the process is largely unstudied. From the many descriptions of water rushing out of the mouths of these whales as they pitch over and roll on the ocean surface, there is no question that inertial and gravitational forces are of paramount importance. The major question concerning this action is how much of the compression of the buccal cavity is due to passive elastic rebound in the stretched tissues of the buccal floor as opposed to active muscle contraction. On the one hand, the older literature (e.g., Carte and Macalister 1868; Lillie 1915; Howell 1930) credits the musculature below the *cavum ventrale,* principally the mylohyoideus, with compressing the pouch. On the other hand, more recent studies of the histology and mechanical properties of the skin, blubber, and muscles all indicate that elastic recoil plays a major role in the return of the buccal floor to its resting position (Slijper 1962; Orton and Brodie 1987). Clearly both play a part (Lambertsen 1983).

Pivorunas (1977) demonstrated that the anterior portion of the pouch has a fibrocartilage skeleton formed as a bifid caudal extension of the mandibular symphysis. This structure gives some rigidity to the buccal floor and should help to elevate the floor, if it is strained during buccal expansion. Lambertsen (1983) suggested that the genioglossus pulls the tongue forward and upward near the end of expulsion. As the tongue comes up, its left and right lobes may be separately wedged between the baleen plates and the central keel of the rostrum. This would force the last remaining water out of the mouth.

Continuous Suction Feeders. For continuous suction-feeding forms with gill slits, the expulsion of water through the gill slits is the compressive half of the oscillating pump cycle (see above). This has been covered above in the section "Transport of Water into the Mouth." The role of the tongue in driving water through the lamellae in ducks and flamingos also has been discussed. In ducks, the topography of the buccal roof and the dorsum of the tongue necessarily directs feeding currents laterally to the marginal lamellae as the tongue is retracted and the upper beak depressed during each feeding cycle. Ciné x-ray analyses have confirmed the exact relationship between tongue movements and the extrusion of water in *Anas platyrhynchos* (Zweers et al. 1977; Kooloos et al. 1989). In flamingos, the tongue and jaw movements are also presumed to control the outflow of water (cf. Jenkin 1957); however, there has been no functional morphological analysis comparable to the work on ducks to test Jenkin's conjectures on this topic.

Intermittent Suction Feeders. The alewife and two *Coregonus* species have been reported to open and close the mouth several times at a rate of approximately two to three times per second, then pause for about 0.5 sec with the mouth closed before resuming feeding (Janssen 1976, 1978). Drenner, O'Brien et al. (1982) described "swallowing" movements that interrupt the feeding of gizzard shad.

The fishes can simply use the upper and lower jaws as a valve to prevent water from exiting anteriorly, or may close a pair of membranous valves (oral valves) that are located in the anterior region of the buccal cavity. With the mouth or oral valves closed, water is drawn through the branchial apparatus to retain food particles. The functional morphology and hydrodynamics of this process during suspension feeding in intermittent suction feeders have not been investigated, but there is no reason to suspect that they differ from those of other suction-feeding fishes. To return the mouth cavity to its resting volume, other suction-feeding species contract the adductor musculature of the jaws and the suspensory apparatus (Liem 1980). Negative pressure is generated in the opercular cavity as the opercular apparatus is abducted, contributing to the posterior flow of water (Lauder 1983).

SEPARATION OF PARTICLES FROM THE WATER

The dimensions of the entrapping structures, and the density and velocity of the food particles, affect entrapment processes for suspension feeders. Retention of particles on filters with a pore size smaller than the particles themselves ("straining" or "sieving") is only one of several possible entrapment mechanisms. Other mechanisms that may operate separately or simultaneously with sieving in vertebrates include direct interception, inertial impaction, and electrostatic entrapment (Rubenstein and Koehl 1977).

LaBarbera (1984) suggested that, based on morphology, sieving is likely to be the major particle-capture mechanism in suspension-feeding fishes and baleen whales. Most suspension feeders capture particles with an efficiency dependent on the size and shape of the particles (Jørgensen 1966). That is consistent with, but does not confirm, sieving as an entrapment mechanism. A sieve with a uniform mesh size should theoretically retain 100% of the particles above a certain size threshold and 0% below that threshold (Rubenstein and Koehl 1977). Few data are available that test this prediction for the gill arch structures of continuous ram-feeding and intermittent suction-feeding fishes.

In teleost suspension feeders and in the paddlefish, each of the anterior four gill arches possesses one or two rows of gill rakers. Where two rows are present, the rakers of one row are directed anterolaterally and those of the other are directed medially or posteromedially. The fifth gill arch usually possesses one row of gill rakers directed anterolaterally. The rakers generally consist of a bony or cartilaginous core covered by epithelium that may contain cuticle-secreting cells, mucus cells, and taste buds (Friedland 1985; Sibbing and Uribe 1985). The number of gill rakers, their length, and the size of the spaces between them may increase with the age and length of the fish (e.g., MacNeill and Brandt 1990; Gibson 1988; Ciechomski 1967; Krefft 1958).

Mummert and Drenner (1986) developed a mechanical-sieve model of filtering efficiency for gizzard shad (an intermittent suction-feeding fish), based on the cumulative frequency distribution of the distances measured between gill rakers. The ingestion rates for different particle sizes, as determined in laboratory feeding experiments, were consistent with the predictions of the model (Mummert and Drenner 1986). Durbin and Durbin (1975) and Friedland et al. (1984) reported that the retention efficiency of menhaden (a continuous ram-feeding fish) increased in a continuous rather than step fashion with the size of the food particles, a result that is not consistent with a sieving mechanism involving a mesh with pores of a single size. They pointed out, however, that detritus and the flocculation of phytoplankton could lead to the retention of some particles smaller than the pore size of the sieve.

From x-ray films of bream (an intermittent suction-feeding fish) with platinum markers implanted in the gill arches, Hoogenboezem et al. (1990) concluded that the distance between adjacent arches was too wide and variable for zooplankters to be sieved by the passive interdigitation of gill rakers on adjacent arches. Additional x-ray films by Hoogenboezem et al. (1991) indicated that 25% of individual *Daphnia* with a 1-mm-diameter iron sphere glued to their carapaces were retained in the channels between adjacent gill rakers on each arch. They proposed a model in which lateral rakers of bream move actively into the channel between medial rakers on the adjacent arch, forming a sieve with an adjustable mesh.

Particles that are small enough to pass between the elements of the filtering array are commonly retained by both invertebrate (Jørgensen 1966) and vertebrate suspension feeders, indicating that entrapment mechanisms other than sieving, such as direct interception and inertial impaction, are operative (Rubenstein and Koehl 1977). Inertial impaction as a particle encounter mechanism may come into play in animals that feed on relatively large, dense particles in high flow velocities (Rubenstein and Koehl 1977), including large fishes that are continuous ram feeders and whales in particular.

The mucus-secreting cells and the copious amounts of mucus found on the branchial elements of lamprey larvae, tadpoles, and some fish species (see, e.g., Hampl et al. 1983; White and Bruton 1983; Weisel 1973; Greenwood 1953) also point to capture mechanisms other than sieving. Food particles observed by Wassersug (1972) in mucus on the branchial food traps of tadpoles certainly could not have been collected by sieving, for those organs are not porous. The small size of tadpoles and ammocoetes means that they perform in a Reynolds number range where viscous forces are relatively significant and prohibit simple sieving (Wassersug 1989). Not surprisingly, none ram feed.

However, the presence of mucus on gill arches does not, of itself, preclude sieving as an entrapment mechanism. Whereas Friedland (1985) found mucus cells in the epithelium of the gill rakers and gill arches of menhaden, they were not present on the smallest units of the branchial apparatus, the branchiospinules on the rakers, which he considered the principal site of prey retention. Consequently, he concluded that sieving and not some form of mucus entrapment was the primary mechanism used in particle capture by the menhaden. Although mucus cells have been noted on the branchial apparatus of paddlefish (Weisel 1973), plankton smaller than the mean space measured between the gill rakers are ingested in a low proportion compared to their concentration in the environment (Rosen and Hales 1981). This led Rosen and Hales to suggest that mucus does not play an important role in paddlefish feeding.

Although gill arch structures have been assumed to be the site of particle retention in suspension-feeding fishes (e.g., Lammens 1985; Mummert and Drenner 1986; MacNeill and Brandt 1990; but see Harrison and Howes 1991), Sanderson et al. (1991) showed that water does not pass between the gill rakers of intermittent suction-feeding blackfish, and that the rakers do not serve as filters. Measurements of flow patterns and water velocities inside the oral cavity of blackfish, made with a fiberoptic endoscope and thermistor flow probe, found that the rakers act as barriers that direct particle-laden water to the mucus-covered roof of the oral cavity, where particles are retained. This filtration mechanism cannot operate in clupeids and engraulids that lack an expansive, mucus-covered oral roof. Further study will determine whether particles are retained on the gill rakers in such species, and whether transport of particles toward the esophagus is mediated by water currents directed passively by the morphology of the branchial apparatus itself during continuous ram feeding.

The problem of determining the filtration mechanism(s) operating at any instant is particularly difficult in intermittent ram feeders and both types of suction feeders because of unsteady flow. These organisms create a current which accelerates from zero or near zero and then decelerates back to that starting point. As the velocity increases, inertial impaction of particles should increase (Rubenstein and Koehl 1977). But as an additional complexity, the filters are flexible in most vertebrate suspension feeders and their pore size is not fixed. Even in those filters that are relatively rigid, such as the gill rakers of fishes and the lamellae of birds, the porosity varies as the gill arches abduct and adduct (Lauder 1986) or the jaws open and close (Kooloos et al. 1989), respectively. Filters in forms such as tadpoles and whales are arranged in such a way that they are compressed by the pressure of the water passing through them, so that their porosity varies with pressure. The pressure, in turn, changes in response to the density of prey and other material on the filters. All of these dynamic factors change the flow at the microscopic level and make it difficult to establish what entrapment mechanism(s) is (are) effective at any instant during vertebrate suspension feeding.

Jørgensen (1983), who was primarily concerned with invertebrates, stated that the Reynolds numbers that apply to the feeding structures of suspension feeders are very low, $<< 1$. Shimeta and Jumars (1991) presented data indicating that the filter elements of some benthic invertebrate suspension feeders may operate at Reynolds numbers from 10 to 40. Compared to invertebrates, vertebrate suspension feeders typically encounter higher flow velocities and possess larger feeding structures ("more porous filters," Jørgensen 1970), and thus may operate at somewhat higher Reynolds numbers. One of the few attempts to calculate a Reynolds number at entrapment surfaces for a vertebrate suspension feeder is that of Friedland (1985) for menhaden. He reported a conservative figure of 2 to 3, using the smallest unit in the feeding apparatus (the branchiospinule) as the relevant length dimension. Vogel (1981) suggested that the baleen whales may be the only suspension feeders operating at a high Reynolds number.

The flow regime around entrapment surfaces for virtually all vertebrate suspension feeders is too poorly known to estimate Reynolds numbers realistically, let alone characterize the specific physical mechanisms involved in particle encounter. Quantitative laboratory investigations of particle encounter and retention, combined with detailed histological, morphological, and fluid dynamic studies, will be needed to solve the problem.

Continuous Ram Feeders. The bones comprising the gill arches of continuous ram feeders may be laterally compressed (Kishinouye 1923); this is carried to an extreme in the paddlefish, which has ceratobranchial and epibranchial elements that are 15–20 mm wide in large specimens but only 1–2 mm thick in cross section (Grande and Bemis 1991). Water must pass between the rakers and the gill arches to reach the gill filaments and to enter the opercular cavity. The tips of the lateral rakers on the first arch abut the side of the oral cavity, and the lateral rakers of each successive arch extend anteriorly to the preceding arch. Continuous ram feeding fishes are characterized by extensive elaboration of the branchial apparatus, including spectacular increases in the length, number, and structural complexity of branchial elements. For example, the rakers of adult mackerel (*Rastrelliger*) are longer than the gill filaments and protrude forward past the corners of the gape when the mouth is open (Collette and Nauen 1983). In addition, denticles or branchiospinules are found on the surfaces of the rakers in many species (Bornbusch 1988; Gibson 1988; Friedland 1985; Collette and Nauen 1983).

There is little information on the extent to which the gill rakers are movable. In the paddlefish, Imms (1904) described muscle fibers on the outside of each raker that attach to the cartilage of the gill arch. He suggested that contraction of these muscle fibers would cause the rakers to be pulled outward at an angle of approximately 60° to the arch. Elastic fibers also attach the basal part of each raker to the arch. Imms (1904) hypothesized that these elastic fibers cause the rakers to lie against the arch when not in use. Matthews and Parker (1950) observed a similar system of muscle fibers and elastic fibers in the basking shark. In a model proposed by Kirchhoff (1958), the rakers of the herring spread and rotate as an elastic membrane at their bases is stretched during mouth opening. This appears to be the only report on the action of such an elastic membrane in teleosts.

In most clupeid and engraulid fishes, a number of gill arches meet in the dorsal midline, allowing the gill slits and rakers to extend further medially than usual. Rows of rakers replace the teeth that are typical in this location (Nelson 1967b). The mediopharyngobranchial is a cartilaginous element present in some of the clupeid fishes that have gill arches meeting in the dorsal midline. According to Nelson (1967b), this element bears rakers and has no apparent homologue in the gill arches of other vertebrates. He also noted that the dorsal attachment of gill arch elements prevents expansion of the pharynx in that area, and tends to be absent in "predaceous" fishes.

In the anchovy *Anchoa*, the gill arches extend far anteroventrally (Chapman 1944a). The hypohyals articulate with the anterior end of the first basibranchial directly behind the symphysis of the lower jaw. There is no glossohyal and, in fact, there is not sufficient space for a tongue. The basibranchials of mackerels, which are very narrow and laterally compressed (Kishinouye 1923), also extend far anteriorly (Matsui 1967). Consequently, the glossohyal is very small, as is the smooth tongue (Kishinouye 1923).

Proliferation of gill rakers, loss of teeth, and development of accessory organs known as epibranchial organs has been a dominant evolutionary theme in clupeid fishes (Nelson 1967a). Epibranchial organs are a pair of diverticula arising from the posterior roof of the pharynx above the esophagus. Small food particles appear to be channeled by gill rakers into the epibranchial organs, where the food is thought to be coalesced into a bolus that is then swallowed. Epibranchial organs are associated with microphagy and have been identified in five of the teleost families listed in tables 2.2 and 2.5. They occur in five groups of "lower" teleosts: the Cypriniformes, Salmoniformes, Gonorynchiformes, Osteoglossiformes, and Clupeiformes (Bertmar et al. 1969). The similarities in the structure and development of the epibranchial organs in these groups led Bertmar et al. (1969) to conclude that these fishes probably derive from a common ancestral group such as pholidophorids. Nelson (1967a), however, attributed the similarities to convergence. Since the functional morphology of these organs relates to the transport of food to the esophagus and involves primarily soft tissue, their structure will not be discussed further.

As in the teleosts, the evolution of continuous ram feeding in elasmobranchs has involved tremendous increases in the length and number of gill rakers (Moss 1981). The comblike gill rakers of the basking shark are arranged in a single series on the edge of each arch, directed anteriorly, as is a strip of hooked denticles (Matthews and Parker 1950, Schnakenbeck 1955). A thick epithelial layer at the bases of the rakers was thought to be the source of much of the abundant mucus found in the stomach (Matthews and Parker 1950).

The whale shark differs from the other two suspension-feeding shark species in that the elements of the feeding apparatus are not restricted to the margins of the internal gill openings (Taylor et al. 1983). Lateral to the five gill arches is a series of parallel compressed plates that connect adjacent arches (Gudger 1941a). These plates have a cartilage core and support a medial spongy tissue grid that is covered with denticles. The mesh of this grid is too fine to permit rapid processing of large volumes of water. Taylor et al. (1983) suggested that this dense screen, combined with a very long, broad, low pharynx and relatively small gill openings, allows the whale shark to generate suction as well as to suspension feed. Small food particles are collected on the feeding apparatus during continuous ram feeding, but intermittent suction feeding is reportedly used to capture fishes while the whale shark remains relatively stationary in a school of feeding fishes (Gudger 1941b). The basking shark does not appear to be capable of suction feeding (Taylor et al. 1983).

Rays in the family Mobulidae possess a series of gill rakers on anterior and posterior surfaces of each of the first four gill arches, and a series on the anterior face of the fifth arch (Bigelow and Schroeder 1953). Each raker is feathered with pinnately arranged protuberances (*Mobula;* MacGinitie 1947), or is composed of overlapping serrated lobes (*Manta;* Bigelow and Schroeder 1953).

The baleen of continuous ram-feeding whales is similar to that of intermittent ram-feeding whales (see below).

Intermittent Ram Feeders. Probably the best-known single feature of any vertebrate suspension feeder is whalebone. Because baleen is keratin of epidermal origin and not strictly part of the skull or skeleton of whales, it will not be discussed here in detail. There are a few general points though that pertain to the relative feeding capabilities and cranial designs of the different species.

The basic morphology of baleen plates, which across species number from 100 to 400 per side (Tomilin 1967; Pivorunas 1979), is summarized in Matthews (1978) and Slijper (1979). Efforts to quantify baleen morphology so that interspecific variation can be correlated with feeding ecology and diet were begun by Nemoto (1959), and extended by Williamson (1973), Pivorunas (1976), and Kawamura (1974, 1978, and other papers cited therein). A good review on this topic remains Nemoto (1970), who offered this concise distinction: "The shape of plates in right, Greenland and pygmy right whales is slender and elastic, and the fringes along the inner margin of the plates are very fine and numerous. The plates of Balaenopteridae whales (blue, fin, humpback, etc.) are short and tough, and have rather rough baleen fringes." The plates in the Greenland right whale (bowhead) may exceed 3 m in length, which is three times the length of the plates in any rorqual. The plates in the latter, however, may be twice as wide as those of the former. Nemoto (1970) estimated that the gross filter area of a 17 m right whale was 13.5 m² compared to only 4.6 m² for a 27 m blue whale.

Matthews (1978) cautioned that there is not a simple correlation between the texture of the baleen fringe and the diets of whales. This is because the fringe is flexible and its characteristics vary in life depending on hydrodynamic factors such as flow direction and water pressure (Pivorunas 1976). Fringe morphology also varies along the length of the baleen plates and from one plate to another along the rostrum. Nevertheless, in light of what is currently known about the diets of whales (e.g., Nerini 1984; Würsig et al. 1985; Ridgway and Harrison 1985; Nelson and Johnson 1987) certain relationships stand out. First, continuous ram-feeding whales have relatively greater filter surface area overall (Kawamura 1974). Secondly, there is a gross relationship between the morphology of the baleen plates, their fringes, and the diets of whales. Those species least likely to take microplankton have stiffer baleen fringes. For example, gray whales, which feed on coarse, abrasive material ram-fed or sucked off the bottom (Ray and Schevill 1974; Nerini 1984; Nelson and Johnson 1987), have stiff, thick, short plates with a coarse, short fringe. At the other extreme, the sei whale, which is the rorqual that has been consistently reported to prefer copepods to larger prey (Kawamura 1974; Watkins and Schevill 1979; Gambell 1985), and even to hunt in a continuous ram-feeding fashion (Nemoto 1970; Mitchell 1974; Gaskin 1976; Krushinskaya 1986), has a finer fringe with both a mean diameter and density per cm of plate more similar to that of balaenid whales than other rorquals.

Continuous Suction Feeders. *Ammocoetes and Tadpoles.* The particle entrapment surfaces of tadpoles and ammocoetes are soft tissue and not part of the skull. Thus, we will not discuss them in detail here other than to emphasize the few features that they have in common.

In both forms the smallest particles are trapped directly in mucus generated by special secretory tissue (for ammocoetes see Mallatt 1979, 1981; for tadpoles, Savage 1952; Kenny 1969b; Wassersug 1972; Wassersug and Rosenberg 1979). In the ammocoete these are the goblet cell fields of the parabranchial chambers located laterally and not, according to Mallatt (1981), the medial endostyle as has been erroneously assumed in much of the older literature. Particles can be trapped anywhere along the mucus cords, but larger particles are more likely to be trapped medially (figs. 2.9, 2.10).

In most tadpoles, the mucus entrapping surfaces are concentrated on the ventral surface of the ventral velum and have been called the branchial food traps by most recent authors (fig. 2.7). In the case of pipids, which lack a ventral velum, the branchial food traps are dorsally facing on the pharyngeal floor above the gill filters (Gradwell 1975; Viertel 1987). In macrophagous forms, the branchial food traps are reduced in size or absent (Wassersug et al. 1981; Lannoo et al. 1987).

In tadpoles, there are papillary fields on the buccal floor and roof that can act as both sieves and funnels (Wassersug 1980; Viertel 1982, 1985; Sokol 1981); they can direct large particles toward the esophagus directly and smaller particles into the pharynx. Particles aggregated in mucus can be caught on the gill filters proper, which extend upward from the gill bars. The mucus, however, comes from the branchial food traps or elsewhere in the mouth since there is little secretory tissue associated with the filters (Kenny 1969a, b). The size and porosity of the gill filters correlate roughly with the size of particles that tadpoles of different species ingest (Wassersug 1980; Wassersug and Heyer 1988) but, as noted above, particles much smaller than the pore size of the filters are commonly ingested. The pore size itself is clearly not static and direct interception seems more important than sieving.

Food and mucus are transported by cilia to the esophagus, but water movements play a motive role as well. The evidence for this is that the

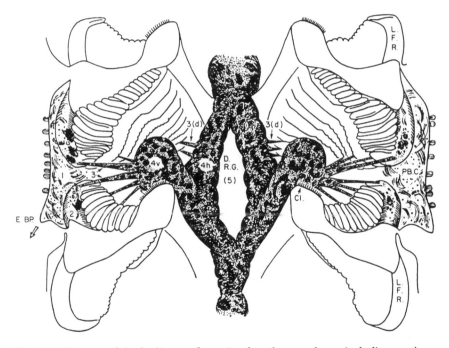

Fig. 2.9. Diagram of the feeding configuration for a lamprey larva, including portions of the mucus complex not visible in Fig. 2.5. The pharynx is shown in frontal hemisection, dorsal half, single gill pouch. Anterior is above. Note the outline of the dorsal ridge under the mucus in the center. Segments of the mucus complex (1–5) are depicted, as is the relative degree of particle aggregation within each. Note how the extreme dorsal gill pouch strands, 3(d), are attached medially to the horizontal band (4h) on the dorsal ridge. L.F.R. = lateral region of gill filament, E.BP. = external branchiopore, D.R.G. = dorsal ridge, CI. = ciliary tract, PB.C. = parabranchial chamber. (From Mallatt 1981, courtesy of the Zoological Society of London)

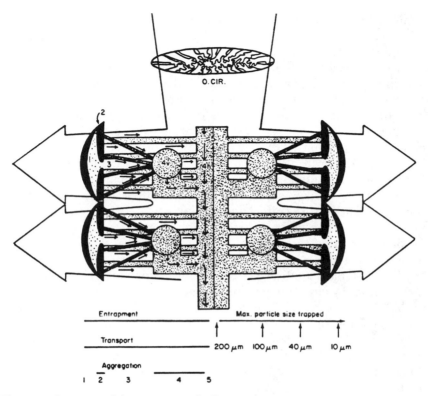

Fig. 2.10. Summary of the ammocoete feeding mechanism. Only the mucus complex (stippled) is shown; its segments are labeled as in fig. 2.9. The very large, unshaded arrows indicate the average path of water flow. For simplicity, only two of the seven gill pouches are shown. Mucus is continually manufactured laterally by the epithelium of the lateral regions of the filaments and the parabranchial chambers (black), then moved medially, then posteriorly, as indicated by small arrows. The three lines at bottom left indicate that while entrapment and transport of particles occur throughout the complex, aggregation occurs only at the lateral regions of the filaments (2) and on the ciliary tracts (4v, h). The line at bottom right indicates that the maximum size of particles trapped decreases from the medial to the lateral parts of the mucus complex. The oral cirri prefilter water entering the pharynx. O.CIR. = oral cirri. (From Mallatt 1981, courtesy of the Zoological Society of London)

ciliary tracts that move the mucus and the goblet cells where the mucus is generated are topographically separated.

Ducks and Flamingos. Until recently the particle capture mechanism for all suspension-feeding birds was presumed to be strictly sieving on lamellae. The fine structure and morphometry of the lamellae in both ducks and flamingos have been studied in great detail (see Crome 1985; Kooloos et al. 1989; Jenkin 1957, and references therein). As with the filters of other suspension-feeding vertebrates, from tadpoles to whales, there is a general relationship between how fine, dense, and numerous the filters of suspension-feeding birds are and the modal size of particles either found in their guts or handled most efficiently by them in the laboratory (Avilova 1978). Unfortunately the pattern is not absolute; the diet of some ducks, but not all, can be predicted from the morphology of their lamellae (Crome 1985; Kooloos et al. 1989). There are two reasons for this imprecision. First, as shown experimentally by Kooloos et al. for ducks and inferred by Jenkin for flamingos, these birds adjust the porosity of their filtering mechanism to the particle size they are feeding on by continuous fine alterations of gape and maxillary elevation. Secondly, some ducks, such as mallards and the tufted duck (*Aythya fuligula*), can maintain feeding efficiency even after fairly extensive ablation of their sieving lamellae (Kooloos et al. 1989), so mechanisms of filtration other than simple sieving must be operating.

Kooloos et al. (1989) suggested that, in addition to sieving, ducks capture particles by inertial impaction secondary to the induction of vortices in their feeding currents. This suggestion is based on a high, but rough, estimate of a Reynolds number of < 2000 at the surfaces where entrapment takes place. Separation of particles by this mechanism, which is a form of centrifugation, requires that the density of the particles be great relative to the water, and particle density was not incorporated in their analysis. Kenny (1969a) criticized vortex separation when it was previously hypothesized by Savage (1952) as a suspension-feeding mechanism for tadpoles. Despite these problems, for the moment there is no better proposal or more sophisticated analysis on how ducks capture particles after lamellar ablation.

The position and orientation of the lamellae on the beaks of both flamingos and ducks, and the fact that they use fine changes in gape to regulate the mesh size of their filters, help explain some of the strange curvatures in the beaks of these birds. The famous, nearly right-angle bend of the beaks in flamingos and the very tight conformity of their jaws mean that a uniform distance across from one jaw to the other can be maintained distal to the bend at any angle of jaw opening (see Jenkin 1957, 466, 489). The bend thus helps maintain uniform spacing of opposing lamellae from the tip of the beaks back to the bend regardless of the gape. Because of the transverse arching of the beaks in ducks the same principle applies, but in a different plane. The facing lamellar surfaces of the upper and lower beaks in ducks are not in the horizontal plane, but are turned slightly vertical. This reorientation helps to maintain a more uniform spacing, as the jaws open, between the lamellae on one surface and those on the other along the length of the facing surfaces (Sanderson and Wassersug 1990).

Intermittent Suction Feeders. In the fishes that are both intermittent suction feeders and continuous ram feeders, the separation of particles from the water is likely to be achieved by the same mechanisms during both suspension-feeding modes. These mechanisms have been described above.

Species in the family Cichlidae have been reported to suspension feed using only intermittent suction. Greenwood (1953) suggested that the gill rakers on the arches of *Oreochromis esculentus* can sieve coarse particles, such as copepods, but are unable to retain phytoplankton. However, phytoplankton may adhere to mucus secreted by abundant mucus cells on the posterior mid-dorsal surface of the oral cavity, the gill arches, and the upper and lower pharyngeal jaws (Greenwood 1953; Northcott and Beveridge 1988). Greenwood (1953) envisioned aggregates of particle-laden mucus becoming entangled in the anterior teeth of the lower pharyngeal jaw, and being raked into the esophagus by subsequent movements of the upper and lower pharyngeal jaws.

Microbranchiospines ("micro-gillrakers") are minute structures in a row posterior to the gill rakers on the lateral faces of the second, third, and fourth gill arches of *Sarotherodon, Tilapia,* and *Oreochromis* species. Each microbranchiospine is approximately 250 μm long and 100 μm wide, with two rows of 8 to 16 teeth (Whitehead 1959). The teeth are approximately 35 μm in length and are spaced at 10μm intervals (Gosse 1955). The points of teeth are curved anteriorly, and they generally meet or overlap the teeth on the adjacent microbranchiospines. Whitehead (1959) hypothesized that microbranchiospines may comb the medial face of the gill filaments on the preceding gill arch, concentrating mucus and preventing the mucus from exiting with the water. Gosse (1955) proposed that the microbranchiospines may function as sieves or may retain particle-laden mucus. However, Beveridge et al. (1988) described well-developed microbranchiospines in a *Tilapia* species that consumes primarily macrophytes and benthic invertebrates rather than suspended particles.

Drenner, Taylor et al. (1984) reported that *Oreochromis aureus* captured particles as small as 7 μm and selectively consumed particles larger than 25 μm while intermittent suction feeding. They suggested that planktivorous cichlids strain particles with gill rakers and may also collect smaller particles on microbranchiospines. To test this hypothesis, Drenner, Vinyard et al. (1987) removed the gill rakers and microbranchiospines of *Sarotherodon galilaeus.* They noted no changes in particle ingestion rates or selectivity resulting from the surgical manipulation. Consequently, the mechanism of particle entrapment and the functions of gill rakers and microbranchiospines have not been established.

Jirasek et al. (1981) and Pichler-Semmelrock (1988) described narrow and dense lamellae, approximately 37 μm wide and 49 μm high, attached perpendicularly to the medial face of each raker in the silver carp. The distance between lamellae ranged from 12 to 26 μm. The lamellae are formed from thin plates of collagenous connective tissue (Hampl et al. 1983). Murphy (1950) described the unusual tufted appearance of the rakers in adult blackfish.

ADDITIONAL EXTANT SUSPENSION FEEDERS

Tables 2.2 through 2.5 give a partial list of the heterogeneous array of vertebrates that can suspension feed. Not included are a few species that are unquestionably suspension feeders, but which do not readily fit our simple four-way classification for suspension-feeding types.

First and foremost is the gray whale, *Eschrichtius robustus* (family Eschrichtiidae). This baleen whale shows a tremendous versatility in feeding, with reports encompassing continuous and intermittent ram feeding, intermittent suction feeding, and suction or ram feeding on benthic prey (Nelson and Johnson 1987; Taylor 1987; Nerini 1984; Ray and Schevill 1974). The gray whale has a small gap separating the baleen plates at the front of the mouth, a feature shared with continuous ram feeders. At the same time it has for its size a large hyoid and a large, muscular tongue, which suggest that it actively pumps water into its mouth. The most common feeding behavior for gray whales is scooping up benthic prey from the ocean floor, leaving trails as they gouge the mud substrate (Nelson and Johnson 1987). What is not clear is whether this action is achieved by ram feeding, suction feeding, or both. Most authors assume that gray whales suck prey off the bottom because the only *E. robustus* specimen observed in captivity (Ray and Schevill 1974) sucked prey off the bottom of its tank. The problem is that that individual was a juvenile and powerful oral suction occurs in all juvenile mammals. Whereas suction feeding is definitional to mammals before weaning, it is not commonly retained after weaning. The gray whale is large enough and swims at a high enough velocity that it is not impossible that it rams through bottom sediments.

Next are the prions. Prions are petrels of the genus *Pachyptila* (family Procellariidae; Warham 1990), which have also been called whale-birds because of the morphological features that they share with right whales (Murphy 1936). There is no question that the three largest species with the broadest bills (*P. desolata, P. vittata,* and *P. salvina*) can subsist on small zooplankton captured without being detected individually (Imber 1981; Prince and Morgan 1987); for example, one 16.0 g gut sample from a Dove prion, *P. desolata,* contained 41,000 copepods (Prince 1980). These species, however, are treated here separately from other suspension-feeding birds because so little is known about their morphology and feeding behavior.

The most conspicuous cranial features of the suspension-feeding *Pachyptila,* in contrast to their non–suspension-feeding congeners, are: a broad bill (extremely so in the aptly named broad-billed prion, *P. vittata*); a wide, muscular tongue; keratinized lamellae descending from the posterior lateral margins of the upper beak; and redundant folds of skin between the lower jaws that allow the buccal floor to expand in a pelicanlike fashion. The lamellae are similar to baleen in that they are closely packed plates, approximately 40 per cm of jaw margin in *P. desolata* (pl. 1c in Prince 1980), and are oriented perpendicular to the margin of the beaks. In *P. vittata* the lamellae number 150 or more per side (Murphy 1936) and reach a maximum length of 3.5 mm.

In lateral view the front half of the beak bows upward whereas the back half bows downward (illustrated in Murphy 1936; Fleming 1941; Prince 1980). As a result, the lamellar fringe at the back of the upper beak descends below the plane of the oral orifice when the mouth is partially open. Theoretically, then, water and food can enter the front of the mouth and be simultaneously strained out the back as the animal swims forward, in continuous ram-feeding fashion. One account of the feeding posture in these prions hints that they may, in fact, continuously ram feed. Ashmole (1971), following Murphy (1936), described these birds as resting on the surface with wings outstretched, bill underwater and propelling themselves forward with their feet. According to Ashmole, since "the power for filtering is provided by motion through the water . . . [this] is a fair analogue to a towed plankton net." On the other hand, they may more commonly feed in intermittent ram or pulse fashion. Murphy (1936) reported that *P. desolata* thrust their heads under water and "scoop for food." We are ignorant of whether the buccal cavity fills passively or actively during this scooping. There are no morphological studies that might give clues to tongue and cranial movements during suspension feeding in *Pachyptila.*

Arguably the most bizarre tadpole in the world is that of the microhylid frog *Otophryne robusta.* It is our final example of a vertebrate that clearly suspension feeds, but does not comfortably fit with either ram or suction feeders. This tadpole has been found shallowly buried in sand only at the bottom of streams in northern South America. It has a spiracular tube that is so long that it can extend above the sand even when the remainder of the larva is concealed. Wassersug and Pyburn (1987) suggested that the *Otophryne* tadpole filter feeds while buried. In a flowing stream the water pressure would necessarily be lower at the exposed tip of the spiracle than at the mouth and, in theory, a current could be drawn through the oral cavity by the Bernoulli effect (cf. Vogel 1988). If this speculation is correct, then the *Otophryne* tadpole would be the first vertebrate capable of filter feeding passively, without either ram feeding or suction feeding. The chondrocranium of *Otophryne* has a plethora of odd features, directly related to its combined fossorial/filter-feeding way of life (see table 1 in Wassersug and Pyburn 1987). These include: laterally expanded and thickened trabecular horns and suprarostral cartilages, to stiffen and brace the front of the snout; expansion and inversion of the muscular process of the palatoquadrate, to form a protective cap of cartilage over the more superficial hyoidean depressor muscles; and expansion of a cartilage lattice lateral to the otic capsule, as a protective cap over the branchial baskets. In general, there is hypertrophy of cranial cartilage which increases cranial density and helps the skull resist deformation during burrowing. The structures involved directly in particle capture (e.g., the filter plates in the branchial baskets and the mucus-secreting branchial food traps), however, differ little from those of *Otophryne*'s microhylid relatives that are obligate midwater suspension feeders.

FOSSIL SUSPENSION FEEDERS

No fossil forms are listed in tables 2.2 through 2.5, but a variety of extinct fish taxa could be added, such as the early teleost family Leptolepidae (Cavender 1970). Mallatt (1984a, b, 1985) argued forcefully that the earliest vertebrates, agnathan forms such as *Astraspis* (Darby 1982), were relatively sessile, benthic suspension feeders. If so, they must have been continuous suction feeders, like ammocoete larvae today. Close fossil relatives of extant forms known to suspension feed also are likely to have been suspension feeders, particularly if they are morphologically similar. Thus, for example, fossil anuran larvae of the extinct family Paleobatrachidae (Spinar 1972), which look very much like midwater, obligate, suspension-feeding pipid tadpoles, such as *Xenopus*, may safely be considered suspension feeders. *Presbyornis*, a charadriiform bird close to the ancestry of ducks, also has been considered a suspension feeder (Olson and Feduccia 1980a).

Several extinct plesiosaurs and pterosaurs have been deemed suspension feeders ostensibly because they had long thin teeth that paleontologists thought must have functioned better as sieves than as piercing/grasping structures. Of these, the pterosaur *Pterodaustro* (Pterodaustriidae) best fits our idea of a suspension-feeding vertebrate. The teeth on the lower jaw of *Pterodaustro* are extremely long, numerous, and closely packed (Bonaparte 1971; Sanchez 1973). They are so thin that to function in piercing prey seems out of the question (fig. 2.11). The teeth are, in fact, so thin that they appear to have been flexible (which is consistent with the observation that the porosity of biological sieves is not immutable in extant suspension feeders). Other putative suspension-feeding fossil reptiles, for example the

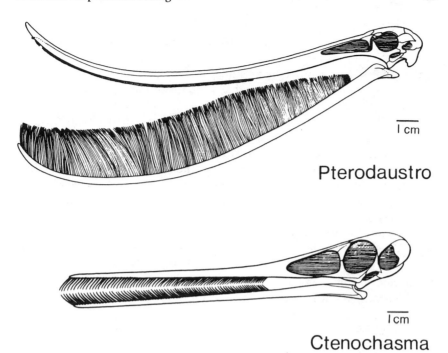

Fig. 2.11. Skulls from two fossil pterosaurs that have been considered suspension feeders. The case for *Ctenochasma* being a suspension feeder is more equivocal than for *Pterodaustro,* whose long, flexible mandibular teeth would seem to preclude grasping individual prey. *Pterodaustro* has been likened to flamingos (Bakker 1986). The teeth would have served as a filter. (From Wellnhofer 1981)

pterosaurs *Ctenochasma* and *Gnathosaurus* (Broili 1924; Sanchez 1973; Wellnhofer 1981) and the plesiosaur *Kimmerosaurus* (Brown 1981), have in comparison much shorter, stouter, more widely spaced teeth. They may have been piscivorous or eaten soft-bodied invertebrates, but we are skeptical that they were obligate suspension feeders.

Pterodaustro was approximately the size of the greater flamingo and shares with it a curved rostrum, although one that curves upward rather than downward (fig. 2.11). Bakker (1986) reconstructed *Pterodaustro* as a flamingo, feeding while standing in shallow water. This posture precludes ram feeding. We do not know whether the hyoid and tongue served as a pump for suction feeding. Since the filter structures (i.e., the teeth) project up from the mandible rather than descend from the skull, the vestibule between them might have been filled by a dipping motion of the lower jaw using either jaw adductors, neck extensors, or both.

PUTATIVE BUT PROBLEMATIC SUSPENSION FEEDERS

The case for many other living and fossil vertebrates being suspension feeders is dubious. Some of the problematic forms include turtles, salamander larvae, avocets, phalaropes, and seals.

Smith (1961) proposed that fleshy papillae called choanal rakers, which extend across the internal nares in the green sea turtle *Chelonia,* could function as strainers. Such structures may serve to protect the internal nares from obstruction, but in and of themselves they do not establish that sea turtles suspension feed and there has been no subsequent study of either the diet or functional morphology in *Chelonia* supporting Smith's hypothesis.

Certain freshwater turtles (e.g., *Podocnemis unifilis, Chrysemys picta, Kinosternon flavescens*) have been observed skimming small particles off the surface of the water (Mahmoud and Klicka 1979). During this behavior, termed neustophagia by Belkin and Gans (1968), the turtle holds its head with the mouth open and the margin of the lower jaw just below the water's surface. This causes a thin film of water to flow into the mouth by gravity. Ciné film analyses indicated a fourfold expansion of pharyngeal volume in *Podocnemis unifilis* when its hyoid was protracted during neustophagia (Belkin and Gans 1968). These turtles, however, do not have any specialized sieving structures at the margins of their mouths or elsewhere in the oropharyngeal cavity. Small particles are entrapped between nearly closed jaws as water is slowly expelled, just as water is expelled when larger prey are caught in the mouth. Given the absence of any true filters, it is not surprising that neustophagia appears to be neither common nor preferred by the few turtles in which it has been observed.

Tilley (1964) speculated that larval tiger salamanders (*Ambystoma tigrinum,* Ambystomatidae) may filter feed. There is no question that they regularly ingest small zooplankton. But despite much recent study of their feeding behavior (e.g., Leff and Bachmann 1986, 1988), no subsequent evidence has come forth indicating that they feed other than by attacking individual prey.

A few extant charadriiform birds with attenuate beaks, such as the American avocet (*Recurvirostra americana,* Recurvirostridae) and phalaropes (Phalaropodidae) take prey individually (Dodson and Egger 1980; Crome 1985) but have morphological features associated with suspension feeding, including papillae on the beak margins or the palate (Olson and Feduccia 1980b; Mahoney and Jehl 1985a). Phalaropes use water's adhesive and cohesive properties to transport a small amount of water containing the prey from the beak tip to the buccal cavity (Rubega 1990). The prey is then apparently held between lingual lumps and posteriorly facing palatal papillae as the remaining water is squeezed out of the mouth (Rubega, in preparation). Based on physiological studies of salt-loading in eared grebes (*Podiceps nigricollis*, Podicipedidae, Podicipediformes) feeding in a hypersaline and alkaline lake, Mahoney and Jehl (1985b) suggested that they also act like suspension feeders by pressing their large, fleshy tongues against the palate to separate prey (brine shrimp and brine flies) from water. The extrusion of water from the mouth is, of course, a component of suspension feeding. However, the issue of whether prey are selected individually, a criterion for suspension feeding, is not addressed by Mahoney and Jehl (1985b).

The crabeater seal, *Lobodon carcinophagus* (Phocidae), which has a diet consisting largely of euphausiacean krill, is often presumed to suspension feed (e.g., King 1972; Taylor 1987; Riedman 1990). This presumption goes back at least to Racovitza's (1900) passing comment that *Lobodon* swims with its mouth open, feeding in a manner similar to baleen whales. The crabeater, however, is a crepuscular forager (King 1983), which makes its feeding activity difficult to observe, and morphological evidence for suspension feeding in the animal is, at best, mixed. *Lobodon* has a proportionally longer, narrower snout and smaller orbits than other phocid seals (King 1972), and a scooplike lower jaw (King 1961). Both upper and lower postcanine teeth are triangular, subequal in size, and adorned with elongate, fingerlike cusps (see fig. 4 in Kooyman 1981). When the jaws are closed, upper and lower teeth occlude in an offset fashion such that a sieve is necessarily formed by the spaces between the cusps. Between the last molar and the coronoid process of the dentary is a bony protuberance which has been interpreted as a guard against prey escaping from the oral cavity posterior to the cheek teeth (King 1961).

It is easy to imagine how water captured with krill could be extruded from the mouth through the spaces between the cusps on *Lobodon*'s teeth. Juvenile crabeater seals feeding on fish in captivity sucked them in individually and ejected excess water from the sides of their mouths (Ross et al. 1976). A similar straining role has been proposed for the far less elaborate cusps on the cheek teeth in the ringed seal, *Phoca hispida* (Frost and Lowry 1981). However, these spaces alone do not establish suspension feeding any more than gill slits do in fishes. In contrast to the filters of virtually all confirmed vertebrate suspension feeders, which are made of soft flexible tissue, the teeth of these seals lack the finely adjustable porosity achieved by typical filters. Although the skulls of mysticete whales are more kinetic than those of odontocete whales (Brodie 1977; Pivorunas 1977), the skull and jaws of *Lobodon* do not appear any more kinetic than in other seals. No specialization of the hyoid, tongue, or other soft tissue of the buccal floor for suspension feeding has been reported so far in this genus. The most extensive observations available to date on *Lobodon* feeding in the wild—merely three sentences reported in Kooyman (1981)—suggest that invertebrate prey are captured one by one. Bonner (1990), however, came to the same conclusion based on an independent interpretation of crabeater seal morphology.

DISCUSSION

Ecomorphological Patterns

Our primary distinction between ram feeding and suction feeding splits the teleost fishes and elasmobranchs into two groups, one of which is placed with whales. Our secondary distinction, between continuous and intermittent feeding, produces some unlikely taxonomic assortments by further dividing the whales (balaenids vs. balaenopterids), and grouping tadpoles with ducks and flamingos. Although this scheme cuts across taxonomic lines, it focuses on biomechanical differences in how water is transported to the entrapping surfaces of suspension feeders. These distinctions have not been emphasized before in literature on suspension-feeding adaptations of vertebrates (see for example fig. 2.12; also Owen 1980; Morton 1967; Taylor 1987), but are important for understanding convergent and nonconvergent cranial designs in these organisms. The distinctions recognize that suspension feeding relates as much to locomotor specializations as to cranial features (see Webb and Buffrénil 1990; Webb 1984, 1988, for a general discussion of the relationship of locomotion to feeding in aquatic vertebrates).

Where locomotion provides the flow to feeding structures (i.e., ram feeding), no cephalic pump is necessary and cranial specializations for suspension feeding—other than the proliferation of filters proper—may be relatively slight. If there is less forward body motion, some cranial adaptations for pumping may be in order (i.e., intermittent suction feeding). Where there is little or no body movement, cranial specializations to ensure adequate flow become essential (i.e., continuous suction feeding). Those latter specializations include not only a lingual or pharyngeal pumping mechanism, but valves to ensure one-way flow. Not surprisingly, those vertebrates that use locomotion totally or partially to deliver water to their feeding structures are best designed for sustained locomotion in the aquatic environment (fishes, whales). Those that feed from a relatively stationary posture and use continuous suction feeding are least designed for sustained aquatic locomotion (birds, lamprey larvae, tadpoles; see Wassersug 1989).

There is some exclusion between cranial designs for continuous ram feeding and those for continuous suction feeding due simply to packing constraints in the vertebrate head. For the ram feeders, maximizing surface

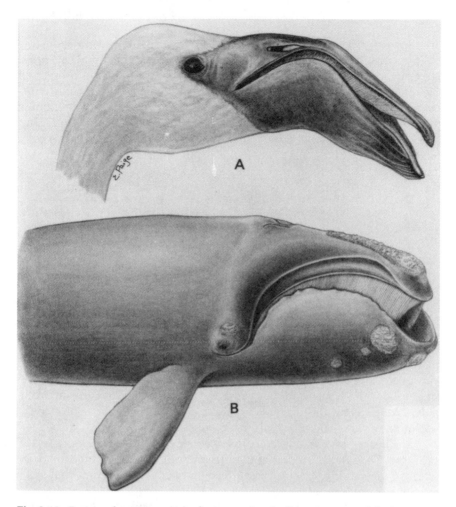

Fig. 2.12. Presumed convergence in the suspension-feeding apparatus of the lesser flamingo, *Phoeniconaias minor,* and the black right whale, *Eubalaena glacialis.* The analogy, however, is superficial. The whale uses continuous ram feeding, whereas the flamingo depends on an oscillating hyoidean suction pump to deliver water to its particle-entrapping surfaces. The whale swims forward as it feeds, whereas the flamingo waves its head from side to side. Water comes in through the front of the mouth in ram-feeding whales through a large gape, whereas it comes in through the side of the mouth in flamingos, through a narrow slit. The flow regimes are not comparable around the filter apparatus of the two animals and it is unlikely that the physical processes used in particle capture are, in fact, the same (see text).

In the right whales only the upper jaw is bowed; the lower jaw is straight in lateral view. This means that at their midpoint the upper and lower jaws are always widely separated, with long baleen plates filling the intervening space. In flamingos the upper and lower jaws have the same arch and are never separated by much distance. The implication of the arch in whales, and the fact that the two jaws do not conform, means extra space for baleen. The implication of the arch for the flamingo is more uniform spacing along the jaws rostral to the bend when the jaws are open. (From Olson and Feduccia 1980b, reprinted by permission of the Smithsonian Institution Press) area for entrapment becomes essential if they are going to process large volumes of water at reasonably low (viz., energy efficient) body velocities. Large buccal volumes and expansive collecting surfaces are in order, and the cross-sectional area of the mouth in these organisms is typically enormous. This large area is achieved, in part, by reducing or never developing the musculoskeletal components that make up the pump in continuous suction-feeding forms. Besides, a buccal pump would be superfluous since feeding usually takes place when the oropharyngeal volume is already maximal. In contrast, in continuous suction feeders, the room available for entrapping surfaces is comparatively reduced to make space for the pump mechanism.

Summary of Morphological and Ecological Features Shared by Vertebrate Suspension Feeders

1. Teeth are reduced or absent (*Pterodaustro* is a specialized exception) and adductor musculature is concomitantly reduced, compared to macrophagous relatives.

2. Forms that lack gill slits—be they bird or mammal—all have their entrapping surfaces on the jaw margins. Deeper placement of entrapping structures within the mouth would require further transport of water and increase the energetic cost of feeding. None rely on mucus entrapment to capture food. Perhaps, with their entrapment surfaces superficial, the loss of mucus to the water would be too great to make that mechanism profitable. Alternatively, this decreased reliance on mucus may be related to the evolution of birds and mammals in a terrestrial environment.

3. Elasmobranchs and cetaceans that suspension feed are large and all ram feed, with the exception of the megamouth shark. Ram feeding is an effective mechanism for suspension feeding only for organisms that swim at high Reynolds numbers.

4. Below a certain minimum body length (approximately 2–5 cm), teleosts do not suspension feed (Sanderson and Cech 1992; but see van der Meeren 1991). Adult suspension-feeding teleosts, and the paddlefish, begin life as juveniles that use suction to capture individual zooplankton (e.g., Michaletz et al. 1982; Durbin 1979). After the transition, these fish may suspension feed on the same type of zooplankton prey that is consumed by juveniles, or they may switch to phytoplankton (Johnson and Vinyard 1987; Moriarty et al. 1973; Cramer and Marzolf 1970; Ciechomski 1967; Bensam 1964). Whereas fishes can discern increasingly smaller prey as they themselves grow larger (Hairston et al. 1982), the ontogenetic shift to suspension feeding cannot be explained by that fact since, by definition, individual prey items are not sensed and attacked during suspension feeding. The ontogenetic shift in feeding habits suggests that the entrapment mechanisms used by larger fishes may not work with the same

efficiency in the low Reynolds number range in which the juvenile fishes necessarily operate.

5. Most suspension-feeding teleost species swim in schools. This is true of the clupeids and engraulids (Blaxter and Hunter 1982), the cyprinid *Orthodon* (Murphy 1950), some species of *Coregonus* (Koelz 1927), and the mackerels (Collette and Nauen 1983). These schools tend to utilize patchy food resources in pelagic habitats.

6. All of the continuous suction feeders that are capable of generating their own suspensions from the bottom material share not so much a common cranial design, as a capability for moving from patch to patch using seasonally available resources. None are permanent residents in the aquatic habitats where they feed; eventually they either metamorphose (tadpoles), emigrate (avians), or do both (lamprey larvae).

7. A common feature of suspension-feeding vertebrates is greater cranial kinesis than in close, macrophagous relatives. This is true whether one compares baleen and toothed whales or tadpoles and frogs. The kinesis appears to be used for fine regulation of suspension-feeding flow rates.

8. Suspension-feeding vertebrates that lack gill slits generate a bidirectional flow; water must both enter and exit through the mouth. After the water surrounding the prey has been accelerated into the oral cavity, it must decelerate in order for the direction of flow to be altered by as much as 180°. Mobile prey may have the opportunity to escape as the flow decelerates. Lauder and Shaffer (1986) presented data on ambystomatid salamanders indicating that bidirectional flow systems are not as successful at capturing elusive prey as are unidirectional flow systems. The tremendously expandable oral cavity of intermittent ram-feeding whales, however, may allow their morphologically bidirectional flow system to become functionally unidirectional, as proposed by Lauder and Shaffer (1986) for the expandable esophagus in turtles. In these cases, the time at which the flow decelerates and reverses can be delayed until the jaws have closed to a gape too small for the escape of prey.

Unsolved Problems

The transport of food captured on oropharyngeal surfaces to the esophagus and the initiation of swallowing are the two least understood steps in suspension feeding by vertebrates. A description of these processes will require a combination of techniques from the disciplines of functional morphology and biomechanics. But even the basic myology of the lingual and pharyngeal regions for most species has not been examined. This problem is glaring for whales, where stomach contents have been repetitively examined, yet the cranial muscles which let those organisms fill their stomachs remain uninvestigated. The two most comprehensive studies of mysticete cranial myology are still Carte and Macalister (1868) and

Schulte (1916), both on *Balaenoptera*. The first is on a small, decomposing specimen and the second on a fetus. That there are errors of omission and interpretation in both of these works has been known for over half a century (Howell 1930). The lingual movements (if it *is* lingual movements) that transport captured food from the baleen to the esophagus are simply not known. The hyoids of baleen whales in general are not large given the size of the heads in these animals. However, those genera known to have either massive tongues (*Eubalaena*) or powerful tongue movements (*Eschrichtius*) do have much larger hyoids (Omura 1964). This suggests that there must be substantive differences among species in the muscles that insert on the hyoid and indirectly work the tongue.

At the other end of the size spectrum, it has been established for some time (Dodd 1950) that cilia carry food from the pharynx down the esophagus in tadpoles. However, what has not been established is how particulate matter gets from a tadpole's gill filters, which lie at the bottom of its pharynx, to the ciliary groove in the lateral pharyngeal wall. Neither the tadpole's branchial food traps nor its gill filters are themselves ciliated. How particulate matter is cleared from the gill rakers of suspension-feeding fishes is essentially the same unsolved problem. From whale to tadpole, and for most suspension feeders in between, this part of the suspension-feeding process remains a mystery.

Another area of major ignorance is the flow regime at the collecting surfaces. The works of Rubenstein and Koehl (1977), Jørgensen (1983), LaBarbera (1984), Shimeta and Jumars (1991), and others on invertebrate suspension feeding have emphasized the complexity of the suspension-feeding process. There are scale effects involved which have rarely been appreciated by biologists studying vertebrate suspension feeding. The entrapment properties of biological filters are affected by flow velocity, pore size, amount of material already collected on the surfaces, etc. All of these factors affect each other and can vary instantaneously in flexible biological filters, like those of vertebrates. Suspension feeding for these animals has a dynamic responsiveness which makes the kinematics and mechanics of the process far more complex than the ballistic capture systems of their toothed, macrophagous relatives. We now know that it is naive to equate suspension feeding with simple sieving, nor can we expect to understand the feeding capability of a suspension feeder by measuring the gross static dimensions of its filters alone. To discover what suspension-feeding mechanisms are operative requires precise hydrodynamic data that are currently lacking.

Our review of the morphology of vertebrate suspension feeders suggests that these data will be difficult to collect. Flow through suspension-feeding structures is not constant for even a few seconds, except possibly for the larger continuous ram feeders, and even there it is altered by the process of entrapment itself. Intermittent ram feeders and both types of suction feeders create a flow of varying velocity. It will be extremely difficult to measure water velocities in these animals to establish the flow regime when and where particle entrapment takes place. Yet such data will be essential, if we are to know even how most vertebrate suspension feeders actually manage to extract particulate matter from the water.

ACKNOWLEDGMENTS

For lots of information about lots of organisms we thank: Marilyn Bachmann, Paul Brodie, Greg M. Cailliet, Joseph J. Cech, Jr., Patrick L. Colin, James P. Collins, Ray W. Drenner, Toby Gaunt, P. Humphry Greenwood, Leon E. Hallacher, Karsten Hartel, Wim Hoogenboezem, Bob Jones, Jan Kooloos, Richard Lambertsen, Robert Lavenberg, Christina Lockyer, Karel Liem, Jon Mallatt, James Mead, C. Hans Nelson, Mary Nerini, Storrs Olson, Lisa Orton, Mark Patterson, August Pivorunas, Jürgen Riess, Barbara Stein, Melanie L. J. Stiassny, David Unwin, Marvalee Wake, Jackie Webb, Peter Wellnhofer, and Gart Zweers. We are particularly grateful to Tracey Earle, Dawn Erickson, Sheila Hubley, and V. Ann King for assistance with literature searches and manuscript preparation. The ratio of fact to fantasy within the manuscript was increased greatly by constructive comments from Paul Brodie, Jan Kooloos, Michael LaBarbera, and August Pivorunas. We also thank the interlibrary loan services of Dalhousie University and the Museum of Comparative Zoology, Harvard University, for providing us with hard copy proof that speculating on suspension-feeding adaptations in vertebrates is an ancient, international enterprise and, in so doing, giving us the material to continue that activity. This review was supported by grant funds from the Natural Science and Engineering Research Council of Canada to RJW. Parts of the manuscript were prepared while SLS was a National Science Foundation Postdoctoral Research Fellow in Environmental Biology (BSR-8800190) in the Department of Wildlife and Fisheries Biology at the University of California, Davis, and a University of California President's Fellow in the Department of Mathematics and the Institute of Theoretical Dynamics, UC Davis.

REFERENCES

Alexander, R. McN. 1967. *Functional Design in Fishes*. A. J. Cain, ed. London: Hutchinson University Library.

Allis, E. P., Jr. 1903. The skull, and the cranial and first spinal muscles and nerves in *Scomber scomber*. Journal of Morphology 18: 45–328, pls. 3–12.

Altig, R., and G. F. Johnston. 1986. Major characteristics of free-living anuran tadpoles. Smithsonian Herpetological Information Service no. 67: 1–75.

Ashmole, N. P. 1971. Seabird ecology and the marine environment. In *Avian Biology*, vol. 1, D. S. Farner and J. R. King, eds. New York: Academic Press, pp. 224–271.

Aubenton, F. d'. 1955. Étude de l'appareil branchiospinal et de l'organe supra-branchial d'*Heterotis niloticus* Ehrenberg 1827. Bulletin de l'Institut français d'Afrique noire (A) 17: 1179–1201.

Avilova, K. V. 1978. On the structure of the filtering and tactile systems of the beak in Anseriformes. Zoologicheskii zhurnal 57 (8): 1210–1217.

Baker, A. N. 1985. Pygmy right whale, *Caperea marginata* (Gray, 1846). In *Handbook of Marine Mammals*, vol. 3, *The Sirenians and Baleen Whales*, S. H. Ridgway and R. Harrison, eds. Orlando, Fla.: Academic Press, pp. 345–354.

Bakker, R. T. 1986. *The Dinosaur Heresies: New Theories Unlocking the Mystery of the Dinosaurs and Their Extinction*. New York: William Morrow and Company.

Batty, R. S., J. H. S. Blaxter, and D. A. Libby. 1986. Herring (*Clupea harengus*) filter-feeding in the dark. Marine Biology 91: 371–375.

Batty, R. S., J. H. S. Blaxter, and J. M. Richard. 1990. Light intensity and the feeding behaviour of herring, *Clupea harengus*. Marine Biology 107: 383–388.

Bayliff. W. H. 1963. The food and feeding habits of the anchoveta, *Cetengraulis mysticetus*, in the Gulf of Panama. Bulletin of the Inter-American Tropical Tuna Commission 7: 397–459.

Beauregard, D. H. 1882. Étude de l'articulation temporo-maxillaire chez les Balaenoptères. Journal de l'anatomie et de la physiologie 18: 16–26.

Belkin, D. A., and C. Gans. 1968. An unusual chelonian feeding niche. Ecology 49 (4): 768–769.

Bensam, P. 1964. Differences in food and feeding adaptations between juveniles and adults of the Indian oil sardine, *Sardinella longiceps* Valenciennes. Indian Journal of Fisheries 11: 377–390.

Bertmar, G., B. G. Kapoor, and R. V. Miller. 1969. Epibranchial organs in lower teleostean fishes—an example of structural adaptation. International Review of General and Experimental Zoology 4: 1–48.

Beveridge, M. C. M., M. Begum, G. N. Frerichs, and S. Millar. 1989. The ingestion of bacteria in suspension by the tilapia *Oreochromis niloticus*. Aquaculture 81: 373–378.

Beveridge, M. C. M., M. R. P. Briggs, M. E. Northcott, and L. G. Ross. 1988. The occurrence, structure, and development of microbranchiospines among the tilapias (Cichlidae: Tilapiini). Canadian Journal of Zoology 66 (11): 2564–2572.

Beveridge, M. C. M., P. K. Sikdar, G. N. Frerichs, and S. Millar. 1991. The ingestion of bacteria in suspension by the common carp *Cyprinus carpio* L. Journal of Fish Biology 39: 825–831.

Bhimachar, B. S., and P. C. George. 1952. Observations on the food and feeding of the Indian mackerel, *Rastrelliger canagurta* (Cuvier). Proceedings of the Indian Academy of Science 36B (3): 105–118.

Bigelow, H. B., and W. C. Schroeder. 1953. *Fishes of the Western North Atlantic*, memoir 1, pt. 2. New Haven, Conn.: Sears Foundation for Marine Research, Yale University.

Blaber, S. J. M. 1979. The biology of filter feeding teleosts in Lake St. Lucia, Zululand, Journal of Fish Biology 15: 37–59.

Blaxter, J. H. S., and J. R. Hunter. 1982. The biology of the clupeoid fishes. Advances in Marine Biology 20: 3–223.

Blay, J., Jr., and K. N. Eyeson. 1982. Feeding activity and food habits of the shad, *Ethmalosa fimbriata* (Bowdich), in the coastal waters of Cape Coast, Ghana. Journal of Fish Biology 21: 403–410.

Bodola, A. 1966. Life history of the gizzard shad, *Dorosoma cepedianum* (Le Sueur), in western Lake Erie. Fishery Bulletin, U.S. 65 (2): 391–425.

Bonaparte, J. F. 1971. Descripción del cráneo y mandibulas de *Pterodaustro guiñazui* (Pterodactyloidea–Pterodaustriidae nov.) de la formación Lagarcito, San Luis, Argentina. Publicaciones, Museo municipal de ciencias naturales de Mar Del Plata 1 (9): 263–272.

Bonner, W. N. 1990. *The Natural History of Seals*. New York: Facts on File.

Bornbusch, A. H. 1988. Gill raker morphologies of anchovies (Teleostei: Engraulidae) from the Rio Orinoco, Venezuela. Copeia (1): 174–182.

Bowen, S. H. 1982. Feeding, digestion and growth—qualitative considerations. In *The Biology and Culture of Tilapias*, R. S. V. Pullin and R. H. Lowe-McConnell, eds. Manila: International Center for Living Aquatic Resources Management, pp. 141–156.

Brodie, P. F. 1977. Form, function, and energetics of cetacea: A discussion. In *Functional Anatomy of Marine Mammals*, vol. 3, R. J. Harrison, ed. New York: Academic Press, pp. 45–56.

Broili, von F. 1924. *Ctenochasma* ist ein Flugsaurier. Sitzungsberichte der Mathematisch-naturwissenschaftliche Klasse: 13–31.

Brown, D. S. 1981. The English Upper Jurassic Plesiosauroidea (Reptilia) and a review of the phylogeny and classification of the Plesiosauria. Bulletin of the British Museum of Natural History, Geology 35(4): 253–347.

Burke, J. S., D. R. Bayne, and H. Rea. 1986. Impact of silver and bighead carps on plankton communities of channel catfish ponds. Aquaculture 55: 59–68.

Byers, S., and G. L. Vinyard. 1990. The effects on the plankton community of filter-feeding Sacramento blackfish, *Orthodon microlepidotus*. Oecologia 83: 352–357.

Carte, A., and A. Macalister. 1868. On the anatomy of *Balaenoptera rostrata*. Philosophical Transactions of the Royal Society of London 158: 201–261.

Cavender, T. M. 1970. A comparison of coregonines and other salmonids with the earliest known teleostean fishes. In *Biology of Coregonid Fishes*, C. C. Lindsey and C. S. Woods, eds. Winnipeg: University of Manitoba Press, pp. 1–32.

Chapman, F. M. 1905. A contribution to the life history of the American Flamingo (*Phoenicopterus ruber*), with remarks upon specimens. Bulletin of the American Museum of Natural History 21: 53–77.

Chapman, W. M. 1944a. The osteology of the Pacific deep-bodied anchovy, *Anchoa compressa*. Journal of Morphology 74: 311–329.

Chapman, W. M. C. 1944b. The comparative osteology of the herring-like fishes (Clupeidae) of California. California Fish and Game 30 (1): 6–21.

Ciechomski, J. Dz., de. 1967. Investigations of food and feeding habits of larvae and juveniles of the Argentine anchovy *Engraulis anchoita*. California Cooperative Oceanic Fisheries Investigations Reports 11: 72–81.

Coles, R. J. 1916. Natural history notes on the devilfish, *Manta birostris* (Walbaum) and *Mobula olfersi* (Muller). Bulletin of the American Museum of Natural History 35: 649–657.

Colin, P. L. 1976. Filter feeding and predation on the eggs of *Thallasoma* sp. by the scombrid fish *Rastrelliger kanagurta*. Copeia (3): 596–597.

Collette, B. B., and C. E. Nauen. 1983. Scombrids of the world. FAO Fisheries Synopsis no. 125 (2): 1–137.

Compagno, L. J. V. 1990. Relationships of the megamouth shark, *Megachasma pelagios* (Lamniformes: Megachasmidae), with comments on its feeding habits. In *Elasmobranchs as Living Resources: Advances in the Biology, Ecology, Systematics, and the Status of the Fisheries*, H. L. Pratt, Jr., S. H. Gruber, and T. Taniuchi, eds. N.p.: National Oceanic and Atmospheric Administration Technical Report, National Marine Fisheries Service 90, pp. 357–379.

Cramer, J. D., and G. R. Marzolf. 1970. Selective predation on zooplankton by gizzard shad. Transactions of the American Fisheries Society 99 (2): 320–332.

Cremer, M. C., and R. O. Smitherman. 1980. Food habits and growth of silver and bighead carp in cages and ponds. Aquaculture 20: 57–64.

Crome, F. H. J. 1985. An experimental investigation of filter-feeding on zooplankton by some specialized waterfowl. Australian Journal of Zoology 33: 849–862.

Crowder, L. B. 1985. Optimal foraging and feeding mode shifts in fishes. Environmental Biology of Fishes 12 (1): 57–62.

Darby, D. G. 1982. The early vertebrate *Astraspis*, habitat based on a lithologic association. Journal of Paleontology 56: 1187–1196.

deJong, F., and G. A. Zweers. 1981. Filterfeeding of flamingos (*Phoenicopterus ruber ruber*). Netherlands Journal of Zoology 31 (3): 612–613.

DeJongh, H. 1968. Functional morphology of the jaw apparatus of larval and metamorphosing *Rana temporaria*. Netherlands Journal of Zoology 18: 1–103.

DeLage, Y. 1886. Histoire du *Balaenoptera musculus* échoué sur la plage de Langrune. Archives de zoologie expérimentale et générale 3 (suppl. 1 m): 1–152.

Denison, R. H. 1937. Anatomy of the head and pelvic fin of the whale shark *Rhineodon*. Bulletin of the American Museum of Natural History 73 (5): 477–515.

Denny, P., D. W. Bowker, and R. G. Bailey. 1978. The importance of the littoral epiphyton as food for commercial fish in the recent African man-made lake, Nyumba ya Mungu reservoir, Tanzania. Biological Journal of the Linnean Society 10: 139–150.

Diamond, J. M. 1985. Filter-feeding on a grand scale. Nature 316: 679–680.

Dodd, J. M. 1950. Ciliary feeding mechanism in anuran larvae. Nature 165: 283.

Dodson, S. L., and D. L. Egger. 1980. Selective feeding of red phalaropes on zooplankton of arctic ponds. Ecology 61 (4): 755–763.

Dorofeyeva, Ye. A., Ye. A. Zinov'yev, V. A. Klyukanov, Yu. S. Reshetnikov, K. A. Savvaitova, and G. Kh. Shaposhnikova. 1980. The present state of research into the phylogeny and classification of Salmonoidei. Journal of Ichthyology 20: 1–20.

Douthwaite, R. J. 1977. Filter-feeding ducks of the Kafue Flats, Zambia, 1971–1973. Ibis 119: 44–66.

Drenner, R. W. 1977. The feeding mechanics of the gizzard shad (*Dorosoma cepedianum*). Ph.D. diss., University of Kansas.

Drenner, R. W., K. D. Hambright, G. L. Vinyard, M. Gophen, and U. Pollingher. 1987. Experimental study of size-selective phytoplankton grazing by a filter-feeding cichlid and the cichlid's effects on plankton community structure. Limnology and Oceanography 32 (5): 1138–1144.

Drenner, R. W., and S. R. McComas. 1980. The roles of zooplankter escape ability and fish size selectivity in the selective feeding and impact of planktivorous fish. In *Evolution and Ecology of Zooplankton Communities,* W. C. Kerfoot, ed. Hanover, N.H.: University Press of New England, pp. 587–593.

Drenner, R. W., J. R. Mummert, F. deNoyelles, Jr., and D. Kettle. 1984. Selective particle ingestion by a filter-feeding fish and its impact on phytoplankton community structure. Limnology and Oceanography 29 (5): 941–948.

Drenner, R. W., W. J. O'Brien, and J. R. Mummert. 1982. Filter-feeding rates of gizzard shad. Transactions of the American Fisheries Society 111: 210–215.

Drenner, R. W., S. B. Taylor, X. Lazzaro, and D. Kettle. 1984. Particle-grazing and plankton community impact of an omnivorous cichlid. Transactions of the American Fisheries Society 113: 397–402.

Drenner, R. W., G. L. Vinyard, M. Gophen, and S. R. McComas. 1982. Feeding behavior of the cichlid, *Sarotherodon galilaeum:* Selective predation on Lake Kinneret zooplankton. Hydrobiologia 87: 17–20.

Drenner, R. W., G. L. Vinyard, K. D. Hambright, and M. Gophen. 1987. Particle ingestion by *Tilapia galilaea* is not affected by removal of gill rakers and microbranchiospines. Transactions of the American Fisheries Society 116: 272–276.

Duellman, W. E., and L. Trueb. 1985. *Biology of Amphibians.* New York: McGraw-Hill.

Durbin, A. G. 1979. Food selection by plankton feeding fishes. In *Predator-Prey Systems in Fisheries Management,* R. H. Stroud and H. Clepper, eds. Washington, D.C.: Sport Fishing Institute, pp. 203–218.

Durbin, A. G., and E. G. Durbin. 1975. Grazing rates of the Atlantic menhaden *Brevoortia tyrannus* as a function of particle size and concentration. Marine Biology 33: 265–277.

Edgar, R. K., and J. G. Hoff. 1976. Grazing of freshwater and estuarine benthic diatoms by adult Atlantic menhaden *Brevoortia tyrannus*. Fishery Bulletin, U.S. 74: 689–693.

Ehlinger, T. J. 1989. Foraging mode switches in the golden shiner (*Notemigonus crysoleucas*). Canadian Journal of Fisheries and Aquatic Sciences 46: 1250–1254.

Engel, S. 1976. Food habits and prey selection of coho salmon (*Oncorhynchus kisutch*) and cisco (*Coregonus artedii*) in relation to zooplankton dynamics in Pallette Lake, Wisconsin. Transactions of the American Fisheries Society 105 (5): 607–614.

Fagade, S. O., and C. I. O. Olaniyan. 1972. The biology of the West African shad

Ethmalosa fimbriata (Bowdich) in the Lagos Lagoon, Nigeria. Journal of Fish Biology 4: 519–533.

Feder, M. E., D. Seale, M. E. Boraas, R. J. Wassersug, and A. G. Gibbs. 1984. Functional conflicts between feeding and gas exchange in suspension-feeding tadpoles, *Xenopus laevis*. Journal of Experimental Biology 110: 91–98.

Fitz, R. B. 1966. Unusual food of a paddlefish (*Polyodon spathula*) in Tennessee. Copeia (2): 356.

Fleming, C. A. 1941. The phylogeny of the prions. Emu, Melbourne 41: 134.

Friedland, K. D. 1985. Functional morphology of the branchial basket structures associated with feeding in the Atlantic menhaden, *Brevoortia tyrannus* (Pisces: Clupeidae). Copeia (4): 1018–1027.

Friedland, K. D., D. W. Ahrenholz, and J. F. Guthrie. 1989. Influence of plankton on distribution patterns of the filter-feeder *Brevoortia tyrannus* (Pisces: Clupeidae). Marine Ecology Progress Series 54: 1–11.

Friedland, K. D., L. W. Haas, and J. V. Merriner. 1984. Filtering rates of the juvenile Atlantic menhaden *Brevoortia tyrannus* (Pisces: Clupeidae), with consideration of the effects of detritus and swimming speed. Marine Biology 84: 109–117.

Frost, K. J., and L. F. Lowry. 1981. Ringed, baikal, and caspian seals—*Phoca hispida, Phoca sibirica,* and *Phoca caspica.* In *Handbook of Marine Mammals,* vol. 2, *Seals,* S. H. Ridgway and R. J. Harrison, eds. New York: Academic Press, pp. 29–54.

Gambell, R. 1985. Sei whale *Balaenoptera borealis* Lesson, 1828. In *Handbook of Marine Mammals,* vol. 3, *The Sirenians and Baleen Whales,* S. H. Ridgway and R. Harrison, eds. Orlando, Fla.: Academic Press, pp. 155–170.

Gaskin, D. E. 1976. The evolution, zoogeography, and ecology of Cetacea. Oceanography and Marine Biology, Annual Review 14: 247–346.

Gibson, R. N. 1988. Development, morphometry, and particle retention capability of the gill rakers in the herring, *Clupea harengus* L. Journal of Fish Biology 32: 949–962.

Gibson, R. N., and I. A. Ezzi. 1985. Effect of particle concentration on filter- and particulate-feeding in the herring *Clupea harengus*. Marine Biology 88: 109–116.

———. 1990. Relative importance of prey size and concentration in determining the feeding behaviour of the herring *Clupea harengus*. Marine Biology 107: 357–362.

Gophen, M., R. W. Drenner, and G. L. Vinyard. 1983. Cichlid stocking and the decline of the Galilee Saint Peter's fish (*Sarotherodon galilaeus*) in Lake Kinneret, Israel. Canadian Journal of Fisheries and Aquatic Sciences 40: 983–986.

Gosse, J. P. 1955. Dispositions speciales de l'appareil branchial des *Tilapia* et *Citharinus.* Société royale zoologique de Belgique, Annales 86: 303–308.

Gradwell, N. 1968. The jaw and hyoidean mechanism of the bullfrog tadpole during aqueous ventilation. Canadian Journal of Zoology 46 (5): 1041–1052.

———. 1971. *Xenopus* tadpole: On the water pumping mechanism. Herpetologica 27: 107–123.

————. 1972a. Gill irrigation in *Rana catesbeiana*. I. On the anatomical basis. Canadian Journal of Zoology 50: 481–499.

————. 1972b. Gill irrigation in *Rana catesbeiana*. II. On the musculoskeletal mechanism. Canadian Journal of Zoology 50: 501–521.

————. 1975. The bearing of filter feeding on the water pumping mechanism of *Xenopus* tadpoles (Anura: Pipidae). Acta zoologica 56: 119–128.

Gradwell, N., and V. M. Pasztor. 1968. Hydrostatic pressures during normal ventilation in the bullfrog tadpole. Canadian Journal of Zoology 46: 1169–1174.

Grande, L., and W. E. Bemis. 1991. Osteology and phylogenetic relationships of fossil and Recent paddlefishes (Polyodontidae) with comments on the interrelationships of Acipenseriformes. Society of Vertebrate Paleontology Memoir I. Journal of Vertebrate Paleontology 11 (suppl. to no. 1): 1–121.

Gras, R. L. Lauzanne, and L. Saint-Jean. 1981. Régime alimentaire et sélection des proies chez les *Brachysynodontis batensoda* (Pisces, Mochocidae) du lac Tchad en période de basses eaux. Revue d'hydrobiologie tropicale 14 (3): 223–231.

Greenwood, P. H. 1953. Feeding mechanism of the cichlid fish, *Tilapia esculenta* Graham. Nature 172 (4370): 207–208.

Gregory, W. K. 1933. Fish skulls: A study of the evolution of natural mechanisms. Transactions of the American Philosophical Society 23: 75–481.

Gudger, E. W. 1935. Maxillary breathing valves in the sharks *Chlamydoselachus* and *Cetorhinus* with notes on breathing valves in thirteen marine teleosts. Journal of Morphology 57: 91–104.

————. 1941a. The feeding organs of the whale shark, *Rhineodon typus*. Journal of Morphology 68: 81–99.

————. 1941b. The food and feeding habits of the whale shark, *Rhineodon typus*. Journal of the Elisha Mitchell Scientific Society 57 (1): 57–72.

Hain, J. H. W., G. R. Carter, S. D. Kraus, C. A. Mayo, and H. E. Winn. 1982. Feeding behavior of the humpback whale, *Megaptera novaeangliae*, in the western North Atlantic. Fishery Bulletin, U.S. 80 (2): 259–268.

Hairston, N. G., Jr., K. T. Li, and S. S. Easter, Jr. 1982. Fish vision and the detection of planktonic prey. Science 218: 1240–1242.

Hall, D. J., and T. J. Ehlinger. 1989. Perturbation, planktivory, and pelagic community structure: The consequence of winterkill in a small lake. Canadian Journal of Fisheries and Aquatic Sciences 46: 2203–2209.

Hallacher, L. E. 1977. On the feeding behavior of the basking shark, *Cetorhinus maximus*. Environmental Biology of Fishes 2 (3): 297–298.

Hampl, A., J. Jirasek, and D. Sirotek. 1983. Growth morphology of the filtering apparatus of silver carp (*Hypophthalmichthys molitrix*). II. Microscopic anatomy. Aquaculture 31: 153–158.

Hand, C. H., and L. Berner, Jr. 1959. Food of the Pacific sardine (*Sardinops caerulea*). Fishery Bulletin, U.S. 60: 175–184.

Harder, W. 1958. The intestine as a diagnostic character in identifying certain clupeoids (Engraulididae, Clupeidae, Dussumieriidae) and as a morphometric character for comparing anchoveta (*Centengraulis mysticetus*) populations. Bulletin of the Inter-American Tropical Tuna Commission 2: 365–388.

Hardisty, M. W. 1981. The skeleton. In *The Biology of Lampreys,* vol. 3, M. W. Hardisty and I. C. Potter, eds. London: Academic Press, pp. 333–376.

Hardisty, M. W., and I. C. Potter, eds. 1971. *The Biology of Lampreys.* New York: Academic Press.

Harrison, I. J., and G. J. Howes. 1991. The pharyngobranchial organ of mugilid fishes: Its structure, variability, ontogeny, possible function, and taxonomic utility. Bulletin of the British Museum of Natural History, Zoology 57 (2): 111–132.

Hatanaka, M., K. Sekino, M. Takahashi, and T. Ichimura. 1957. Growth and food consumption in young mackerel, *Pneumatophorus japonicus* (Houttuyn). Tohoku Journal of Agricultural Research 7: 351–368.

Hlohowskyj, C. P., M. M. Coburn, and T. M. Cavender. 1989. Comparison of a pharyngeal filtering apparatus in seven species of the herbivorous cyprinid genus, *Hybognathus* (Pisces: Cyprinidae). Copeia (1): 172–183.

Hobson, E. S. 1963. Selective feeding by the gafftopsail pompano, *Trachinotus rhodopus* (Gill), in mixed schools of herring and anchovies in the Gulf of California. Copeia (3): 595–596.

Holanov, S. H., and J. C. Tash. 1978. Particulate and filter feeding in threadfin shad, *Dorosoma petenense,* at different light intensities. Journal of Fish Biology 13: 619–625.

Hoogenboezem, W., J. G. M. van den Boogaart, F. A. Sibbing, E. H. R. R. Lammens, A. Terlouw, and J. W. M. Osse. 1991. A new model of particle retention and branchial sieve adjustment in filter-feeding bream (*Abramis brama,* Cyprinidae). Canadian Journal of Fisheries and Aquatic Sciences 48: 7–18.

Hoogenboezem, W., E. H. R. R. Lammens, Y. van Vugt, and J. W. M. Osse. 1992. A model for switching between particulate-feeding and filter-feeding in the common bream, *Abramis brama.* Environmental Biology of Fishes 33: 13–21.

Hoogenboezem, W., F. A. Sibbing, J. W. M. Osse, J. G. M. van den Boogaart, E. H. R. R. Lammens, and A. Terlouw. 1990. X-ray measurements of gill-arch movements in filter-feeding bream, *Abramis brama* (Cyprinidae). Journal of Fish Biology 36: 47–58.

Howell, A. B. 1930. *Aquatic Mammals: Their Adaptations to Life in the Water.* Springfield, Ill.: Charles C. Thomas, Publisher.

Hughes, G. M. 1960a. A comparative study of gill ventilation in marine teleosts. Journal of Experimental Biology 37: 28–45.

———. 1960b. The mechanism of gill ventilation in the dogfish and skate. Journal of Experimental Biology 37: 11–27.

Hunter, J. R., and H. Dorr. 1982. Thresholds for filter feeding in northern anchovy, *Engraulis mordax.* California Cooperative Oceanic Fisheries Investigations Reports 23: 198–204.

Hurlbert, S. H., W. Loayza, and T. Moreno. 1986. Fish-flamingo-plankton interactions in the Peruvian Andes. Limnology and Oceanography 31 (3): 457–468.

Imber, M. J. 1981. Diets of storm petrels *Pelagodroma* and *Garrodia* and of prions (Procellariiformes): Ecological separation and bill morphology. In *Proceedings of the Symposium on Birds of the Sea and Shore, 1979,* J. Cooper, ed. Cape Town: African Seabird Group, pp. 63–68.

Imms, A. D. 1904. Notes on the gill-rakers of the spoonbill sturgeon, *Polyodon spathula*. Proceedings of the Zoological Society of London 2: 22–35.

Iwata, K. 1976. Morphological and physiological studies on the phytoplankton feeders in cyprinid fishes. I. Developmental changes of feeding organs and ingestion rates in kawachibuna (*Carassius auratus cuvieri*), silver carp (*Hypophthalmichthys molitrix*) and nigorobuna (*C. auratus grandoculis*). Japanese Journal of Limnology 37 (4): 135–147.

James, A. G. 1987. Feeding ecology, diet and field-based studies on feeding selectivity of the Cape anchovy *Engraulis capensis* Gilchrist. South African Journal of Marine Science 5: 673–692.

———. 1988. Are clupeid microphagists herbivorous or omnivorous? A review of the diets of some commercially important clupeids. South African Journal of Marine Science 7: 161–177.

James, A. G., and K. P. Findlay. 1989. Effect of particle size and concentration on feeding behaviour, selectivity and rates of food ingestion by the Cape anchovy *Engraulis capensis*. Marine Ecology Progress Series 50: 275–294.

Janssen, J. 1976. Feeding modes and prey size selection in the alewife (*Alosa pseudoharengus*). Journal of the Fisheries Research Board of Canada 33: 1972–1975.

———. 1978. Feeding-behavior repertoire of the alewife, *Alosa pseudoharengus,* and the ciscoes *Coregonus hoyi* and *C. artedii*. Journal of the Fisheries Research Board of Canada 35: 249–253.

Jenkin, P. M. 1957. The filter-feeding and food of flamingoes (Phoenicopteri). Philosophical Transactions of the Royal Society of London B 240: 401–493.

Jennings, D. P. 1988. Bighead carp (*Hypophthalmichthys nobilis*): A biological synopsis. U.S. Fish and Wildlife Service, Biological Report 88 (29).

Jirasek, J., A. Hampl, and D. Sirotek. 1981. Growth morphology of the filtering apparatus of silver carp (*Hypophthalmichthys molitrix*). I. Gross anatomy state. Aquaculture 26: 41–48.

Johnson, P. C., and G. L. Vinyard. 1987. Filter-feeding behavior and particle retention efficiency of Sacramento blackfish. Transactions of the American Fisheries Society 116: 634–640.

Jollie, M. 1982. What are the "Calcichordata"? and the larger question of the origin of Chordates. Zoological Journal of the Linnean Society 75: 167–188.

Jørgensen, C. B. 1966. *Biology of Suspension Feeding*. Oxford: Pergamon Press.

———. 1970. Introduction. In *Marine Food Chains,* J. H. Steele, ed. Berkeley: University of California Press, pp. 193–195.

———. 1975. Comparative physiology of suspension feeding. Annual Review of Physiology 37: 57–79.

———. 1983. Fluid mechanical aspects of suspension feeding. Marine Ecology Progress Series 11: 89–103.

Jurasz, C. M., and V. P. Jurasz. 1979. Feeding modes of the humpback whale, *Megaptera novaeangliae,* in Southeast Alaska. Scientific Reports of the Whales Research Institute 31: 69–83.

Kawamura, A. 1974. Food and feeding ecology in the southern sei whale. Scientific Reports of the Whales Research Institute 26: 25–144.

————. 1978. On the baleen filter area in the South Pacific Bryde's whales. Scientific Reports of the Whales Research Institute 30: 291–300.

Kellogg, R. 1928. The history of whales—their adaptation to life in the water. Quarterly Review of Biology 3 (1): 29–76.

Kenny, J. S. 1969a. Feeding mechanisms in anuran larvae. Journal of Zoology, London 157: 225–246.

————. 1969b. Pharyngeal mucous secreting epithelia of anuran larvae. Acta zoologica 50: 143–153.

King, D. P. F., and P. R. Macleod. 1976. Comparison of the food and the filtering mechanism of pilchard Sardinops ocellata and anchovy Engraulis capensis off South West Africa, 1971–1972. Sea Fisheries Branch Investigational Report no. 111. Department of Industries, Republic of South Africa.

King, J. E. 1961. The feeding mechanism and jaws of the crabeater seal (Lobodon carcinophagus). Mammalia 25: 462–466.

————. 1972. Observations on phocid skulls. In Functional Anatomy of Marine Mammals, R. J. Harrison, ed. London: Academic Press, pp. 81–115.

————. 1983. Seals of the World, 2d ed. Ithaca, N.Y.: British Museum (of Natural History) and Cornell University Press.

Kirchhoff, H. 1958. Funktionell-anatomische Untersuchung des Visceralapparates von Clupea harengus L. Zoologische Jahrbücher, Abteilung für Anatomie und Ontogenie der Tiere 76: 461–540.

Kishinouye, K. 1923. Contributions to the comparative study of the so-called scombroid fishes. Journal of the College of Agriculture, Imperial University of Tokyo 8: 293–473.

Koelz, W. 1927. Coregonid fishes of the Great Lakes. Bulletin of the Bureau of Fisheries 43 (2): 297–643.

Kooloos, J. G. M. 1986. A conveyer-belt model for pecking in the mallard (Anas platyrhynchos L.). Netherlands Journal of Zoology 36 (1): 47–87.

Kooloos, J. G. M., A. R. Kraaijeveld, G. E. J. Langenbach, and G. A. Zweers. 1989. Comparative mechanics of filter-feeding in Anas platyrhynchos, Anas clypeata and Aythya fuligula (Aves, Anseriformes). Zoomorphology 108: 269–290.

Kooloos, J. G. M., and G. A. Zweers. 1991. Integration of pecking, filter feeding, and drinking mechanisms in waterfowl. Acta biotheoretica 39: 107–140.

Kooyman, G. L. 1981. Crabeater seal—Lobodon carcinophagus. In Handbook of Marine Mammals, vol. 2, Seals, S. H. Ridgway and R. J. Harrison, eds. New York: Academic Press, pp. 221–236.

Krefft, G. 1958. Counting of gill rakers as a method of morphological herring investigations. Rapports et procès-verbaux des réunions, Conseil international pour l'exploration de la mer 143: 22–25.

Krushinskaya, N. L. 1986. The behaviour of cetaceans. In Investigations of Cetacea, vol. 19, G. Pilleri, ed. Berne, Switzerland: University of Berne, pp. 115–220.

Kutkuhn, J. H. 1958. Utilization of plankton by juvenile gizzard shad in a shallow prairie lake. Transactions of the American Fisheries Society 87: 80–103.

Kuznetsov, Ye. A. 1977. Consumption of bacteria by the silver carp (Hypophthalmichthys molitrix). Journal of Ichthyology 17: 398–403.

LaBarbera, M. 1984. Feeding currents and particle capture mechanisms in suspension feeding animals. American Zoologist 24: 71–84.

————. 1990. Principles of design of fluid transport systems in zoology. Science 249: 992–1000.

Lambertsen, R. H. 1983. Internal mechanism of rorqual feeding. Journal of Mammalogy 64 (1): 76–88.

Lammens, E. H. R. R. 1985. A test of a model for planktivorous filter feeding by bream *Abramis brama*. Environmental Biology of Fishes 13: 289–296.

Lannoo, M. J., D. S. Townsend, and R. J. Wassersug. 1987. Larval life in the leaves: Arboreal tadpole types, with special attention to the morphology, ecology, and behavior of the oophagous *Osteopilus brunneus* (Hylidae) larva. Fieldiana: Zoology, n.s. 38: 1–31.

Last, J. M. 1989. The food of herring, *Clupea harengus,* in the North Sea, 1983–1986. Journal of Fish Biology 34: 489–501.

Lauder, G. V. 1980. Hydrodynamics of prey capture by teleost fishes. In *Biofluid Mechanics,* vol. 2, D. J. Schneck, ed. New York: Plenum Press, pp. 161–181.

————. 1983. Prey capture hydrodynamics in fishes: Experimental tests of two models. Journal of Experimental Biology 104: 1–13.

————. 1986. Aquatic prey capture in fishes: Experimental and theoretical approaches. Journal of Experimental Biology 125: 411–416.

Lauder, G. V., Jr., and L. E. Lanyon. 1980. Functional anatomy of feeding in the bluegill sunfish, *Lepomis macrochirus: In vivo* measurement of bone strain. Journal of Experimental Biology 84: 33–55.

Lauder, G. V., and H. B. Shaffer. 1986. Functional design of the feeding mechanism in lower vertebrates: Unidirectional and bidirectional flow systems in the tiger salamander. Zoological Journal of the Linnean Society 88: 277–290.

Lavenberg, R. J. 1991. Megamania: The continuing saga of megamouth sharks. Terra 30 (1): 30–39.

Lazzaro, X. 1987. A review of planktivorous fishes: Their evolution, feeding behaviours, selectivities, and impacts. Hydrobiologia 146: 97–167.

Leff, L. G., and M. D. Bachmann. 1986. Ontogenetic changes in predatory behavior of larval tiger salamanders (*Ambystoma tigrinum*). Canadian Journal of Zoology 64: 1337–1344.

————. 1988. Basis of selective predation by the aquatic larvae of the salamander, *Ambystoma tigrinum*. Freshwater Biology 19: 87–94.

Leong, R. J. H., and C. P. O'Connell. 1969. A laboratory study of particulate and filter feeding of the northern anchovy (*Engraulis mordax*). Journal of the Fisheries Research Board of Canada 26 (3): 557–582.

Liem, K. F. 1980. Acquisition of energy by teleosts: Adaptive mechanisms and evolutionary patterns. In *Environmental Physiology of Fishes,* M. A. Ali, ed. New York: Plenum Press, pp. 299–334.

Lillie, D. G. 1915. *Cetacea.* British Antarctic ("Terra Nova") expedition of 1910. Natural history report. Zoology (Publications of the British Museum of Natural History, London) 1 (3): 85–125.

Loukashkin, A. S. 1970. On the diet and feeding behavior of the northern anchovy, *Engraulis mordax* (Girard). Proceedings of the California Academy of Sciences 37 (13): 419–458.

McDonald, M. E. 1987. Interactions between a phytoplanktivorous fish, *Oreo-*

chromis aureus, and two unialgal forage populations. Environmental Biology of Fishes 18 (3): 229–234.

MacGinitie, G. E. 1947. Notes on the devilfish, *Mobula lucasana,* and its parasites. Copeia (4): 276–278.

MacNeill, D. B., and S. B. Brandt. 1990. Ontogenetic shifts in gill-raker morphology and predicted prey capture efficiency of the alewife, *Alosa pseudoharengus.* Copeia (1): 164–171.

Mahmoud, I. Y., and J. Klicka. 1979. Feeding, drinking, and excretion. In *Turtles: Perspectives and Research,* M. Harless and H. Morlock, eds. New York: John Wiley and Sons, pp. 229–243.

Mahoney, S. A., and J. R. Jehl, Jr., 1985a. Adaptations of migratory shorebirds to highly saline and alkaline lakes: Wilson's phalarope and American avocet. Condor 87: 520–527.

———. 1985b. Avoidance of salt-loading by a diving bird at a hypersaline and alkaline lake: Eared grebe. Condor 87: 389–397.

Maitipe, P., and S. S. De Silva. 1985. Switches between zoophagy, phytophagy and detritivory of *Sarotherodon mossambicus* (Peters) populations in twelve manmade Sri Lankan lakes. Journal of Fish Biology 26: 49–61.

Mallatt, J. 1979. Surface morphology and functions of pharyngeal structures in the larval lamprey *Petromyzon marinus.* Journal of Morphology 162 (2): 249–274.

———. 1981. The suspension feeding mechanism of the larval lamprey *Petromyzon marinus.* Journal of Zoology, London 194: 103–142.

———. 1982. Pumping rates and particle retention efficiencies of the larval lamprey, an unusual suspension feeder. Biological Bulletin 163: 197–210.

———. 1984a. Early vertebrate evolution: Pharyngeal structure and the origin of gnathostomes. Journal of Zoology, London 204: 169–183.

———. 1984b. Feeding ecology of the earliest vertebrates. Zoological Journal of the Linnean Society 82: 261–272.

———. 1985. Reconstructing the life cycle and the feeding of ancestral vertebrates. In *Evolutionary Biology of Primitive Fishes,* R. E. Foreman, A. Gorbman, J. M. Dodd, and R. Olsson, eds. New York: Plenum Press, pp. 59–68.

Matsui, T. 1967. Review of the mackerel genera *Scomber* and *Rastelliger* with description of a new species of *Rastrelliger.* Copeia (1): 71–83.

Matthews, L. H. 1978. *The Natural History of the Whale.* New York: Columbia University Press.

Matthews, L. H., and H. W. Parker. 1950. Notes on the anatomy and biology of the basking shark (*Cetorhinus maximus* [Gunner]). Proceedings of the Zoological Society, London 120: 535–576.

Michaletz, P. H., C. F. Rabeni, W. W. Taylor, and T. R. Russell. 1982. Feeding ecology and growth of young-of-the-year paddlefish in hatchery ponds. Transactions of the American Fisheries Society 111: 700–709.

Mikhman, A. S., and L. V. Tomanovich. 1977. The feeding of the Azov anchovy, *Engraulis encrasicholus maeoticus.* Journal of Ichthyology 17 (2): 240–244.

Miller, G. S., Jr. 1923. The telescoping of the cetacean skull. Smithsonian Miscellaneous Collections 76 (5): 1–55.

Miller, R. R. 1960. Systematics and biology of the gizzard shad (*Dorosoma cepedianum*) and related fishes. Fishery Bulletin, U.S. 60: 371–392.

Miller, R. V. 1967. Food of the threadfin shad, *Dorosoma petenense*, in Lake Chicot, Arkansas. Transactions of the American Fisheries Society 96 (3): 243–246.

Mitchell, E. 1974. Trophic relationships and competition for food in northwest Atlantic whales. Proceedings of the Canadian Society of Zoologists, Annual Meeting: 123–133.

Monod, T. 1961. *Brevoortia* Gill 1861 et *Ethmalosa* Regan 1917. Bulletin de l'Institut français d'Afrique noire (A) 23: 506–547.

Moona, J. C. 1959. Studies on the cranial osteology of Indian clupeoid fishes. I. The skull of *Hilsa ilisha* (Ham.). Agra University Journal of Research 8: 53–71.

Moriarty, C. M., and D. J. W. Moriarty. 1973. Quantitative estimation of the daily ingestion of phytoplankton by *Tilapia nilotica* and *Haplochromis nigripinnis* in Lake George, Uganda. Journal of Zoology, London 171: 15–23.

Moriarty, D. J. W., J. P. E. C. Darlington, I. G. Dunn, C. M. Moriarty, and M. P. Tevlin. 1973. Feeding and grazing in Lake George, Uganda. Proceedings of the Royal Society of London B 184: 299–319.

Morton, J. 1967. *Guts: The Form and Function of the Digestive System*. Institute of Biology, Studies in Biology, no. 7. New York: St. Martin's Press.

Moss, S. A. 1972. The feeding mechanism of sharks of the family Carcharhinidae. Journal of Zoology, London 167: 423–436.

———. 1977. Feeding mechanisms in sharks. American Zoologist 17: 355–364.

———. 1981. Shark feeding mechanisms. Oceanus 24 (4): 23–29.

Muller, M., and J. W. M. Osse. 1984. Hydrodynamics of suction feeding in fish. Transactions of the Zoological Society of London 37: 51–135.

Mummert, J. R., and R. W. Drenner. 1986. Effect of fish size on the filtering efficiency and selective particle ingestion of a filter-feeding clupeid. Transactions of the American Fisheries Society 115: 522–528.

Murphy, G. I. 1950. The life history of the greaser blackfish (*Orthodon microlepidotus*) of Clear Lake, Lake County, California. California Fish and Game 36 (1): 119–133.

Murphy, R. C. 1936. *Oceanic Birds of South America*, vol. 1. New York: Macmillan.

Nelson, C. H., and K. R. Johnson. 1987. Whales and walruses as tillers of the sea floor. Scientific American 112–117.

Nelson, G. J. 1967a. Epibranchial organs in lower teleostean fishes. Journal of Zoology, London 153: 71–89.

———. 1967b. Gill arches of teleostean fishes of the family Clupeidae. Copeia (2): 389–399.

———. 1973. Relationships of clupeomorphs, with remarks on the structure of the lower jaw in fishes. In *Interrelationships of Fishes*, P. H. Greenwood, R. S. Miles, and C. Patterson, eds. London: Academic Press.

Nemoto, T. 1959. Food of baleen whales with reference to whale movements. Scientific Reports of the Whales Research Institute 14: 149–290.

————. 1970. Feeding pattern of baleen whales in the ocean. In *Marine Food Chains,* J. H. Steele, ed. Berkeley: University of California Press, pp. 241–252.

Nerini, M. 1984. A review of gray whale feeding ecology. In *The Gray Whale,* M. L. Jones, S. Leatherwood, and S. Swartz, eds. Orlando, Fla.: Academic Press, pp. 423–450.

Norden, C. R. 1961. Comparative osteology of representative salmonid fishes, with particular reference to the grayling (*Thymallus arcticus*) and its phylogeny. Journal of the Fisheries Research Board of Canada 18: 679–791.

Northcott, M. E., and M. C. M. Beveridge. 1988. The development and structure of pharyngeal apparatus associated with filter feeding in tilapias (*Oreochromis niloticus*). Journal of Zoology, London 215: 133–149.

Northcott, M. E., M. C. M. Beveridge, and L. G. Ross. 1991. A laboratory investigation of the filtration and ingestion rates of the tilapia, *Oreochromis niloticus,* feeding on two species of blue-green algae. Environmental Biology of Fishes 31: 75–85.

Northcutt, R. G., and C. Gans. 1983. The genesis of neural crest and epidermal placodes: A reinterpretation of vertebrate origins. Quarterly Review of Biology 58: 1–28.

Notarbartolo-di-Sciara, G. 1988. Natural history of the rays of the genus *Mobula* in the Gulf of California. Fishery Bulletin, U.S. 86 (1): 45–66.

O'Connell, C. P., and J. R. Zweifel. 1972. A laboratory study of particulate and filter feeding of the Pacific mackerel, *Scomber japonicus.* Fishery Bulletin, U.S. 70 (3): 973–981.

Odum, W. E. 1970. Utilization of the direct grazing and plant detritus food chains by the striped mullet *Mugil cephalus.* In *Marine Food Chains,* J. H. Steele, ed. Berkeley, University of California Press, pp. 222–240.

Olson, S. L., and A. Feduccia. 1980a. *Presbyornis* and the origin of the Anseriformes (Aves: Charadriomorphae). Smithsonian Contributions to Zoology no. 323.

————. 1980b. Relationships and evolution of flamingos (Aves: Phoenicopteridae). Smithsonian Contributions to Zoology no. 316.

Omura, H. 1964. A systematic study of the hyoid bones in the baleen whales. Scientific Reports of the Whales Research Institute 18: 149–170.

Orton, L. S., and P. F. Brodie. 1987. Engulfing mechanics of fin whales. Canadian Journal of Zoology 65: 2898–2907.

Owen, J. 1980. *Feeding Strategy.* Chicago: University of Chicago Press.

Pepin, P., J. A. Koslow, and S. Pearre, Jr. 1988. Laboratory study of foraging by Atlantic mackerel, *Scomber scombrus,* on natural zooplankton assemblages. Canadian Journal of Fisheries and Aquatic Sciences 45: 879–887.

Perrin, J. B. 1870. Notes on the anatomy of *Balaenoptera rostrata.* Proceedings of the Zoological Society of London: 805–817.

Philippart, J-Cl., and J-Cl. Ruwet. 1982. Ecology and distribution of tilapias. In *The Biology and Culture of Tilapias.* R. S. V. Pullin and R. H. Lowe-McConnell, eds. Manila: International Center for Living Aquatic Resources Management, pp. 15–59.

Phillips, J. B. 1942. Osteology of the sardine (*Sardinops caerulea*). Journal of Morphology 70: 463–500.

Pichler-Semmelrock, V. F. 1988. The influence of growth on the construction of the gill-filters and the nutritional intake of the silver carp (*Hypophthalmichthys molitrix* VAL. (Teleostei, Osteichthyes). Zoologischer Anzeiger 221 (5/6): 267–280.

Pierce, R. J., T. E. Wissing, and B. A. Megrey. 1981. Aspects of the feeding ecology of gizzard shad in Acton Lake, Ohio. Transactions of the American Fisheries Society 110: 391–395.

Pivorunas, A. 1976. A mathematical consideration on the function of baleen plates and their fringes. Scientific Reports of the Whales Research Institute 28: 37–55.

————. 1977. The fibrocartilage skeleton and related structures of the ventral pouch of balaenopterid whales. Journal of Morphology 151 (2): 299–314.

————. 1979. The feeding mechanisms of baleen whales. American Scientist 67 (4): 432–440.

Prince, P. A. 1980. The food and feeding ecology of Blue petrel (*Halobaena caerulea*) and Dove prion (*Pachyptila desolata*). Journal of Zoology, London 190: 59–76.

Prince, P. A., and R. A. Morgan. 1987. Diet and feeding ecology of Procellariiformes. In *Seabirds: Feeding Ecology and Role in Marine Ecosystems*, J. P. Croxall, ed. Cambridge: Cambridge University Press, pp. 135–172.

Racovitza, E. G. 1900. La vie des animaux et des plantes dans l'Antarctique. Bulletin de la Société Belge de géographie, Brussels 24: 177–230.

Radcliffe, L. 1914. The sharks and rays of Beaufort, North Carolina. Bulletin of the United States Bureau of Fisheries, Washington 34: 239–284, pls. 38–49.

Rao, K. V. N., and K. P. Rao. 1957. Differences in the food of the young and the adult Indian mackerel, *Rastrelliger kanagurta* (Cuv.). Nature 180 (4588): 711–712.

Ray, G. C., and W. E. Schevill. 1974. Feeding of a captive gray whale, *Eschrichtius robustus*. Marine Fisheries Review 36 (4): 31–38.

Reeves, R. R., and S. Leatherwood. 1985. Bowhead whale—*Balaena mysticetus*. In *Handbook of Marine Mammals*, vol. 3, *The Sirenians and Baleen Whales*, S. H. Ridgway and R. Harrison, eds. Orlando, Fla.: Academic Press, pp. 305–344.

Reinthal, P. N. 1990a. The feeding habits of a group of herbivorous rock-dwelling cichlid fishes (Cichlidae: Perciformes) from Lake Malawi, Africa. Environmental Biology of Fishes 27: 215–233.

————. 1990b. Morphological analyses of the neurocranium of a group of rock-dwelling cichlid fishes (Cichlidae: Perciformes) from Lake Malawi, Africa. Zoological Journal of the Linnean Society 98: 123–139.

Ridewood, W. G. 1904. On the cranial osteology of the clupeoid fishes. Proceedings of the Zoological Society of London 2: 448–493.

Ridgway, S. H., and R. Harrison, eds. 1985. *Handbook of Marine Mammals*, vol. 3, *The Sirenians and Baleen Whales*. Orlando, Fla.: Academic Press.

Riedman, M. 1990. *The Pinnipeds: Seals, Sea Lions, and Walruses*. Berkeley: University of California Press.

Robotham, P. W. J. 1982. An analysis of a specialized feeding mechanism of the spined loach, *Cobitis taenia* (L.), and a description of the related structures. Journal of Fish Biology 20: 173–181.

Rosen, R. A., and D. C. Hales. 1981. Feeding of paddlefish, *Polyodon spathula.* Copeia (2): 441–455.

Ross, G. J. B., F. Ryan, G. S. Saayman, and J. Skinner. 1976. Observations on two captive crabeater seals at Port Elizabeth Oceanarium. International Zoo Yearbook 16: 160–164.

Rovainen, C. M., and M. H. Schieber. 1975. Ventilation in larval lampreys. Journal of Comparative Physiology 104: 188–203.

Rubega, M. 1990. Prey transport by phalaropes using surface tension: A novel solution to the problems of planktivory. American Zoologist 30 (4): 102A.

Rubenstein, D. I., and M. A. R. Koehl. 1977. The mechanisms of filter feeding: Some theoretical considerations. American Naturalist 111: 981–994.

Runge, J. A., P. Pepin, and W. Silvert. 1987. Feeding behavior of the Atlantic mackerel *Scomber scombrus* on the hydromedusa *Aglantha digitale.* Marine Biology 94: 329–333.

Sanchez, T. M. 1973. Redescripción del cráneo y mandíbulas de *Pterodaustro guiñazui* Bonaparte (Pterodactyloidea, Pterodaustriidae). Ameghiniana 10 (4): 313–325.

Sanderson, S. L., and J. J. Cech, Jr. 1992. Energetic cost of suspension feeding versus particulate feeding by juvenile Sacramento blackfish. Transactions of the American Fisheries Society 121: 149–157.

Sanderson, S. L., J. J. Cech, Jr., and M. R. Patterson. 1991. Fluid dynamics in suspension-feeding blackfish. Science 251: 1346–1348.

Sanderson, S. L., and R. Wassersug. 1990. Suspension-feeding vertebrates. Scientific American 262 (3): 96–101.

Satel, S. L., and R. J. Wassersug. 1981. On the relative sizes of buccal floor depressor and elevator musculature in tadpoles. Copeia (1): 129–137.

Savage, R. M. 1952. Ecological, physiological, and anatomical observations on some species of Anuran tadpoles. Proceedings of the Zoological Society of London 122: 467–514.

Schnakenbeck, V. W. 1955. Der kiemenreusenapparat vom riesenhai (*Cetorhinus maximus*). Zoologischer Anzeiger 154 (5/6): 99–108.

Schulte, H. von W. 1916. The sei whale (*Balaenoptera borealis* Lesson): Anatomy of a foetus of *Balaenoptera borealis.* Monographs of the Pacific Cetacea. Memoirs of the American Museum of Natural History, n.s. 1: 389–499.

Seale, D. B. 1980. Influence of amphibian larvae on primary production, nutrient flux, and competition in a pond ecosystem. Ecology 61 (6): 1531–1550.

———. 1982. Obligate and facultative suspension feeding in anuran larvae: Feeding regulation in *Xenopus* and *Rana.* Biological Bulletin 162 (2): 214–231.

Seale, D. B., and N. Beckvar. 1980. The comparative ability of anuran larvae (genera: *Hyla, Bufo,* and *Rana*) to injest suspended blue-green algae. Copeia (3): 495–503.

Seale, D. B., K. Hoff, and R. Wassersug. 1982. *Xenopus laevis* larvae (Amphibia, Anura) as model suspension feeders. Hydrobiologia 87: 161–169.

Seale, D. B., and R. J. Wassersug. 1979. Suspension feeding dynamics of anuran larvae related to their functional morphology. Oecologia 39: 259–272.

Sears, R. 1983. A glimpse of blue whales feeding in the gulf of St. Lawrence. Whale-watcher (Fall): 12–14.

Severtzov, A. S. 1969. Food seizing mechanism of anuran larvae. Doklady Akademii Nauk SSSR 187: 211–214. Translation.

Shimeta, J., and P. A. Jumars. 1991. Physical mechanisms and rates of particle capture by suspension-feeders. Oceanography and Marine Biology Annual Review 29: 191–257.

Sibbing, F. A. 1988. Specializations and limitations in the utilization of food resources by the carp, *Cyprinus carpio:* A study of oral food processing. Environmental Biology of Fishes 22 (3): 161–178.

Sibbing, F. A., and R. Uribe. 1985. Regional specializations in the oro-pharyngeal wall and food processing in the carp (*Cyprinus carpio* L.). Netherlands Journal of Zoology 35 (3): 377–422.

Slijper, E. J. 1962. *Whales.* London: Hutchinson.

———. 1979. *Whales.* Ithaca, N.Y.: Cornell University Press.

Smith, H. M. 1961. Function of the choanal rakers of the green sea turtle. Herpetologica 17 (9): 214.

Sokol, O. M. 1981. The filter apparatus of larval *Pelodytes punctatus* (Amphibia: Anura). Amphibia-Reptilia 2: 195–208.

Spataru, P., and M. Zorn. 1978. Food and feeding habits of *Tilapia aurea* (Steindachner) (Cichlidae) in Lake Kinneret (Israel). Aquaculture 13: 67–79.

Spinar, Z. V. 1972. *Tertiary Frogs from Central Europe.* The Hague: Dr. W. Junk N.V. Publishers.

Starostka, V. J., and R. L. Applegate. 1970. Food selectivity of bigmouth buffalo, *Ictiobus cyprinellus,* in Lake Poinsett, South Dakota. Transactions of the American Fisheries Society 99 (3): 571–576.

Stone, H. H., and G. R. Daborn. 1987. Diet of alewives, *Alosa pseudoharengus,* and blueback herring, *A. aestivalis* (Pisces: Clupeidae), in Minas Basin, Nova Scotia, a turbid, macrotidal estuary. Environmental Biology of Fishes 19: 55–67.

Storro-Patterson, R. 1981. Great gulping blue whales. Oceans 14: 16–23.

Strickler, J. R. 1975. Intra- and interspecific information flow among planktonic copepods: Receptors. Verhandlungen der Internationale Vereinigung für theoretische und angewandte Limnologie 19: 2951–2958.

Taylor, L. R., L. J. V. Compagno, and P. J. Struhsaker. 1983. Megamouth—a new species, genus, and family of lamnoid shark (*Megachasma pelagios,* family Megachasmidae) from the Hawaiian Islands. Proceedings of the California Academy of Sciences 43 (8): 87–110.

Taylor, M. A. 1987. How tetrapods feed in water: A functional analysis by paradigm. Zoological Journal of the Linnean Society 91 (2): 171–195.

Tilley, S. G. 1964. A quantitative study of shrinkage in the digestive tract of the tiger salamander (*Ambystoma tigrinum* Green) during metamorphosis. Journal of the Ohio Herpetological Society 4 (4): 81–85.

Tomilin, A. G. 1967. *Cetacea: Mammals of the U.S.S.R. and Adjacent Countries,* vol. 9. Jerusalem: Israel Program for Scientific Translations.

True, F. W. 1904. The whalebone whale of the western north Atlantic. Smithsonian Contributions to Knowledge 33: 1–332.

Uchida, S. 1983. On the morphology of the whale shark, *Rhincodon thypus* Smith. Aquabiology 5 (2): 93–101.

Van Beneden, P.-J. 1882. Sur l'articulation temporo-maxillaire chez les Cétacés. Archives de biologie 3: 669–678.

van der Meeren, T. 1991. Algae as first food for cod larvae, *Gadus morhua* L.: Filter feeding or ingestion by accident? Journal of Fish Biology 39: 225–237.

Vanderploeg, H. A. 1990. Feeding mechanisms and particle selection in suspension-feeding zooplankton. In *The Biology of Particles in Aquatic Systems,* R. S. Wotton, ed. Boca Raton: CRC Press, pp. 183–212.

Viertel, B. 1982. The oral cavities of Central European anuran larvae (Amphibia): Morphology, ontogenesis, and generic diagnosis. Amphibia-Reptilia 4: 327–360.

———. 1985. The filter apparatus of *Rana temporaria* and *Bufo bufo* larvae (Amphibia, Anura). Zoomorphology 105: 345–355.

———. 1987. The filter apparatus of *Xenopus laevis, Bombina variegata,* and *Bufo calamita* (Amphibia, Anura): A comparison of different larval types. Zoologische Jahrbücher, Anatomie 115: 425–452.

———. 1990. Suspension feeding of anuran larvae at low concentrations of *Chlorella* algae (Amphibia, Anura). Oecologia 85: 167–177.

Vinyard, G. L., R. W. Drenner, M. Gophen, U. Pollingher, D. L. Winkelman, and K. D. Hambright. 1988. An experimental study of the plankton community impacts of two omnivorous filter-feeding cichlids, *Tilapia galilaea* and *Tilapia aurea*. Canadian Journal of Fisheries and Aquatic Sciences 45: 685–690.

Vladykov, V. D. 1970. Pearl tubercles and certain cranial peculiarities useful in the taxonomy of coregonid genera. In *Biology of Coregonid Fishes,* C. C. Lindsey and C. S. Woods, eds. Winnipeg: University of Manitoba Press, pp. 167–193.

Vogel, S. 1981. *Life in Moving Fluids: The Physical Biology of Flow.* Boston: Willard Grant Press, 352 pp.

———. 1988. How organisms use flow-induced pressures. American Scientist 76: 28–34.

Wallace, J. B., and R. W. Merritt. 1980. Filter-feeding ecology of aquatic insects. Annual Review of Entomology 25: 103–132.

Warham, J. 1990. *The Petrels: Their Ecology and Breeding Systems.* London: Academic Press.

Wassersug, R. J. 1972. The mechanism of ultraplanktonic entrapment in anuran larvae. Journal of Morphology 137 (3): 279–288.

———. 1975. The adaptive significance of the tadpole stage with comments on the maintenance of complex life cycles in anurans. American Zoologist 15: 405–417.

———. 1980. Internal oral features of larvae from eight anuran families: Functional, systematic, evolutionary, and ecological considerations. Miscellaneous Publications of the University of Kansas Museum of Natural History, no. 68: 1–146.

———. 1989. Locomotion in amphibian larvae (or "Why aren't tadpoles built like fishes?"). American Zoologist 29: 65–84.

Wassersug, R., K. Frogner, and R. Inger. 1981. Adaptations for life in treeholes by rhacophorid tadpoles from Thailand. Journal of Herpetology 15 (1): 41–52.

Wassersug, R. J., and W. R. Heyer. 1988. A survey of internal oral features of lep-
todactyloid larvae (Amphibia: Anura). Smithsonian Contributions to Zoology
457: 1–99.
Wassersug, R., and K. Hoff. 1979. A comparative study of the buccal pumping
mechanism of tadpoles. Biological Journal of the Linnean Society 12: 225–259.
———. 1982. Developmental changes in the orientation of the anuran jaw suspension: A preliminary exploration into the evolution of metamorphosis. Evolutionary Biology 15: 223–246.
Wassersug, R. J., and A. M. Murphy. 1987. Aerial respiration facilitates growth in
suspension-feeding anuran larvae (Xenopus laevis). Experimental Biology 46:
141–147.
Wassersug, R. J., and W. F. Pyburn. 1987. The biology of the Pe-ret' toad, Otophryne robusta (Microhylidae), with special consideration of its fossorial larva
and systematic relationships. Zoological Journal of the Linnean Society 91:
137–169.
Wassersug, R., and K. Rosenberg. 1979. Surface anatomy of the branchial food
traps of tadpoles: A comparative study. Journal of Morphology 159: 393–426.
Watkins, W. A., and W. E. Schevill. 1979. Aerial observation of feeding behavior
in four baleen whales: Eubalaena glacialis, Balaenoptera borealis, Megaptera
novaeangliae, and Balaenoptera physalus. Journal of Mammalogy 60 (1):
155–163.
Webb, P. 1984. Body form, locomotion and foraging in aquatic vertebrates. American Zoologist 24: 107–120.
———. 1988. Simple physical principles and vertebrate aquatic locomotion. Amer-
ican Zoologist 28: 709–725.
Webb, P. W., and V. de Buffrénil. 1990. Locomotion in the biology of large aquatic
vertebrates. Transactions of the American Fisheries Society 119: 629–641.
Weed, A. C. 1925. Feeding the paddlefish. Copeia 146: 67–68.
Weihs, D. 1980. Hydrodynamics of suction feeding of fish in motion. Journal of
Fish Biology 16: 425–433.
Weisel, G. F. 1973. Anatomy and histology of the digestive system of the paddlefish
(Polyodon spathula). Journal of Morphology 140: 243–256.
Wellnhofer, P. 1981. Flugsaurier—Als die Saurier fliegen lernten. Freunde der Bay-
erischen Staatssammlung für Paläontologie und historische Geologie, Mün-
chen, pp. 1–6.
White, E. G. 1930. The whale shark, Rhineodon typus: Description of the skeletal
parts and classification based on the Marathon specimen captured in 1923.
Bulletin of the American Museum of Natural History 61 (4): 129–160.
White, P. N., and M. N. Bruton. 1983. Food and feeding mechanisms of Gilchris-
tella aestuarius (Pisces: Clupeidae). South African Journal of Zoology 18:
31–36.
Whitehead, P. J. 1959. Feeding mechanism of Tilapia nigra. Nature 184 (4697):
1509–1510.
Whitehead, P. J. P. 1985. Clupeoid fishes of the world (suborder Clupeoidei). FAO
Fisheries Synopsis no. 125 (7): 1–303.
Williamson, G. R. 1973. Counting and measuring baleen and ventral grooves of
whales. Scientific Reports of the Whales Research Institute 25: 279–292.

Worthy, G. A. J., and J. P. Hickie. 1986. Relative brain size in marine mammals. American Naturalist 128 (4): 445–459.

Wotton, R. S. 1990. Methods for capturing particles in benthic animals. In *The Biology of Particles in Aquatic Systems,* R. S. Wotton, ed. Boca Raton: CRC Press, pp. 161–182.

Würsig, B., E. M. Dorsey, W. J. Richardson, C. W. Clark, and R. Payne. 1985. Normal behavior of bowheads, 1980–84. In *Behavior, Disturbance Responses, and Distribution of Bowhead Whales Balaena mysticetus in the Eastern Beaufort Sea, 1980–84,* J. Richardson, ed. U.S. Minerals Management Service, pp. 14–88.

Youson, J. H. 1981. The alimentary canal. In *The Biology of Lampreys,* vol. 3, M. W. Hardisty and I. C. Potter, eds. London: Academic Press, pp. 95–190.

Zweers, G. A. 1974. Structure, movement, and myography of the feeding apparatus of the mallard (*Anas platyrhynchos* L.): A study in functional anatomy. Netherlands Journal of Zoology 24 (4): 323–467.

Zweers, G. A., A. F. Ch. Gerritsen, and P. J. van Kranenburg-Voogd. 1977. Mechanics of feeding of the mallard (*Anas platyrhynchos* L.; Aves, Anseriformes). In *Contributions to Vertebrate Evolution,* vol. 3, M. K. Hecht and F. S. Szalay, eds. New York: S. Karger.

3

Design of Feeding Systems in Aquatic Vertebrates: Major Patterns and Their Evolutionary Interpretations

GEORGE V. LAUDER AND H. BRADLEY SHAFFER

INTRODUCTION

A MAJOR GOAL OF RESEARCH in functional morphology should be to produce general concepts and define patterns of structural and functional evolution. However, few general concepts have been identified from the study of structure and function of the vertebrate skull. The lack of concepts has not been due to any deficiency in the empirical data base. On the contrary, functional morphologists have been extremely successful in their descriptions of skull structure and function in vertebrates. As evidenced by these volumes on the vertebrate skull (Hanken and Hall 1993), many investigators have documented the diversity of skull morphology. In general, the major patterns of skull morphology are understood, although controversies exist on some aspects of skull structure (such as the extent of segmental organization of the skull).

To a lesser extent, functional patterns of vertebrate skull diversity have also been documented. While growth in our comparative knowledge of skull function has been relatively slow (perhaps in part owing to the complex nature of functional analyses and the relatively recent application of quantitative experimental techniques), a great deal is now known about skull function in individual vertebrate clades (Chondrichthyes: Frazzetta and Prange 1987; Moss 1972, 1977; Actinopterygii: Alexander 1967; Lauder 1980a, 1982; Liem 1970; Actinistia: Lauder 1980b; Dipnoi: Bemis 1987; Bemis and Lauder 1986; Amphibia: Bemis et al. 1983; Cundall et al. 1987; Druner 1904; Erdman and Cundall 1984; Findeis and Bemis 1990; Gans and Gorniak 1982; Lauder and Shaffer 1985, 1986; Lombard and Wake 1977; Ozeti and Wake 1969; Shaffer and Lauder 1985a, b; Reilly and Lauder 1989, 1990c; and Amniota: Bock 1964; Crompton et al. 1977; Gans et al. 1978; Smith and Hylander 1985; Weijs and Dantuma 1981).

Despite this growth in our basic knowledge of skull structure and function, there have been few attempts to summarize the key ideas that have emerged from all this research. In consequence, virtually none of the generalities derived from research on vertebrate skull structure and function are available to workers in fields such as systematics, neurophysiology, evolutionary biology, population biology, and ecology.

Our goal in this paper is to provide a summary and analysis of the key conclusions derived from studies of form and function in the skull of aquatic vertebrates. We will make no attempt to review the many specific studies, as several volumes have provided substantial overviews of skull structure and function (Hildebrand et al. 1985; Kluge 1977). Also, we will limit ourselves to considering the head and feeding system in lower vertebrates (fishes and amphibians), and will not address aquatic feeding in amniotes (see Jenkin 1957; Lambertsen 1983; Pivorunas 1979; Zweers 1974). Filter feeding and feeding methods in other clades are covered elsewhere in this volume.

This chapter is divided into three parts. First, we consider major results of general interest that have been derived from research on the skull of aquatic vertebrates over the past twenty years: we have identified four dominant concepts that have emerged from the current data available on feeding systems. Second, we discuss the importance and evolutionary significance of each of the four major concepts. Finally, we address future directions of research on skull structure and function in aquatic vertebrates.

KEY CONCEPTS

Concept 1
Biomechanical patterns of aquatic prey capture are evolutionarily conservative.

A key conclusion of comparative studies on feeding mechanics in lower vertebrates is that many of the biomechanical mechanisms used in prey capture are highly conserved evolutionarily. That is, many biomechanical patterns in the skull are found throughout lower vertebrates, and have been retained across the aquatic-terrestrial transition in vertebrate evolution (Reilly and Lauder 1990a). This conservatism in functional systems across a broad range of vertebrate clades occurs despite the remarkable diversity in skull shape and gross morphology, as well as in habitats occupied by lower vertebrates. For example, taxa as diverse in morphology, life history, and ecology as axolotls, trout, lungfish, and nurse sharks all share common biomechanical mechanisms for opening the mouth.

The conservation of biomechanical systems applies primarily to the musculoskeletal mechanisms used to control the initial capture of prey by suction feeding (Alexander 1967; Lauder 1980a, 1985b; Liem 1970). Suction feeding is the process of aquatic prey capture whereby the mouth

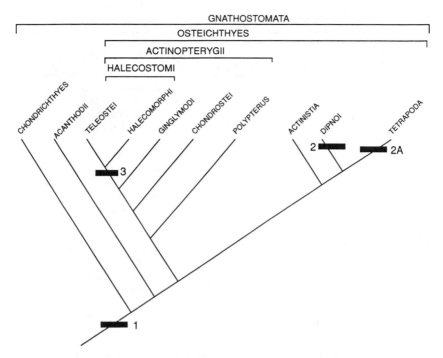

Fig. 3.1. A cladogram of lower vertebrate lineages with key functional and morphological characters relating to the skull and feeding mechanism mapped onto it. Functional aspects of skull design associated with characters denoted by the black bars (and representing specializations of the clades above the bars) are listed in table 3.1. As discussed in the text, lungfishes (Dipnoi) and tetrapods have independently acquired a depressor mandibulae muscle that functions as a second mandibular depression mechanism during feeding (characters 2 and 2A).

cavity is rapidly expanded, resulting in a negative (suction) pressure inside the oral cavity relative to the surrounding water (Lauder 1985a). This intraoral negative pressure creates a flow of water into the mouth that carries the prey within reach of the jaws. Suction feeding is a process proposed to have originated with the jawed vertebrates, and represents the dominant feeding mode in virtually all modern aquatic vertebrates.

Figure 3.1 and table 3.1 outline the major biomechanical pathways in osteichthyan fishes, and several of the major innovations in skull biomechanics in selected lineages are noted. There is still a paucity of experimental data on chondrichthyans, and thus the biomechanical basis of the feeding system in this clade has not been well worked out. The key biomechanical system that is retained throughout anamniotic vertebrates is the musculoskeletal apparatus controlling mouth opening. In lower vertebrate clades, the primary mechanism mediating mandibular depression in-

TABLE 3.1 Morphological and functional novelties in the feeding mechanism of vertebrates

Phylogenetic level for biomechanical novelties	Character in fig. 3.1*	Description of characters
Gnathostomata	1	i. Mandibular depression mechanism involving the hypaxialis and sternohyoideus muscles, the mandibulohyoid ligament, and posterodorsal rotation of the proximal end of the hyoid around the articulation with the interhyal bone or cartilage
		ii. Antero-posterior sequence of skull bone movement during suction feeding
		iii. Unidirectional flow of water through the buccal cavity during suction feeding
		iv. Elevation of the skull by the epaxial muscles
		v. Suction feeding as a prey-capture system
Dipnoi + Tetrapoda	2 and 2A	i. Mandibular depression mechanism involving a depressor mandibulae muscle (arising from the visceral musculature of the hyoid arch) that originates on the skull and inserts posterior to the jaw joint on the mandible
Halecostomi	3	i. Mandibular depression mechanism involving the levator operculi and opercular series (fig. 3.2), and a novel ligament, the interoperculomandibular ligament

* Characters listed are keyed to the black bars on the cladogram in figure 3.1.

volves the ventral body and hyoid musculature and the hyoid apparatus. In salamanders and fishes (Lauder 1980a; Liem 1970; Lauder and Shaffer 1985), contraction of the hypaxial and sternohyoideus (= rectus cervicis) muscles causes a posteroventral translation of the hyoid arch. This movement causes the posterodorsal aspect of the hyoid to apply tension to the mandibulohyoid ligament. Because the mandibulohyoid ligament attaches to the mandible ventral to the axis of rotation of the quadratomandibular joint, the lower jaw is depressed. The major structural units involved in this system are diagramed in figure 3.2. This biomechanical pathway is present in all lower vertebrate clades, including taxa as diverse as coelacanths, salamanders, trout, sharks, and lungfishes. It thus forms the fundamental component of skull design in vertebrates.

Three other aspects of skull function appear to be conserved across lower vertebrate clades (table 3.1; fig. 3.1). First, in all groups studied experimentally, there is a specific timing of skull bone movement during prey capture (Lauder 1979, 1980a; Lauder and Shaffer 1985). As the mouth opens and reaches peak gape, the hyoid is moving posteroventrally and is the major contributor to the increase in buccal cavity volume. Peak hyoid depression occurs after maximum gape is reached, and this is in turn followed by expansion of the posterior (opercular) region of the skull.

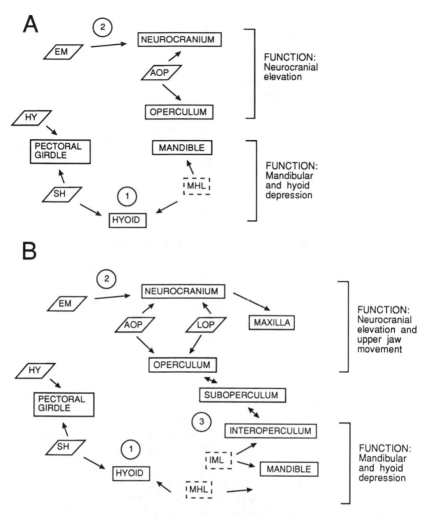

Fig. 3.2. Schematic diagram of the major structural components in the skull of ray-finned fishes at two phylogenetic levels. A. The primitive condition for ray-finned fishes (Actinopterygii, fig. 3.1). B. The primitive condition for the Halecostomi (fig. 3.1). This figure illustrates the addition of a novel biomechanical pathway (no. 3) to the two primitive systems (nos. 1 and 2). The new biomechanical pathway is added to the structural configuration of the head without modifying the primitive pattern, and the function of mandibular and hyoid depression in halecostome fishes is achieved via two biomechanical pathways. Solid rectangles represent bony elements; dashed rectangles, ligaments; parallelograms, muscles. Solid arrows extend from the muscle to the bone of insertion, and double-headed arrows indicate ligamentous connections between bones. Abbreviations: AOP, adductor operculi muscle; EM, epaxial muscles; HY, hypaxial muscles; IML, interoperculomandibular ligament; LOP, levator operculi muscle; MHL, mandibulohyoid ligament; SH, sternohyoideus muscle.

There is thus a consistent anterior-to-posterior sequence in timing of head movements during feeding.

Second, the flow of water into the mouth during suction is predominantly unidirectional, owing to the resistance of the gill bars to water flow at the back of the head. In both fishes and salamanders (Lauder 1985b; Lauder and Shaffer 1985), the branchial apparatus forms a dynamic resistance to water flow during feeding. As the mouth opens and water enters the buccal cavity, the gill arches at the back of the mouth cavity are adducted, preventing water influx from the back of the head. As peak gape is reached, the gill bars begin to abduct, allowing water drawn into the mouth to exit posteriorly. This dynamic resistance of the gill apparatus is fundamental to the suction-feeding mechanism, and is postulated to have been present in early osteichthyan fishes. No data are available on the nature of the gill resistance during feeding by sharks, and it is thus not yet possible to say whether a dynamic gill resistance is primitive for gnathostomes.

Third, in all clades studied experimentally, a key aspect of feeding biomechanics is elevation of the cranium by the epaxial muscles. Cranial elevation contributes to the increase in gape and to the increase in buccal volume.

There are two important corollaries to concept 1.

Corollary 1: *Major innovations in skull design related to initial prey capture typically occur by adding on functional/design features to those primitively present, not by changing existing biomechanical mechanisms.* Two examples of this phenomenon are shown in figure 3.1. Early ray-finned fishes possess only one mechanism of mandibular depression, the hypaxialis–sternohyoideus–hyoid apparatus–mandible coupling (fig. 3.1, character 1). However, halecostome fishes (the Halecostomi contain the family Amiidae and the teleost fishes, as well as several fossil taxa; fig. 3.1) possess a second biomechanical system for depressing the mandible, the levator operculi–opercular apparatus–mandible system (fig. 3.1, character 3; Lauder 1979, 1980a). Figure 3.2 diagrammatically illustrates the transformation in the structural network of the head from the primitive actinopterygian condition to the halecostome configuration. Note that the addition of a novel biomechanical system, the levator operculi coupling (fig. 3.2B: pathway 3), occurs while retaining all of the elements in the original system (fig. 3.2A: pathways 1 and 2). The new mechanism for lower-jaw depression utilizes several bony components of the head that are primitive for ray-finned fishes, such as the operculum (fig. 3.2A). The levator operculi and the ligamentous connection of the interoperculum to the mandible are novelties at the halecostome level (fig. 3.1, character 3; fig. 3.2B; table 3.1) that are *added on* to the primitive structural configuration of the feeding mechanism (with minimal modification to the primitive system).

A second example is provided by lungfishes and salamanders, which also possess a novel mandibular depression mechanism: a biomechanically independent system that does not disrupt function of the hyoid-based depression mechanism. Lungfishes and salamanders have independently acquired a depressor mandibulae muscle (Bemis 1987; Bemis and Lauder 1986) that inserts directly on the lower jaw (fig. 3.1, characters 2 and 2A). In both lungfishes and salamanders this muscle has been demonstrated to function in concert with the primitive mandibulohyoid system (Bemis and Lauder 1986; Lauder and Shaffer 1985) to mediate mouth opening. Thus, in these clades a second novel muscular biomechanical mechanism has been added onto the primitive mouth opening system without modification of the original system.

Corollary 2: *Jaw muscle activity patterns (motor patterns) among closely related taxa may be phylogenetically conserved, and phylogenetic changes in feeding behavior within these clades is then a consequence primarily of changes in the design of peripheral morphology.*

Recent quantitative analyses of the jaw muscle activity patterns used during initial prey capture and in prey processing by lower vertebrates have shown that there tend to be relatively few interspecific differences in motor patterns, despite significant differences in feeding behavior and performance among these species (Lauder 1991; Sanderson 1988; Shaffer and Lauder 1985a; Wainwright and Lauder 1986; Wainwright 1989).

For example, Wainwright and Lauder (1986) studied the motor pattern of the jaw muscles in four genera in the family Centrarchidae (a clade of endemic North American fishes that includes the bass, *Micropterus,* and sunfishes, *Lepomis*). The four genera differ considerably in head shape and mouth size and have different natural feeding habits and abilities. Only one of the eleven electromyographic variables measured showed any significant difference among genera, indicating that the pattern of muscle activity used during feeding is very similar among the genera. Similar conservatism among closely related species has been found in the feeding motor pattern in ambystomatid salamanders (Shaffer and Lauder 1985a), and haemulid and labrid fishes (Sanderson, 1988).

Concept 2
Functional characters differ in their levels of intraspecific and interspecific variation.

Functional characters differ in their levels of variation, with those most important to suction-feeding performance exhibiting the greatest interspecific variation and the least intraspecific variation.

While the previous section suggests that certain general movement and muscle activity patterns are conserved across most suction-feeding verte-brates, recent detailed studies of variation within and among closely re-lated species emphasize that interesting patterns of variability occur in some functional characters. In particular, certain movement and muscle activity patterns appear to be relatively stereotyped within species, and yet differ among related taxa. Others show the exact opposite pattern, with virtually all variation occurring within species, and species means exhibit-ing little or no differentiation. A key point in these population level analy-ses of suction feeding is the role of individual variation within species, and how it shapes the opportunity for selection to act on functional characters and their morphological constituents.

Detailed descriptions of populational variation in functional systems have been carried out in aquatic salamanders (Shaffer and Lauder 1985a, b; Lauder and Shaffer 1985, 1986) and fishes (Sanderson 1988; Wain-wright 1986; Wainwright and Lauder 1986). While these studies cover only a small fraction of the morphological, taxonomic, and behavioral variation found in aquatic suction feeding, several patterns are emerging.

Perhaps most important is the lack of a one-to-one relationship be-tween morphological divergence and functional output. In nontransform-ing ambystomatid salamanders (the axolotl, *Ambystoma mexicanum*, and its relatives), there is a great deal of variation in head size and shape (Shaf-fer 1984; Lauder and Shaffer 1985). However, when three morphologi-cally divergent species were quantitatively tested for variation in kinematic variables (Shaffer and Lauder 1985b), similar functional divergence was not observed. Rather, functional variables display a range of variation, from maximum hyoid depression, where virtually all (90%) of the pheno-typic variance is attributable to differentiation among species, to maximal cranial elevation, where an estimated 22% of the variance is attributable to among-species differences, and most (63%) is at the level of variation among trials of the same individual (table 3.2). These results emphasize the crucial importance of experimental verification of functional hypothe-ses based on morphology alone; they also stress the necessity of quanti-fying variation in *function* within species before general conclusions on divergence among species may be drawn (Lauder 1990).

A general trend that is emerging is that functional characters most important in generating suction during feeding show the least variation within species, and tend to differentiate closely related taxa. For virtually all suction-feeding vertebrates, the hyoid apparatus acts as the primary pump involved in generating negative pressures within the buccal cavity (Lauder 1985a). Thus, patterns of hyoid movement and electromyographic activ-ity in its associated musculature (the rectus cervicus or sternohyoideus)

TABLE 3.2 Patterns of variation in the feeding mechanism of three species of ambystomatid salamanders (genus *Ambystoma*)

Kinematic variable in the feeding mechanism	Percentage of total variance			Mean value of the variable for each species		
	Among species	Among individuals within species	Among trials within individuals	*A. dumerilii*	*A. mexicanum*	*A. ordinarium*
Cranial elevation (in degrees)	22	15**	63	45.5	32.6	38.1
Maximum hyoid depression (in cm)	90**	6**	4	2.8	1.9	1.8
Maximum gape (in cm)	63**	16**	21	2.1	1.5	1.2
Time to maximum gape (in ms)	39*	19**	42	46.7	33.8	38.0
Time to maximum hyoid depression (in ms)	69**	15**	16	52.5	28.2	38.0
Total gape cycle time (in ms)	38*	18**	44	88.0	69.7	73.0

Source: Shaffer and Lauder (1985b).
Note: These three species are the most morphologically divergent in the family (Shaffer 1984). Six kinematic variables were digitized from high-speed films of feedings for several individuals in each species.
 * Significant at the 0.05 level.
** Significant at the 0.01 level.

TABLE 3.3 Patterns of variation in the feeding mechanism of two species of ambystomatid salamanders (genus *Ambystoma*).

Electromyographic variable in the feeding mechanism	Percentage of total variance				Mean value of the variable for each species (in ms)	
	Among species	Among individuals within species	Among days within individuals	Among trials within days	A. dumerilii	A. mexicanum
Onset time difference between the depressor mandibulae and sternohyoideus muscles	51**	13	6**	30	2.80	−2.11
Onset time difference between the depressor mandibulae and adductor mandibulae internus muscles	7	4	2	87	0.45	−1.94
Duration of activity in the depressor mandibulae muscle	0	40*	15**	45	67.7	59.0
Duration of activity in the sternohyoideus muscle	25	33**	2	40	39.1	66.1
Duration of activity in the adductor mandibulae internus muscle	0	27	24**	49	116.5	98.1

Source: These data are abstracted from Shaffer and Lauder (1985a).
Note: Eleven electromyographic variables were digitized from recordings of cranial muscle activity during prey capture for several individuals in each species (five are shown here). Data are shown for three muscles: the depressor mandibulae (a muscle that contributes to mouth opening by depressing the mandible), the sternohyoideus (a muscle that causes both lower-jaw depression and buccal volume expansion), and the adductor mandibulae internus (one of the jaw-closing muscles).
* Significant at the 0.05 level.
** Significant at the 0.01 level.

consistently differentiate species of ambystomatid salamanders (table 3.3; Shaffer and Lauder 1985a, b; Lauder and Shaffer 1985) and centrarchid sunfishes (Wainwright and Lauder 1986). Interestingly, this is the only muscle showing significant electromyographic variation among species, and therefore a relatively stereotyped behavior within taxa, in these studies. All other muscles and kinematic variables demonstrate consistently high levels of variation among conspecific individuals and large amounts of within-individual variation. However, the mean values of congeneric species are often very similar to each other.

Unfortunately, we have virtually no information on how these levels of functional variation are related to morphological variation in the bones and muscles of the head. For head width, the only variable so far considered in salamanders, within-species correlations with mean values of kinematic variables range from 0.21 to 0.63, suggesting that morphometric and functional variation at the individual level may be related. Species means are even more highly correlated, with average head width and kinematic variable correlations ranging from 0.54 to 0.96 (Shaffer and Lauder 1985b).

Concept 3
Environmental transitions affect kinematic and EMG patterns, but these changes are not a direct consequence of the biophysics of the media.

Significant differences in feeding and breathing behavior are observed as vertebrates shift from water to air, but the patterns of cranial bone movement and muscle function used during the manipulation of prey in the two media are remarkably similar.

A central concern in functional analyses of morphology is the extent to which the physical environment sets limits to, or constrains, the functional performance attained with a given morphology. The transition from water to air has been emphasized as a particularly important one in vertebrates as so many species have shifted, both ontogenetically and phylogenetically, from aquatic to terrestrial lifestyles. In particular, amphibians, turtles, and a few fishes have both aquatic and terrestrial life history phases, and functional analyses of feeding by these organisms in water and on land have allowed a preliminary examination of the biophysical constraints imposed by these two very different media on the structure and function of the skull (Bramble and Wake 1985). Additionally, comparisons between aquatic and aerial respiration have illuminated the extent to which the same structures may serve dual functional roles in lower vertebrates (Liem 1985, 1987).

One conclusion to emerge from these studies has been the overall conservatism of movement and muscle activity patterns that may be used during respiration and prey manipulation in different environments. In

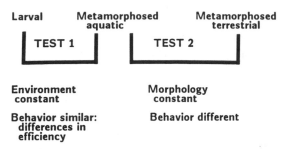

Fig. 3.3. Conceptual design of the experimental comparisons used in analyses of the effect of the environment on skull function by Lauder and Shaffer (1988) and Shaffer and Lauder (1988). The tiger salamander, *Ambystoma tigrinum*, was used as an experimental animal to investigate both the influence of the medium (water versus air) and the effect of morphological transformations at metamorphosis on skull function. Because metamorphosed animals will still feed in the water, we were able to conduct two sets of comparisons (tests). Test 1 involves comparing feeding behavior and muscle activity between larval and metamorphosed animals feeding in the water (termed the metamorphosed aquatic stage): the environment is constant, but the morphology is different. Test 2 involves comparing metamorphosed aquatic individuals with metamorphosed individuals feeding on land: morphology is constant but the feeding environment has changed. From Lauder and Shaffer (1986).

our work on the salamander *Ambystoma tigrinum*, we have used an experimental design that allows us to partition the variation in feeding kinematics and electromyographic muscle activity into distinct components reflecting the morphological changes at metamorphosis and the environmental transitions associated with feeding in the water and on land (fig. 3.3). This general design provides information on two aspects of the functional transition from aquatic suction to terrestrial lingual feeding. First, by comparing variation in function between larval and metamorphosed animals feeding in the water (fig. 3.3; test 1) we were able to assess the effect of morphological changes at metamorphosis alone on feeding function (the presence of the aquatic environment is a constant). Second, comparing metamorphosed animals feeding in the water and on land documents the magnitude of the functional shifts associated with the change in environment that occurs at metamorphosis (fig. 3.3: test 2). Partitioning the overall variation in feeding kinematics and muscle function into environmental and morphological components allows us to quantify the degree to which a given change in morphology of the skull and hyobranchial skeleton necessitates a change in function.

Figures 3.4 and 3.5 illustrate some of the morphological changes that occur during metamorphosis. Externally, the gills are lost, the gill slits close, the head narrows, and the eyes move to a more anterodorsal loca-

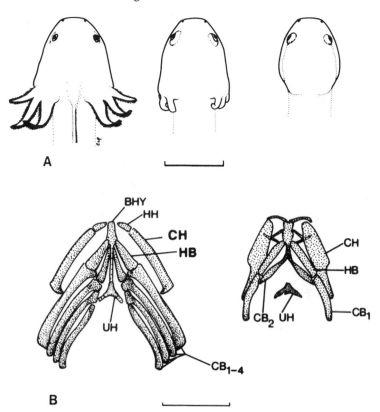

Fig. 3.4. A. Three dorsal views of the head of *Ambystoma tigrinum*. The left panel shows the head of a larva, the middle panel the head of an individual in the middle of metamorphosis, and the right panel the head of a metamorphosed individual. B. The hyobranchial apparatus of larva (on the left) and an adult (on the right) *Ambystoma tigrinum*. Note the major morphological changes that occur at metamorphosis: loss of ceratobranchials 2, 3, and 4, and extensive alterations in shape of the hyoid and branchial arches. Scale bars = 1.0 cm. Abbreviations: BHY, Basihyal cartilage; CB_{1-4}, Ceratobranchial bones 1 through 4; CH, Ceratohyal cartilage; BH, Hypobranchial cartilage; HH, Hypohyal cartilage; UH, Urohyal. Modified from Lauder and Shaffer (1988).

tion (fig. 3.4A). Changes in the skull at metamorphosis include the loss of the palatine and alterations in shape of the vomer, pterygoid, and prearticular bones. Many changes occur in the hyobranchial apparatus (fig. 3.4B). For example, the posterior ceratobranchials are lost, most hyobranchial skeletal elements change shape, the radials form, and a glandular tongue with lingual sinuses develops (see Duellman and Trueb 1986; Lauder and Reilly 1990; Reilly and Lauder 1989, 1990b; Yamasaki 1956). A great many changes also take place in the muscular system of the head (fig. 3.5):

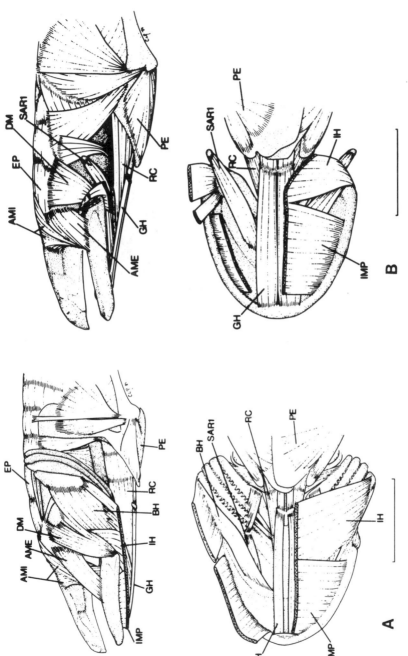

Fig. 3.5. A. Dorsal and ventral views of the muscles of the head of a larval *Ambystoma tigrinum*. Note the ventral branchial muscles and particularly the large branchiohyoideus muscle. B. Dorsal and ventral views of the muscles of the head of an adult *Ambystoma tigrinum*. Note the lack of gill bars and the branchiohyoideus muscle, and the subarcualis rectus 1 muscle that attaches to the distal end of ceratobranchial 1. Scale bars = 1.0 cm. Abbreviations: AME, Adductor mandibulae externus muscle; AMI, Adductor mandibulae internus muscle; BH, Branchiohyoideus muscle; DM, Depressor mandibulae muscle; EP, Epaxial muscles; GH, Geniohyoideus muscle; IH, Interhyoideus muscle; IMP, Intermandibularis posterior muscle; PE, Pectoralis muscle; RC, Rectus cervicis muscle; SAR1, Subarcualis rectus 1 muscle. Modified from Lauder and Shaffer (1988).

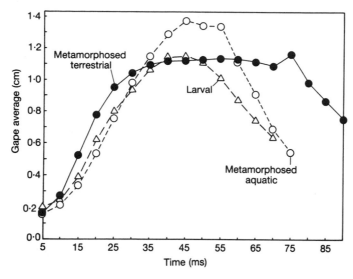

Fig. 3.6. Graph of the average pattern of mouth opening (gape) with respect to time for three individuals feeding as larvae, as metamorphosed animals in the water, and as metamorphosed individuals on land. Each point represents the mean gape distance for each time interval measured from high-speed films of feeding. There are no statistically significant differences among the three curves, although there is a tendency for terrestrial feedings to be longer in duration. Similar results were obtained for most other kinematic variables. Modified from Shaffer and Lauder (1988).

tongue muscles are formed, many gill arch muscles (such as the larval branchiohyoideus) are lost, and the subarcualis rectus 1 muscle elongates and moves its insertion to the distal end of ceratobranchial 1 (fig. 3.5). Given the extensive morphological changes at metamorphosis, one might predict that major functional transformations occur also.

The primary conclusion from both kinematic (Shaffer and Lauder 1988) and electromyographic (Lauder and Shaffer 1988; Reilly and Lauder 1990c) studies of feeding in salamanders is that while feeding *mode* changes across environments, many functional components of the feeding act are retained from the larval ontogenetic stage. For our kinematic data, there were no detectable differences between larval and metamophosed animals feeding in the water (figs. 3.6, 3.7), suggesting that the morphological changes at metamorphosis do not necessitate a shift in function. That is, both larval and metamorphosed animals can suction feed, and the metamorphosed animals retain the larval patterns of muscle activity and bone movement when they do feed by suction in the water. Feeding performance is reduced (with metamorphosed individuals capturing fewer prey; Lauder and Shaffer 1986), suggesting that the morphological

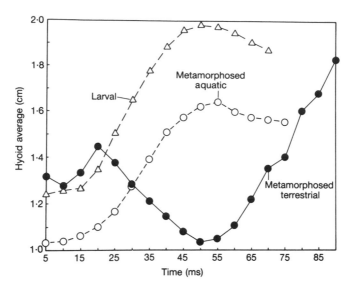

Fig. 3.7. Graph of the average pattern of hyoid depression with respect to time for three individuals feeding as larvae, as metamorphosed animals in the water, and as metamorphosed individuals on land. Each point represents the mean hyoid distance for each time interval measured from high-speed films of feeding (Shaffer and Lauder 1988). Note the close similarity of the larval and metamorphosed aquatic curves (offset vertically owing to morphological changes at metamorphosis) and the radical change in hyoid kinematics during terrestrial feedings: for this variable there is a major effect of the environment on feeding behavior. Modified from Shaffer and Lauder (1988).

changes (especially in the hyobranchial apparatus) have a profound influence on feeding ability. The muscle activity patterns used by larval and metamorphosed ambystomatid salamanders feeding in the water are not significantly different when motor pattern variables are compared using a MANOVA (Lauder and Shaffer 1988).

When metamorphosed animals feed on land, many kinematic and muscle activity patterns change as feeding mode shifts entirely from suction to lingual protrusion (Lauder and Shaffer 1988; Shaffer and Lauder 1988; Reilly and Lauder 1990c). For kinematic data, the variable showing the most pronounced shift is hyoid excursion (fig. 3.7), which changes from continuous abduction during the prey-capture phase of suction feeding in larvae, to protraction followed by retraction associated with tongue protrusion in adults (Shaffer and Lauder 1988). Muscle activity patterns exhibit a more complex pattern of change, with activity on land being longer in duration than in aquatic feedings (see Lauder and Shaffer 1988: epaxial muscles, rectus cervicis, and the adductor mandibulae externus).

The muscle activity patterns of metamorphosed animals feeding in the water and land (fig. 3.3: test 2) do show a significant overall effect of the environmental shift on motor pattern (Lauder and Shaffer 1988), with a significant MANOVA testing the global hypothesis of mean differences in muscle activity ($P = 0.014$) across environments.

These changes in electromyographic pattern are striking for two reasons. First, this pattern provides an example of a change in the motor pattern across environments. Second, the changes in the motor pattern represent a change in the *opposite* direction to that predicted on the basis of the biophysical properties of air and water alone, since muscles are active for a longer period in a less viscous medium (air). The longer durations of muscle activity on land compared to water may function to increase the duration of the gape cycle (allowing time for tongue extension and retraction), but the changes in motor pattern cannot be attributed to differences in resistance of the two media.

Following the initial capture of prey by ambystomatid salamanders, a series of discrete prey transport events occurs in which the prey is moved posteriorly in the mouth toward the esophagus for swallowing (Reilly and Lauder 1990a, 1991). Prey transport involves the use of a complex motor pattern in head muscles and a relatively stereotyped pattern of bone movement. Reilly and Lauder (1991) have hypothesized that the process of terrestrial prey transport in ambystomatid salamanders utilizes a kinematic and electromyographic pattern similar to the processes of aquatic prey capture and transport. In this view, the major behavioral novelty in salamander feeding is the process of terrestrial prey capture by tongue projection, with the other three behaviors (terrestrial prey transport, aquatic prey capture, aquatic prey transport) all being similar despite differences in environment between water and land.

Liem (1980, 1985, 1987), in his work on respiratory ventilation in air-breathing fishes, has conducted a set of interesting investigations on the effect of switching respiratory media on functional patterns in the head. His studies show many parallels with the results from ambystomatid salamanders discussed above. Liem identified triphasic and quadruphasic air ventilation as to the two basic patterns in advanced teleosts. Both patterns involve gulping a bubble of air at the surface and extracting oxygen by passing the air across a highly modified first epibranchial bone (Liem 1985). Using both pressure profiles and electromyographic data, Liem showed that the triphasic mode is very similar to prey capture during aquatic suction feeding; in this case, the "prey" is an air bubble. Similarly, in quadruphasic air ventilation, muscle activity and pressure profiles are identical to those used in coughing, a widespread response to novel aquatic environments in many teleosts. Thus, the "new" function of air ventilation is achieved by using a conservative motor pattern for a new environment, while retaining the original function in the aquatic environment (Liem 1985; Gans 1970).

Concept 4
Unidirectional and bidirectional feeding systems are the two basic skull designs in aquatic vertebrates.

Feeding mechanisms in aquatic vertebrates can be divided into two fundamental hydrodynamic categories: unidirectional and bidirectional flow systems. Unidirectional flow systems are used during feeding by most fishes, larval salamanders, and some tadpoles (Ruibal and Thomas 1988; Wassersug and Hoff 1979). The feeding mechanism is said to be unidirectional because water drawn into the mouth during suction feeding passes through the buccal cavity to exit posteriorly between the gill bars and out the opercular opening. Flow is thus from anterior to posterior and travels in one direction.

In bidirectional flow systems, water drawn into the mouth anteriorly as the gape increases and buccal volume expands is expelled through the mouth as the jaws close. Thus, water both enters and leaves through the mouth, and flow during feeding is bidirectional. Aquatic vertebrates that feed with bidirectional flow systems include turtles, frogs, completely metamorphosed salamanders, and some mammals.

Relative to the considerable body of research on unidirectional flow systems (e.g., Alexander 1969, 1970; Lauder 1980c; Lauder and Clark 1984; Lauder and Shaffer 1985; Liem 1978), there are very few studies of feeding in vertebrates with bidirectional flow. Most of the research on prey capture and skull function in aquatic vertebrates has focused on fishes (e.g., Grobecker and Pietsch 1979; Lauder 1985b; Liem 1970; Osse 1969), and this has to some extent overshadowed the significant differences between these two fundamental suction-feeding systems. Indeed, it is remarkable that more attention has not been devoted to aquatic feeding in turtles and frogs, two groups that exemplify bidirectional feeding systems.

In an effort to investigate the functional significance of the difference between unidirectional and bidirectional feeding systems in vertebrates, Lauder and Shaffer (1986) and Lauder and Reilly (1988) studied the functional morphology of prey capture in salamanders. Salamanders, both by the ontogenetic changes that occur in the feeding mechanism and because of their amenability to experimental manipulation, make an excellent system in which to investigate the functional implications of different feeding designs.

Figure 3.8 illustrates the ontogenetic transformation between larval *Ambystoma tigrinum*, which possess a unidirectional feeding system, and

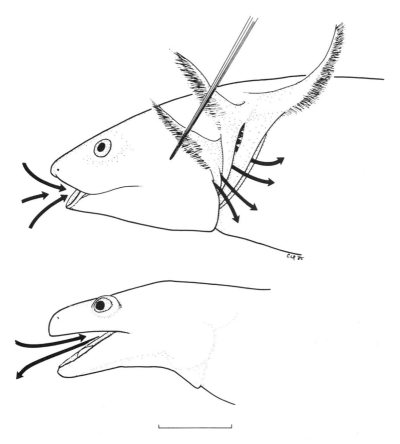

Fig. 3.8. Basic hydrodynamic design of the feeding mechanism in a larval tiger salamander, *Ambystoma tigrinum* (upper panel), and a metamorphosed individual (lower panel). Arrows indicate the direction of water flow in and out of the mouth during feeding. In larvae, gill slits are present and water that enters the mouth during suction feeding is expelled posteriorly out the gill slits. At metamorphosis the gill slits are lost, and adults feeding in the water must expel water anteriorly in a bidirectional flow regime. This transformation from a unidirectional to a bidirectional design of the feeding system during ontogeny has served as an experimental system for investigating the functional significance of the two designs in vertebrates. From Lauder and Shaffer (1986).

the bidirectional system of completely metamorphosed individuals. Larvae possess an extensive branchial apparatus with posterior gill openings (Lauder and Shaffer 1985, 1986) that allow water to exit posteriorly from the buccal cavity. At metamorphosis, the branchial apparatus is greatly reduced (Reilly 1986, 1987), the external gills are lost, and the gill slits close, converting the feeding system to a bidirectional flow regime (Reilly and Lauder 1988b).

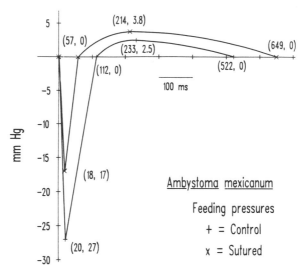

Fig. 3.9. Average pattern of buccal pressure change during feeding in normal axolotls (*Ambystoma mexicanum*) and in individuals which have had the gill slits sutured closed. Buccal pressure (in mm Hg) is given on the y-axis and time on the x-axis; coordinates indicate the time and pressure for various points on the curve. Note that suturing the gill slits reduces the negative buccal pressure and increases the positive portion of the pressure waveform. From Lauder and Reilly (1988).

Lauder and Shafer (1986) measured buccal cavity pressures in larval and metamorphosed *Ambystoma tigrinum* feeding in the water to determine the functional consequences of the ontogenetic shift from unidirectional to bidirectional feeding. They found that metamorphosed individuals generated significantly different buccal pressure curves, and specifically, that the amount of negative pressure produced declined after metamorphosis. This was correlated with a decrease in feeding performance by metamorphosed individuals: larval *Ambystoma tigrinum* were more effective at capturing freely swimming prey than were adults.

Lauder and Reilly (1988) specifically investigated changes in buccal pressure profiles that accompany the experimental transformation from a unidirectional to a bidirectional feeding system in *Ambystoma mexicanum* (with no change in morphology). By suturing the posterior gill openings, they experimentally converted individuals with a unidirectional feeding system into bidirectional feeding systems and compared buccal pressures and feeding performance in control and experimentally sutured individuals. The results of these experiments are summarized in figure 3.9, which shows that suturing the gill slits causes a decrease in negative pressure, and an increase in the positive portion of the pressure waveform. Because water cannot flow posteriorly out of the mouth and is entering at a high velocity due to hyoid expansion, a larger positive pressure is created in bidirectional feeding systems. The reduction in negative pressure magnitude and duration (fig. 3.9) correlates with a dramatic reduction in feeding performance: sutured (bidirectional) individuals captured freely moving prey 5% of the time, while control (unidirectional) individuals captured prey 56% of the time.

The conclusion from these studies is that, all other things being equal, unidirectional feeding systems are more efficient than bidirectional systems, primarily because of the reduction in buccal pressure generated during feeding and the correlated increase in positive (backflow) pressure in bidirectional feeding systems.

Although these results on feeding systems in salamanders provide a basis for an understanding of the functional significance of unidirectional and bidirectional feeding systems, our knowledge of the diversity of such feeding systems among vertebrates is still woefully inadequate. With the exception of the preliminary reports by Bramble (1973), Shafland (1968), and Weisgram (1982), there are no studies of bidirectional aquatic feeding systems in frogs and turtles. Many lineages of fishes and salamanders possess reduced opercular openings that may have the effect of converting a primitively unidirectional feeding system into a bidirectional feeding system. Also, many of the specializations that occur in the feeding systems of turtles, such as the highly distensible esophagus, may function to circumvent the constraints of bidirectional feeding systems. The esophagus could function to store water drawn into the mouth and greatly delay the reversal of flow, thus effectively converting the feeding system into a unidirectional design. The functional consequences of these morphological transformations have yet to be investigated.

EVOLUTIONARY IMPLICATIONS AND PREDICTIONS: A DISCUSSION OF THE FOUR CONCEPTS

The four major concepts that emerge from research on aquatic vertebrate feeding systems invite explanation and analysis in the context of comparative and historical biology. What are the implications, predictions, and avenues for future research that emerge from these concepts?

Discussion of Concept 1
Evolutionary conservation of biomechanical patterns

The demonstration that certain critical biomechanical features of the feeding system in lower vertebrates are highly conserved may not appear especially noteworthy at first. After all, in phylogenetic terms this conclusion amounts merely to documenting gnathostome or osteichthyan characters with little homoplasy. However, we emphasize several important features of concept 1 that point to its wider significance in comparative biology.

First, the number of synapomorphies for the Osteichthyes is not large (Lauder and Liem 1983), and complex morphological features that define major clades are rare and of critical importance in testing hypotheses of monophyly. Second, there are comparatively few biomechanical synapomorphies available for any vertebrate clade, and those provided by the feeding mechanism of lower vertebrates provide some of the best-documented examples to date of the use of biomechanical characters in phylogenetic analysis (also see Emerson 1982; Lauder 1983b; and Liem 1974, 1979 for other examples). Third, while morphological systems are widely used in phylogenetic analysis, only recently have historical patterns of functional transformation been studied in a rigorous manner (see Lauder 1990 for a review). If we are to understand the evolution of form *and* function, then we must attempt to identify functional characters and use them in a phylogenetic context. The research that underlies concept 1 attempts to do just this. Finally, the mere demonstration that certain complex biomechanical features of the vertebrate skull have been retained throughout hundreds of millions of years of divergent evolution in gross morphology is noteworthy. Very few other complex features of skull design have proven to be so invariant, and such highly conservative features point to interesting biological problems of functional constraint and versatility in relation to the evolution of morphological designs.

Why have biomechanical patterns in the skull, such as the relative timing of head movements or muscle activity patterns (table 3.1; fig. 3.1), been retained throughout lower vertebrate evolution? Two possible hypotheses (not necessarily mutually exclusive) might explain this result. First, the constraints of feeding in an aquatic medium that is 900 times as dense and 80 times as viscous as air may severely limit the range of functional solutions to the problem of obtaining prey from the water. If there is only one sequence of movements that will effectively work to extract quickly moving prey from water, then after the origin of such a system, perhaps at the base of the Gnathostomata, it may have been retained throughout all subsequent cladogenetic events. In this view, extrinsic (environmental) constraints on the design of the skull have limited the expression of functional diversity.

The second hypothesis states that conservative morphological substrates constrain function so that head kinematics and muscle activity patterns are preserved. In this view, conservative functional patterns are retained because of their close link to morphological features. These morphological features may themselves be retained as a result of developmental links with other skull features, and not because of any a priori functional requirements. For example, the muscle activity pattern used during feeding might be conserved because of the difficulty of changing the morphological substrate for these functional characters: the complex neural circuitry that drives the jaw muscles. Thus, intrinsic (structural) constraints on the design of the skull may have limited the expression of functional diversity. It is also possible that changes in the central nervous system may occur that are masked by changes in peripheral morphology so that the final behavior stays the same even though changes have occurred at several levels.

It is our view that both hypotheses are needed to fully explain the historical pattern of conservative biomechanical features in the lower vertebrate skull. The results of experiments on unidirectional and bidirectional feeding systems in salamanders (Lauder and Shaffer 1986; Lauder and Reilly 1988) have shown unequivocally that unidirectional feeding systems outperform bidirectional systems (all other things being equal), when both feeding modes exist in closely related taxa sharing the same basic anatomical design. Our interpretation of these results is that certain extrinsic (hydrodynamic) constraints exist on skull design.

On the other hand, there is no a priori reason why the timing of muscle activity and kinematic patterns could not have been modified to a greater extent than has been observed. An example of a cranial muscle activity pattern that has been altered during cladogenesis is provided by Lauder (1983a, c). While this case study demonstrates that motor patterns can be modified, it focused on a chewing behavior that takes place over a relatively long period of time (on the order of seconds to minutes) and presumably involves considerable sensory feedback during execution of the behavior. Neuronal circuitry that drives behaviors of this type may be more malleable over evolutionary time than circuitry that drives initial prey capture (a behavior that occurs in 10 to 150 msec, is noncyclical, and does not involve sensory feedback during its execution). Thus, the hypothesis that functional features of the feeding mechanism have been retained because of intrinsic structural constraints holds that complex, preprogrammed behaviors (and their associated motor and kinematic patterns) are likely to be evolutionarily conservative owing to the difficulties of modifying complex circuitry. This hypothesis has yet to be tested, but is one possible explanation for the conservatism in functional features of the lower vertebrate skull.

The question of conservative motor patterns is important, for it directly addresses the issue of how one explains behavioral and functional transformations in animals. How does behavior evolve: by alterations in central nervous output to the musculature, or by reorganization of peripheral musculoskeletal design so that conservative motor patterns have a different effect (Lauder 1986)? The data obtained so far from quantitative

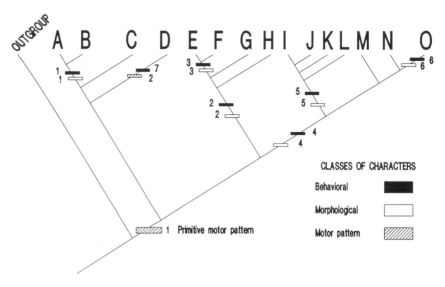

Fig. 3.10. Hypothetical cladogram of species A to O showing the phylogenetic pattern of morphological, motor pattern, and behavioral/performance characters if behavioral evolution is largely a consequence of changes in peripheral morphology and not of alterations in muscle activity patterns. Thus, all species in the clade retain the primitive pattern of muscle activity (hatched bar 1), while some species have acquired behavioral novelties (black bars 1 to 6). Alterations in the topology of the musculoskeletal system have occurred in those species that possess behavioral novelties (open bars 1 to 6). Note that a novel aspect of the motor pattern (hatched bar 2) is present in species D along with a behavioral novelty (black bar 7). It is important that the morphological characters analyzed be related (by a causal biomechanical model and experiments) to the behaviors being mapped onto the cladogram, so that a *causal* link is established between the morphological changes and the behavioral novelties (Lauder, 1991).

analyses of jaw muscle motor patterns indicate that motor patterns may be phylogenetically (historically) conservative and that peripheral musculo-skeletal reorganization is often the basis for differences in feeding behavior.

There are a variety of ways in which one might attempt to explain changes in the behavior and behavioral performance of animals. For example, if two species differ in the pattern of jaw bone movement during feeding, these kinematic differences might be due to distinctions in the pattern of jaw muscle activity between the species. Alternatively, the topology of the musculoskeletal system could differ between the species so that a given muscle, activated by the central nervous system in exactly the same way in both species, has a different effect because of differences in the lever arms of the muscle (Lauder, 1991).

Figure 3.10 shows an example of an expected phylogenetic pattern to the transformation of peripheral morphology, motor patterns, and behavior, if motor patterns are historically conserved during behavioral evolution. Under these conditions, congruence between morphological novelties and behavioral novelties will be high, while novelties in motor patterns should be rare and plesiomorphic to alterations in peripheral morphology and behavior.

The extent to which this view of motor patterns as conservative evolutionary units can be extended to other vertebrates (or to larger clades of more distantly related taxa) is as yet unknown because of the scarcity of quantitative analyses of muscle activity variation. Testing the generality of this hypothesis will be an important avenue for future research in functional and evolutionary morphology.

Discussion of Concept 2
Functional characters vary in their levels of intraspecific and interspecific variation

This result, stemming from population-level analyses of functional characters, is in our opinion one of the most important and potentially general results to emerge from recent functional studies on lower vertebrate feeding. Two findings in particular deserve further mention: the generally high levels of stereotyped behavior in hyoid movement patterns within species of suction-feeding vertebrates, and the high levels of among-individual variation in virtually all other functional characters examined to date.

That the hyoid has repeatedly been identified as the key functional unit in suction feeding (e.g., Lauder 1985c) suggests that this structure and its associated musculature may be under strong selection in nature. Current evidence indicates that movement of the hyoid apparatus determines the velocity of water entering the buccal cavity, and hyoid function is predicted to be related to the size and activity level of prey that may be captured. Unfortunately, there are no studies explicitly linking prey-capture performance to either intra- or interspecific variation in hyoid morphology, and such analyses are critical for future formulations of hypotheses on the reduced intraspecific variation in hyoid function (see Arnold [1983, 1986] for a general discussion of this research program). However, one reasonable interpretation of this pattern postulates strong stabilizing selection on hyoid function, and therefore feeding performance. Such stabilizing selection will tend to reduce both phenotypic and additive genetic variance in hyoid characters (Falconer 1981), leading to the observed pattern of stereotyped responses within species, and relatively great variation among taxa.

If this scenario is correct, then several predictions follow from population genetic and evolutionary theory. First, the heritability (defined as V_A/V_T where V_A is the additive genetic variance, and V_T is the total phenotypic variance; Falconer 1981) of functional characteristics of the hyoid should be less than that of other, less strongly selected characters such as maximum gape, head lift, etc. The extent of this difference in heritabilities will depend on the intensity of selection on these characters and their polygenic mutation rates (Lande 1976; Turelli 1984). However, as long as mutation rates are roughly equivalent in both sets of characters, strong selection should reduce the additive genetic variance. In addition, if morphological variation in hyoid elements is responsible for variation in functional output, one should find reduced morphometric variation, and lower heritability estimates, in these characters as well. This prediction may prove especially useful since studies of morphometric variation are far easier to accomplish than corresponding functional analyses.

A final prediction involves measuring either functional or morphological variability in several characters early and late in ontogeny in a single cohort of animals. If strong stabilizing or directional selection is actively maintaining reduced variation in hyoid or other strongly selected characters, then one should find a reduction in phenotypic variance (and possibly a shift in population mean) as a cohort is exposed to these selection pressures over time (Arnold 1986). This research program is especially important since it involves actively measuring fitness effects on functional characters in a natural situation.

An additional and extremely important consideration is the functional and genetic correlations of different sets of characters. As Lande (1979) and many subsequent authors have emphasized, selection does not operate on single characters, and the correlated responses to selection on one character may effect the mean and variance of others. This may be especially true for functional "complexes" of characters, like those associated with different aspects of the feeding mechanism during underwater prey capture. Although no definitive work on the correlations (genetic or phenotypic) of characters important in underwater suction feeding has been carried out, such correlations have been shown to be important components of variance in other studies. Several studies have demonstrated large phenotypic and genetic correlations between morphological and functional components of locomotion (Garland 1988; Tsuji et al. 1989), although metamorphosis can apparently decouple such correlations, at least in the one amphibian studied so far (Shaffer et al. 1991). In the most complete analysis of a vertebrate known to us, Cheverud (1982) showed that phenotypic correlations among characters within the same "functional set" were large compared to such character correlations between functional sets. Interestingly, this difference in correlation structure was not found at the genetic level, suggesting that the patterns may reflect selection shaping the multivariate character distribution rather than underlying genetic covariances.

Whether or not considerations such as the genetic correlations of characters are important in understanding the patterns of variation and divergence among aquatic vertebrates remains almost completely unknown, as does the fundamental relationship between morphological and functional variation. However, on the basis of a single study, it is known that genetic correlations of morphometric characters in the head can be extremely high in ambystomatid salamanders (Shaffer 1986). Obviously, the generality of this result requires further empirical testing, but it at least raises the possibility that selection on one part of a functional complex may have cascading effects on other aspects of skull morphology (e.g., Emerson 1988).

Discussion of Concept 3
Environmental transitions affect kinematic and EMG patterns, but these changes are not a direct consequence of the biophysics of the media

The limited data available on the biophysical constraints associated with aquatic versus terrestrial feeding provide two primary results. First, while many aspects of motor control (as summarized by electromyograms) and kinematic output are highly conservative, they are not totally fixed. Just as suction-feeding fishes modulate muscle activity patterns with different prey types (Wainwright and Lauder 1986), salamanders modulate certain aspects of the feeding act depending on the environment. Second, this modulation is not explainable simply in terms of the physical properties of water and air as fluids with different densities and viscosities. Given this result, we are then faced with explaining the functional differences across environments that we do find. In particular, why is the duration of feeding longer in air, where resistance to movement is less than in water? Since the opposite trend follows from purely biophysical considerations (and, in a sense, might be considered a null hypothesis), there does seem to be a phenomenon in need of explanation.

Before these trends can be investigated, we need a much larger series of studies describing feeding on land and in the water. Our work on one population of *Ambystoma tigrinum* is the only quantitative assessment of kinematic and electromyographic variation across environments to date; future studies on air-breathing fishes (e.g., Liem 1985, 1987) and turtles (e.g., Bramble and Wake 1985) may reflect similar patterns. The study of other salamander families would greatly add to our understanding of the generality of these patterns, especially in the newts (Salamandridae), where the life history of many species necessitates metamorphosed adults returning to the water for long periods of time (Duellman and Trueb 1986; Reilly 1986). Quantitative assessments of kinematic patterns in the primitive salamander family Hynobiidae would also be of interest in testing the generality of this result across the phylogenetic diversity of urodeles. Additional work on turtles and crocodilians is also crucial, since some species can feed on land and in water (Gans 1969; Bramble and Wake 1985).

These taxa should be particularly useful in testing the tenet of Bramble and Wake (1985, 232) that "the major functional and biomechanical distinctions between aquatic and terrestrial feeding stem mainly from morphological differences reflecting adaptation to the physical properties of the two fluids," since the same morphology is used in both media.

The currently available data suggest at least two hypotheses concerning the impact of different physical environments on feeding mechanics. First, some muscle activity patterns may change as a result of differential recruitment of muscles in water and on land. Most electromyographic analyses consider only relatively crude measures of muscle activity (such as onset, offset, amplitude, and integrated activity), and the quantitative assessment of recruitment or power output of muscles (or parts of muscles) has not been a primary focus of most studies. The results of Lauder and Shaffer (1988), while useful as an indicator of environmental effects on feeding function in one species (*Ambystoma tigrinum*), need to be compared to other quantitative studies of feeding function across environments in other taxa.

Second, primarily terrestrial metamorphosed individuals may simply not perform well in the water, and may in fact be overcompensating for physical differences in the two media by truncating the strike early in the more viscous aquatic environment. If the pattern seen in *A. tigrinum* reflects poorly coordinated feeding activity in the water, then it should not constitute a general trend in other urodele taxa; additional comparative data on species that routinely feed in the water after metamorphosis will help resolve this issue.

Discussion of Concept 4
Unidirectional and bidirectional feeding systems are the two basic skull designs in aquatic vertebrates

The results obtained on the relative efficiency of unidirectional and bidirectional feeding mechanisms in salamanders suggest several hypotheses regarding the evolution of suction feeding in aquatic vertebrates. However, discussion of historical patterns of the transformation of feeding designs must, at this point, be highly speculative, as not even the rudimentary bases for a historical analysis are currently available.

To our knowledge, all secondarily aquatic lower vertebrates possess a bidirectional feeding system. The transformation to terrestrial life involves the loss of branchial arches and associated posterior openings to the gill cavity, and these openings are never regained with the transition back to the aquatic environment. Thus, there has been no ontogenetic or phylogenetic morphological transformation from a bidirectional to a unidirectional feeding design. The sole exception to this pattern appears to be nontransforming salamanders, in which lineages with a derived unidirectional adult form have evolved from bidirectional ancestors. However, the paedomorphic mechanism by which this transformation occurs involves the truncation of development in the normal bidirectional adult, not a transformation from a bidirectional to unidirectional system (Shaffer 1984). The scarcity of bidirectional-to-unidirectional transformations indicates that the loss or severe reduction of the branchial apparatus and the acquisition of a terrestrial respiratory system (Wake 1982) may constrain the nature and extent of morphological reorganization that can occur in the posterior region of the head.

If, as indicated by current data (e.g., Lauder and Reilly 1988; Lauder and Shaffer 1986; Reilly and Lauder 1988b), unidirectional designs are more efficient than bidirectional systems in capturing prey (when the morphology of other head features is held constant), lineages that have reinvaded the aquatic environment either have suffered a competitive disadvantage in feeding or have evolved morphological and functional systems to circumvent the hydrodynamic disadvantages of bidirectional systems. (However, in areas with little competition for food, as in fish-free ponds of the central and western United States where adult *Ambystoma tigrinum* feed routinely [Miller and Larsen 1986; Reese 1969], there may be little selection for an increase in aquatic feeding efficiency.)

The hypothesis that morphological specializations have accumulated in secondarily aquatic lineages to mitigate the deleterious effects of a bidirectional feeding system could be tested with a corroborated phylogenetic hypothesis of a secondarily aquatic lineage with a concomitant functional analysis of the living taxa in the clade. Basal taxa, which generally possess plesiomorphic character states for that clade, would be predicted to possess reduced feeding performance when compared to more derived taxa. These derived taxa would be predicted to have acquired morphological and functional novelties that aid in circumventing the hydrodynamic constraints of bidirectional feeding systems. Examples of such potential novelties include forming a distensible posterior region of the buccal cavity to mitigate the increase in positive pressure, increasing the lever arm of the hyoid apparatus and the cross-sectional area of muscles depressing the hyoid (such as the rectus cervicis), and lengthening the buccal cavity.

Confidence that such observed changes were causally related to changing function of the feeding mechanism would be increased by two observations. The first is the occurrence of multiple lineages, each of which has independently become secondarily aquatic. If each lineage exhibits similar morphological modifications, and those changes are specifically those predicted on the basis of functional analyses of uni- and bidirectional feeding systems (Lauder and Shaffer 1986; Lauder and Reilly 1988), then this convergence suggests a causal link between changes in the morphology and feeding function. The second observation is an experimental test of the significance of the morphological modifications. To demonstrate the causal basis of the phylogenetic correlation between the changes in morphology and feeding system design, experimental modification of derived clades in a secondarily aquatic lineage is needed. Reduced feeding performance is expected when morphological changes that increase the effectiveness of bidirectional feeding systems are eliminated experimentally.

Taken together, these phylogenetic and experimental functional data would make a strong argument for the constraints of the aquatic medium on the design of the vertebrate skull. Turtles would appear to provide the best possibilities for testing this hypothesis, but as yet few data are available.

CONCLUSIONS AND DIRECTIONS FOR FUTURE RESEARCH

Throughout this chapter, we have emphasized certain directions for future research on the functional design of the aquatic vertebrate skull. In this final section, we discuss two new avenues that we feel will be critical in further investigating the evolution of the skull, and in linking morphological and functional studies with current theoretical work in evolutionary biology.

First, what are the links, both phenotypically and genetically, between form and function? There are three prerequisites for evolution by natural selection: there must be phenotypic variation in natural populations, it must be heritable, and variants must confer differential fitness. We have stressed the individual variation component of much of our functional work; it appears to be generally true that there is considerable variation among individuals in functional attributes. However, the extent to which this variation is based on additive genetic variation that can respond to selection, as opposed to learning or other environmentally induced variation, is completely unknown. In addition, the relationship between fine-scale morphometric variation, which often has a heritable basis, and functional output remains unknown. This is true both at the phenotypic and genetic levels; yet, understanding these relationships is crucial for modeling the evolution of functional characters.

To forge the links between functional, morphological, and population genetic levels of analysis requires a research strategy that is different from those generally employed by morphologists. Within-population sample sizes must be large if correlations between morphometric variation and functional output at the individual level are to be determined (Jayne and Bennett 1990; Shaffer et al. 1991). Furthermore, for an understanding of the genetic basis of the relationship between morphological variation and functional response, animals from a known pedigree must be available. While these are large orders, they are feasible for a wide range of aquatic vertebrates. Fishes and aquatic salamanders in particular have had sufficient descriptive work done to document the accessibility of phenotypic variation at the individual level; the next phase requires the integration of these results with phenotypic and genetic analyses of population variation in morphology.

Second, the concept of constraints has been much discussed in the recent literature in evolutionary biology (e.g., Raup and Jablonski 1986; Maynard Smith et al. 1985). However, there are very few examples of precisely identified constraints on any morphological feature for which it is possible to say unequivocally why (in the causal sense) the proposed constraint has limited pathways of historical differentiation. The aquatic vertebrate skull provides an ideal system to study such constraints, several of which have been proposed in this chapter. Some strengths of the lower vertebrate skull as a model system are that: (1) a solid phylogenetic foundation exists for formulating and testing historical arguments, (2) the biomechanics of skull function is now reasonably well established, and (3) the discipline of biomechanics provides (through its use of physical laws and mechanical models) a method of precisely quantifying and defining performance curves. The aquatic vertebrate skull may be the first system in which the concept of a functional and historical constraint can be quantified and its effect on performance clearly documented.

These two avenues are by no means an exhaustive survey of future directions in the study of functional design of aquatic vertebrate skulls. However, they represent new paths targeted at integrating functional and comparative morphology into the mainstream of evolutionary biology. We feel that this integration is one of the key directions for future research, and we emphasize the importance of moving functional studies toward their proper place as a central discipline in evolutionary biology.

ACKNOWLEDGMENTS

We thank Steve Reilly, Peter Wainwright, Chris Sanford, Jim Clark, and the editors for many helpful comments on the manuscript. Figures 3.4 and 3.5 were drawn by Clara Richardson. This research was supported by National Science Foundation grants BSR 85-20305 and DCB 87-21010 to GVL, and grants BSR 85-19211 and 90–18686 to HBS.

BIBLIOGRAPHY

Alexander, R. McN. 1967. *Functional design in fishes*. London: Hutchinson.
———. 1969. Mechanics of the feeding action of a cyprinid fish. Journal of Zoology, London 159: 1–15.
———. 1970. Mechanics of the feeding action of various teleost fishes. Journal of Zoology, London 162: 145–156.

Arnold, S. J. 1983. Morphology, performance, and fitness. American Zoologist 23: 347–361.

———. 1986. Laboratory and field approaches to the study of adaptation. In *Predator-Prey Relationships: Perspectives and Approaches from the Study of Lower Vertebrates*, M. E. Feder and G. V. Lauder, eds. Chicago: University of Chicago Press, pp. 157–179.

Bemis, W. E. 1987. Feeding systems of living Dipnoi: Anatomy and function. Journal of Morphology suppl. 1: 249–275.

Bemis, W. E., and G. V. Lauder. 1986. Morphology and function of the feeding apparatus of the lungfish, *Lepidosiren paradoxa*. Journal of Morphology 187: 81–108.

Bemis, W. E., K. Schwenk, and M. H. Wake. 1983. Morphology and function of the feeding apparatus in *Dermophis mexicanus* (Amphibia: Gymnophiona). Zoological Journal of the Linnean Society 77: 75–96.

Bock, W. J. 1964. Kinetics of the avian skull. Journal of Morphology 114: 1–42.

Bramble, D. M. 1973. Media dependent feeding in turtles. American Zoologist 13: 1342.

Bramble, D. M., and D. B. Wake. 1985. Feeding mechanisms of lower tetrapods. In *Functional Vertebrate Morphology*, M. Hildebrand, D. M. Bramble, K. F. Liem, and D. B. Wake, eds. Cambridge: Harvard University Press, pp. 230–261.

Cheverud, J. M. 1982. Phenotypic, genetic, and environmental morphological integration in the cranium. Evolution 36: 499–516.

Crompton, A. W., A. J. Thexton, P. Parker, and K. Hiiemae. 1977. The activity of the jaw and hyoid musculature in the Virginia opossum, *Didelphis virginiana*. In *The Biology of Marsupials*, B. Stonehouse and G. Gilmore, eds. New York: MacMillan, pp. 287–305.

Cundall, D., J. Lorenz-Elwood, and J. D. Grooves. 1987. Asymmetric suction feeding in primitive salamanders. Experientia 43: 1229–1231.

Druner, L. 1904. Studien zur Anatomie der Zungenbein, Kiemenbogen—und Kehlkopfmusculatur der Urodelen, II. Thiel zoologische anatomie 19: 361–690.

Duellman, W. E., and L. Trueb. 1986. *Biology of Amphibians*. New York: McGraw Hill.

Emerson, S. 1982. Frog postcranial morphology: Identification of a functional complex. Copeia: 603–613.

———. 1988. Testing for historical patterns of change: A case study with frog pectoral girdles. Paleobiology 14: 174–186.

Erdman, S., and D. Cundall. 1984. The feeding apparatus of the salamander *Amphiuma tridactylum:* Morphology and behavior. Journal of Morphology 181: 175–204.

Falconer, D. S. 1981. *Introduction to Quantitative Genetics*. London: Longman.

Findeis, E. K., and W. E. Bemis. 1990. Functional morphology of tongue projection in *Taricha torosa* (Urodela: Salamandridae). Zoological Journal of the Linnean Society of London 99: 129–157.

Frazzetta, T. H., and C. D. Prange. 1987. Movements of cephalic components during feeding in some requium sharks (Carcharhiniformes: Carcharhinidae). Copeia: 979–993.

Gans, C. 1969. Comments on inertial feeding. Copeia: 855–857.

———. 1970. Strategy and sequence in the evolution of the external gas exchangers of ectothermal vertebrates. Forma et Functio 3: 61–104.

Gans, C., F. DeVree, and G. C. Gorniak. 1978. Analysis of mammalian masticatory mechanisms: Progress and problems. Zentralblatt für veterinaermedizin, Reihe C, Anatomia, Histologia, Embryologia 7: 226–244.

Gans, C., and G. C. Gorniak. 1982. Functional morphology of lingual protrusion in marine toads (*Bufo marinus*). American Journal of Anatomy 163: 195–222.

Garland, T. 1988. Genetic basis of activity metabolism. I. Inheritance of speed, stamina, and antipredator displays in the garter snake *Thamnophis sirtalis*. Evolution 42: 335–350.

Grobecker, D. B., and T. W. Pietsch. 1979. High-speed cinematographic evidence for ultrafast feeding in antennariid anglerfish. Science 205: 1161–1162.

Hanken, J., and B. K. Hall. 1993. *The Vertebrate Skull*, vols. 1–3. Chicago: University of Chicago Press.

Hildebrand, M., D. M. Bramble, K. F. Liem, and D. B. Wake, eds. 1985. *Functional Vertebrate Morphology*. Cambridge: Harvard University Press.

Jayne, B. C., and A. F. Bennett. 1990. Scaling of speed and endurance in garter snakes: A comparison of cross-sectional and longitudinal allometries. Journal of Zoology, London 220: 257–277.

Jenkin, P. M. 1957. The filter-feeding and food of flamingoes (Phaenicopteri). Philosophical Transactions of the Royal Society of London B 240: 401–493.

Kluge, A. 1977. *Chordate structure and function*. New York: Macmillan.

Lambertsen, R. H. 1983. Internal mechanism of rorqual feeding. Journal of Mammalogy 64: 76–88.

Lande, R. 1976. The maintenance of genetic variability by mutation in a polygenic character with linked loci. Genetics Research, Cambridge 26: 221–235.

———. 1979. Quantitative genetic analysis of multivariate evolution, applied to brain: body size allometry. Evolution 33: 402–416.

Larsen, J. H., and D. J. Guthrie. 1975. The feeding system of terrestrial tiger salamanders (*Ambystoma tigrinum melanostictum* Baird). Journal of Morphology 147: 137–154.

Lauder, G. V. 1979. Feeding mechanisms in primitive teleosts and in the halecomorph fish *Amia calva*. Journal of Zoology, London 187: 543–578.

———. 1980a. Evolution of the feeding mechanism in primitive actinopterygian fishes: A functional anatomical analysis of *Polypterus, Lepisosteus*, and *Amia*. Journal of Morphology 163: 283–317.

———. 1980b. The role of the hyoid apparatus in the feeding mechanism of the living coelacanth, *Latimeria chalumnae*. Copeia: 1–9.

———. 1980c. The suction feeding mechanism in sunfishes (*Lepomis*): An experimental analysis. Journal of Experimental Biology 88: 49–72.

———. 1982. Patterns of evolution in the feeding mechanism of actinopterygian fishes. American Zoologist 22: 275–285.

———. 1983a. Functional and morphological bases of trophic specialization in sunfishes (Teleostei: Centrarchidae). Journal of Morphology 178: 1–21.

———. 1983b. Functional design and evolution of the pharyngeal jaw apparatus in euteleostean fishes. Zoological Journal of the Linnean Society 77: 1–38.

———. 1983c. Neuromuscular patterns and the origin of trophic specialization in fishes. Science 219: 1235–1237.

———. 1985a. Aquatic feeding in lower vertebrates. In *Functional Vertebrate Morphology*, M. Hildebrand, D. Bramble, K. F. Liem, and D. B. Wake, eds. Cambridge: Harvard University Press, pp. 210–229.

———. 1985b. Functional morphology of the feeding mechanism in lower vertebrates. In *Functional Morphology of Vertebrates*, H.-R. Duncker and G. Fleischer, eds. New York: Springer Verlag, pp. 179–188.

———. 1986. Homology, analogy, and the evolution of behavior. In *The Evolution of Behavior*, M. Nitecki and J. Kitchell, eds. London: Oxford University Press, pp. 9–40.

———. 1990. Functional morphology and systematics: Studying functional patterns in an historical context. Annual Review of Ecology and Systematics 21: 317–340.

———. 1991. Biomechanics and evolution. In *Biomechanics in Evolution*. J. M. V. Rayner, ed. Cambridge: Cambridge University Press, pp. 1–19.

Lauder, G. V., and B. Clark. 1984. Water flow patterns during prey capture by teleost fishes. Journal of Experimental Biology 113: 143–150.

Lauder, G. V., and K. F. Liem. 1983. The evolution and interrelationships of the actinopterygian fishes. Bulletin of the Museum of Comparative Zoology, Harvard 150: 95–197.

Lauder, G. V., and S. M. Reilly. 1988. Functional design of the feeding mechanism in salamanders: Causal bases of ontogenetic changes in function. Journal of Experimental Bilogy 134: 219–233.

———. 1990. Metamorphosis of the feeding mechanism in tiger salamanders: The ontogeny of cranial muscle mass. Journal of Zoology, London 222: 59–74.

Lauder, G. V., and H. B. Shaffer. 1985. Functional morphology of the feeding mechanism in aquatic ambystomatid salamanders. Journal of Morphology 185: 297–326.

———. 1986. Functional design of the feeding mechanism in lower vertebrates: Unidirectional and bidirectional flow systems in the tiger salamander. Zoological Journal of the Linnean Society 88: 277–290.

———. 1988. The ontogeny of functional design in the tiger salamander (*Ambystoma tigrinum*): Are motor patterns conserved during major morphological transformations? Journal of Morphology 197: 249–268.

Liem, K. F. 1970. Comparative functional anatomy of the Nandidae (Pisces, Teleostei). Fieldiana: Zoology 56: 1–166.

———. 1974. Evolutionary strategies and morphological innovations: Cichlid pharyngeal jaws. Systematic Zoology 22: 424–441.

———. 1978. Modulatory multiplicity in the functional repertoire of the feeding mechanism in cichlid fishes. I. Piscivores. Journal of Morphology 158: 323–360.

———. 1979. Modulatory multiplicity in the feeding mechanism in cichlid fishes, as exemplified by the invertebrate pickers of Lake Tanganyika. Journal of Zoology, London 189: 93–125.

————. 1980. Adaptive significance of intra- and interspecific differences in the feeding repertoires of cichlid fishes. American Zoologist 20: 295–314.

————. 1985. Ventilation. In *Functional Vertebrate Morphology*, M. Hildebrand, D. Bramble, K. F. Liem, and D. B. Wake, eds., Cambridge: Harvard University Press, pp. 185–209.

————. 1987. Functional design of the air ventilation apparatus and overland excursions by teleosts. Fieldiana: Zoology, n.s. 37.

Lombard, R. E., and D. B. Wake. 1977. Tongue evolution in the lungless salamanders, family Plethodontidae. II. Function and evolutionary diversity. Journal of Morphology 153: 39–80.

————. 1986. Tongue evolution in the lungless salamanders, family Plethodontidae. IV. Phylogeny of plethodontid salamanders and the evolution of feeding dynamics. Systematic Zoology 35: 532–551.

Maynard Smith, J., R. Burian, S. Kauffman, P. Alberch, J. Campbell, B. Goodwin, R. Lande, D. Raup, and L. Wolpert. 1985. Developmental constraints and evolution. Quarterly Review of Biology 60: 265–287.

Miller, B. T., and J. H. Larsen. 1986. Feeding habits of metamorphosed *Ambystoma tigrinum melanostictum* in ponds of high pH (> 9). Great Basin Naturalist 46: 299–301.

Moss, S. A. 1972. The feeding mechanism of sharks of the family Carcharhinidae. Journal of Zoology, London 167: 423–436.

————. 1977. Feeding mechanisms in sharks. American Zoologist 17: 355–364.

Osse, J. 1969. Functional morphology of the head of the perch (*Perca fluviatilis* L.): An electromyographic study. Netherlands Journal of Zoology 19: 289–392.

Ozeti, N., and D. B. Wake. 1969. The morphology and evolution of the tongue and associated structures in salamanders and newts (family Salamandridae). Copeia: 91–123.

Pivorunas, A. 1979. The feeding mechanisms of baleen whales. American Scientist 67: 432–440.

Raup, D., and D. Jablonski. 1986. *Patterns and Processes in the History of Life.* Berlin: Springer-Verlag.

Reese, R. W. 1969. *The Taxonomy and Ecology of the Tiger Salamander (Ambystoma tigrinum) of Colorado.* Ph.D. diss., University of Colorado.

Reilly, S. M. 1986. Ontogeny of cranial ossification in the eastern newt, *Notophthalmus viridescens*, and its relationship to metamorphosis and neoteny. Journal of Morphology 188: 315–326.

————. 1987. Ontogeny of the hyobranchial apparatus in the salamanders *Ambystoma talpoideum* (Ambystomatidae) and *Notophthalmus viridescens* (Salamandridae): The ecological morphology of two neotenic strategies. Journal of Morphology 191: 205–214.

Reilly, S. M., and G. V. Lauder. 1988a. Atavisms and the homology of hyobranchial elements in lower vertebrates. Journal of Morphology 195: 237–245.

————. 1988b. Ontogeny of aquatic feeding performance in the eastern newt, *Notophthalmus viridescens* (Salamandridae). Copeia: 87–91.

————. 1989. Kinetics of tongue projection in *Ambystoma tigrinum:* Quantitative kinematics, muscle function, and evolutionary hypotheses. Journal of Morphology 199: 223–243.

———. 1990a. The evolution of tetrapod feeding behavior: Kinematic homologies in prey transport. Evolution 44: 1542–1557.

———. 1990b. Metamorphosis of cranial design in tiger salamanders (*Ambystoma tigrinum*): A morphometric analysis of ontogenetic change. Journal of Morphology 204: 121–137.

———. 1990c. The strike of the tiger salamander: Quantitative electromyography and muscle function during prey capture. Journal of Comparative Physiology A 167: 827–839.

———. 1991. Prey transport in the tiger salamander: Quantitative electromyography and muscle function in tetrapods. Journal of Experimental Zoology. 200: 1–17.

Ruibal, R., and E. Thomas. 1988. The obligate carnivorous larvae of the frog, *Lepidobatrachus laevis* (Leptodactylidae). *Copeia:* 591–604.

Sanderson, S. L. 1988. Variation in neuromuscular activity during prey capture by trophic specialists and generalists (Pisces: Labridae). Brain Behavior and Evolution 32: 257–268.

Schaefer, S. A., and G. V. Lauder. 1986. Historical transformation of functional design: Evolutionary morphology of the feeding mechanism in loricarioid catfishes. Systematic Zoology 35: 489–508.

Shaffer, H. B. 1984. Evolution in a paedomorphic lineage. II. Allometry and form in the Mexican ambystomatid salamanders. Evolution 38: 1207–1218.

———. 1986. The utility of quantitative genetic parameter estimates in character weighting. Systematic Zoology 35: 124–134.

Shaffer, H. B., C. C. Austin, and R. B. Huey. 1991. The consequences of metamorphosis on salamander (*Ambystoma*) locomotor performance. Physiological Zoology 64: 212–231.

Shaffer, H. B., and G. V. Lauder. 1985a. Aquatic prey capture in ambystomatid salamanders: Patterns of variation in muscle activity. Journal of Morphology 183: 273–284.

———. 1985b. Patterns of variation in aquatic ambystomatid salamanders: Kinematics of the feeding mechanism. Evolution 39: 83–92.

———. 1988. The ontogeny of functional design: Metamorphosis of feeding behavior in the tiger salamander (*Ambystoma tigrinum*). Journal of Zoology, London 216: 437–454.

Shafland, J. L. 1968. *Functional and Anatomical Convergence in Body Form and Feeding Behavior in Three Diverse Species of Freshwater Bottom Dwelling Vertebrates*. Ph.D. diss. University of Chicago.

Smith, K. K., and W. L. Hylander. 1985. Strain gauge measurement of mesokinetic movement in the lizard *Varanus exanthematicus*. Journal of Experimental Biology 114: 53–70.

Tsuji, J. S., and R. B. Huey, F. H. van Berkum, T. Garland, and R. G. Shaw. 1989. Locomotor performance of hatchling fence lizards (*Sceloporus occidentalis*): Quantitative genetics and morphometric correlates. Functional Ecology 3: 240–252.

Turelli, M. 1984. Heritable genetic variation via mutation-selection balance: Lerch's Zeta meets the abdominal bristle. Theoretical Population Biology 25: 138–193.

Wainwright, P. 1986. Motor correlates of learning behavior: Feeding on novel prey by pumpkinseed sunfish (*Lepomis gibbosus*). Journal of Experimental Biology 126: 237–247.

———. 1989. Prey processing in haemulid fishes: Patterns of variation in pharyngeal jaw muscle activity. Journal of Experimental Biology 141: 359–375.

Wainwright, P., and G. V. Lauder. 1986. Feeding biology of sunfishes: Patterns of variation in prey capture. Zoological Journal of the Linnean Society 88: 217–228.

Wake, D. B. 1982. Functional and developmental constraints and opportunities in the evolution of feeding systems in urodeles. In *Environmental Adaptation and Evolution*, D. Mossakowski and G. Roth, eds. New York: G. Fischer, pp. 51–66.

Wassersug, R., and K. Hoff. 1979. A comparative study of the buccal pumping mechanism of tadpoles. Biological Journal of the Linnean Society of London 12: 225–259.

Weijs, W. A., and R. Dantuma. 1981. Functional anatomy of the masticatory apparatus in the rabbit (*Oryctolagus cuniculus* L.). Netherlands Journal of Zoology 31: 99–147.

Weisgram, J. 1982. *Claudius angustatus* (Kinosternidae)—Nahrungsaufnahme. Wiss Film 28: 28–35.

Yamasaki, F. 1956. Uber die Entwicklung der Zunge von *Hynobius retardatus* Dunn. Sapporo Medical Journal 10: 1–34.

Zweers, G. A. 1974. Structure, movement, and myography of the feeding apparatus of the mallard (*Anas platyrhynchos* L.): A study in functional anatomy. Netherlands Journal of Zoology 24: 323–467.

4

The Form of the Feeding Apparatus in Terrestrial Vertebrates: Studies of Adaptation and Constraint

KATHLEEN K. SMITH

INTRODUCTION

THE SKULL OF TERRESTRIAL VERTEBRATES exhibits tremendous diversity in form and function. Some of this diversity reflects the multiple roles played by the skull: feeding, housing of sense organs, protecting the central nervous system and, in some cases, functioning in locomotion or social displays. Much of the diversity reflects features related to feeding. As a feeding organ the skull is important in obtaining, processing, and ingesting food. It is therefore subject to a number of specific mechanical requirements, and all vertebrates exhibit some adaptations to meet the requirements of feeding. On the other hand, the skull exhibits a common basic pattern across all terrestrial vertebrates. The tetrapod skull in early development is remarkably similar, and the same major bone, muscle, and nerve groups are present in all groups. This similarity is often attributed to common developmental patterns. Further, recognizable patterns characterize each major vertebrate taxon. These patterns are often attributed to phylogenetic constraints. What are the relative roles of adaptive modification and phylogenetic or developmental heritage in patterning cranial form in terrestrial vertebrates?

This question, the relative roles of adaptation and constraint in determining form, is a central question in evolutionary morphology. In recent decades, the assumption that an animal's form reflects adaptation to specific requirements of its way of life has dominated functional morphological studies. Approaches and assumptions about adaptation have varied among vertebrate morphologists. Most commonly, form and function relations are identified and hypotheses are constructed about the adaptive basis of those relations. These hypotheses are then tested by comparative studies. At its best, such a comparative approach includes: (1) a morphological and behavioral analysis, including significant information on how the structure functions and what role the structure plays in the animal's natural environment, (2) an analysis of the phylogenetic context of the morphology, (3) a presentation of a specific model of function, (4) the construction of hypotheses about the relation between function and performance, (5) predictions about morphological diversity based on the functional model and known behavioral differences between animals, and (6) testing of predictions with comparative data.

If the comparative data contradict the explanatory hypotheses, then an argument of adaptation is insufficient to explain the observed pattern of diversity. If the same form/function relation evolves repeatedly and convergently, it is parsimonious to assume that the morphology is to some extent due to the processes of natural selection. It is particularly significant if it can be shown that there is design or functional convergence irrespective of whether the specific morphological features are homologous. Components of this methodology may be found explicitly or implicitly in many studies (e.g., Arnold 1983; Clutton-Brock and Harvey 1979; Dullemeijer 1968, 1974; Dullemeijer and Barel 1976; Gans 1968, 1974, 1988; Greene 1983, 1986; Hylander 1979; Kay 1984; Kay and Cartmill 1977; Liem 1978; Lombard and Wake 1976, 1977; Savitsky 1980, 1983; Smith 1984, 1986).

In the past decade focus has been on constraint as an alternative explanation of form. A number of specific sources of constraint have been suggested (e.g., Alberch 1980; Gould 1980; Gould and Lewontin 1979; Maynard Smith et al. 1985 and references therein). Physical processes and mechanical properties are thought to restrict diversity or make some kinds of form impossible and impose *physical constraints* (see, e.g., Alexander 1985). Compromise between competing demands of multiple function has been suggested as a source of *selective* or *compromise constraints* because an individual is not "decomposable into independent and separately optimized parts" (Gould and Lewontin 1979, 591). *Phylogenetic constraints* arise because evolutionary change in a particular lineage is possible only within the functional and genetic context of the ancestors of the lineage. A particular "choice" made by an ancestor may make the appearance of some forms more likely than others in the descendants (see, e.g., Mayr 1983). Finally, *developmental constraints* may produce a bias in variation from several sources, including basic mechanisms of morphogenesis or epigenetic interactions that restrict the independent differentiation and development of certain systems (see, e.g., Alberch 1980; Maynard Smith et al. 1985).

It is increasingly recognized that adaptation and constraint are not alternative explanations but instead are, to a large extent, alternative questions. An emphasis on constraint focuses attention on the limits to diversity, the unity of animals, and the emptiness of large portions of potential "morphospace" (e.g., Alberch 1980; Gould 1980; Maynard Smith et al. 1985). An emphasis on adaptation focuses attention on the existing diversity of form and the reasons for the observed diversity. Both approaches are necessary to explain the determinants of form. In this chapter I will review studies of the diversity of skull form which contain hypotheses for both the generation of and limits on diversity. Thus, I seek to present studies that recognize both adaptation and constraint.

In this chapter I will not attempt to mold the feeding system of terrestrial vertebrates into a single model, as in the course of such modeling, an understanding of the diversity or specialization within each group is lost. Such discussions by necessity must take either a generalized or hypothetical representative. The focus here is on the analysis of existing diversity and will proceed into two steps. First, I will discuss the major specializations within four groups of terrestrial amniotes—lizards, snakes, birds, and mammals—with three major goals: (1) to provide information on the basic form and function of the skull in feeding in these groups, (2) to discuss the pattern of diversification of the feeding apparatus within each group, and (3) to provide an introduction to the methods that various workers have used to study form and function as illustrated by case studies. Second I will compare the patterns of diversification within each of the four groups. The focus of the chapter is on patterns of diversification rather than on functional or morphological studies of individual species, because ultimately questions on adaptation or constraint are questions of diversity. This chapter is not a comparative review of feeding behavior, but of the relation between skull, tooth, and masticatory muscle morphology and feeding activities. There is little discussion of the tongue, hyoid, and pharynx, although these latter morphological features are of central significance in the trophic adaptations of terrestrial vertebrates (see Smith 1984; Smith 1992). Finally, this is not a review of morphological detail, as such presentations are in earlier volumes of this series (Novacek 1993; Rieppel 1993; Zusi 1993).

STUDIES OF VERTEBRATE SKULLS

The Skull in Lizards

The skull of lizards is often taken as a primitive model for amniotes. A number of features, such as a partially ossified neurocranium (occipital segment) that is connected to the ossified dermal skeleton via relatively mobile junctions, and the existence of a number of independent segments separated by joints or zones of mobility (fig. 4.1), characterize the skull in lizards. The separation of the neurocranium and dermal skeleton and some sort of intracranial mobility is primitive in therapsids, archosaurs, and lepidosaurs (Romer 1956). The existence of mobile joints within the skull is termed cranial kinesis, and speculations on the functional significance of

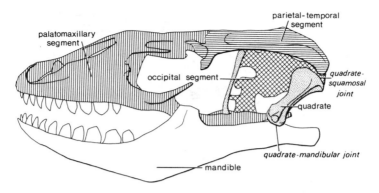

Fig. 4.1. The lizard skull (*Varanus exanthematicus*), with the major segments of the skull labeled. The mesokinetic joint is the junction between the palatomaxillary and parietal-temporal segments. Streptostyly involves movement of the quadrate relative to the rest of the skull, and metakinesis involves movement of the occipital relative to the rest of the cranium. Reprinted with permission from Smith (1982).

the kinetic apparatus in vertebrates have spanned a century and a half (see Frazzetta [1962] and Smith [1982] for early references). The focus of previous functional studies on the cranium of lizards has been largely on the function of the kinetic apparatus, with some attention paid to the jaws and teeth. These studies will be briefly summarized below.

Cranial Kinesis in Lizards. The most commonly cited model for the function of the lizard kinetic apparatus is that of Frazzetta (1962), although elements of this model go back to the work of Versluys (1910, 1912). Frazzetta proposes that the kinetic apparatus in lizards operates as a four-bar crank so that movements of all elements operate in unison (Fig. 4.2). Three distinct types of kinesis are proposed for lizards: metakinesis, or movement of the occipital segment relative to the dermal skeleton; meso-kinesis, or movement of the palato-maxillary segment relative to other segments; and streptostyly, movement of the quadrate relative to the rest of the skull. Frazzetta suggests that during jaw opening, significant and regular lifting or protraction of the snout occurs at the mesokinetic joint. The snout is lowered or retracted during jaw closing.

In the years since Frazzetta's paper was published, numerous other studies of kinesis have appeared. These papers take a number of approaches, including (1) examinations of fossil lepidosaurs and the evolution of the kinetic apparatus (Carroll 1976; Frazzetta 1986; Robinson 1967, 1973), (2) mechanical and functional analyses of lizard skulls and jaw muscles (Alexander and Sinclair 1987; Dalrymple 1979; Frazzetta 1983; Gomes and Gasc 1973; Hofer 1960; Iordansky 1966, 1970; Rieppel 1978 a, b; Rieppel and Labhardt 1979; Smith 1980a, b), or (3) use of an

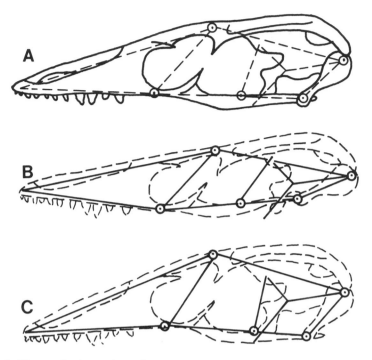

Fig. 4.2. The quadratic crank mechanism in *Varanus* as modeled by Frazzetta. A. Resting state. B. Snout protracted. C. Snout retracted. Redrawn from Frazzetta (1962).

experimental technique to attempt to measure directly movements or activity of jaw muscles (Condon 1987; Gans and De Vree 1987; Gans et al. 1985; Impey 1967; Smith 1982; Smith and Hylander 1985; Throckmorton 1976; Throckmorton and Clarke 1981).

No general consensus concerning lizard cranial kinesis has emerged. For example, a number of authors have expressed doubts that the above model of kinesis applies to all lizards (e.g., Bradley 1903; Dalrymple 1979; Gans 1961; Gans and De Vree 1987; Haas 1973; Hofer 1960; Smith 1982; Smith and Hylander 1985; Throckmorton and Clarke 1981). There are contrary results on direct measurements of the timing and extent of movement, even within the same species. Most studies have focused on *Varanus* (Boltt and Ewer 1964; Condon 1987; Impey 1967; Rieppel 1979; Smith 1982; Smith and Hylander 1985), although Frazzetta's original cinematographic work is on *Gerrhonotus* (1962, 1983). Smith (1980a) examines *Ctenosaura, Tupinambis,* and *Uromastyx* and observes no movement except movements of the quadrate (streptostyly). Throckmorton (1976; Throckmorton and Clarke 1981) focuses on *Iguana, Uromastyx,* and *Am-*

phibolurus; his results do not confirm the quadratic crank model. Gans and De Vree (1987) observe limited kinetic movement in *Trachydosaurus.*

Adaptive Significance of Cranial Kinesis. A number of hypotheses for the adaptive significance of cranial kinesis in lizards have been proposed. Frazzetta (1962, 1983) proposes that "kinesis could be explained by its provision in allowing the upper jaws to close downward as the mandibles move upward, to insure nearly simultaneous contact with the prey. This would avoid premature collision by the lower jaw alone, before the prey was secured and prevent the quarry from being deflected out of seizing range by the very apparatus designed to capture it" (1983, 228). Other hypotheses for the adaptive significance of cranial kinesis in lizards are summarized by Frazzetta (1962) and for the most part rejected. Iordansky (1966) proposes that retraction of the upper jaw allows the net direction of bite forces to be directed posteriorly rather than anteriorly during hard biting. Boltt and Ewer (1964) and Rieppel (1979) hypothesize that the functional significance of kinesis is that it allows the release of recurved teeth from prey. Rieppel argues that varanid lizards are adapted to feed on large prey and that in handling large prey a recurved tooth is advantageous. Mesokinesis allows the tip of a recurved tooth to engage the prey at the most efficient angle.

There are two fundamental problems with the above hypotheses on the adaptive significance of cranial kinesis in lizards. The first is that without a consensus on the mechanics and mechanical significance of the cranial apparatus, it is difficult to form convincing hypotheses on its adaptive significance. The second is that there are few broad-based comparative analyses of lizard cranial form. The hypotheses therefore do not address the diversity of the cranial apparatus and have not tested hypotheses comparatively. For example, Rieppel's analysis applies to only a few species of lizards. Comparative tests are likely to be fruitful because there is variation in the kinetic apparatus. Gekkonids, for example, have very loosely constructed skulls. Articulations between intracranial segments are notably weak, and deformations may be easily produced by manipulations of wet specimens. Retraction of the snout during biting is easily observed. On the other hand, in many agamids, iguanids, and macroteiids the connections within the palate are firm, as is the connection in the postorbital or supratemporal region. Mesokinesis is unlikely in these species. Streptostyly is exceedingly well developed in the Agamidae (Throckmorton 1976; Throckmorton and Clark 1981). Adaptive hypotheses could be tested by a comparison of intracranial mobility and diet in relation to independently corroborated phylogenies. Thus far, this has been done in only a few studies and on a small scale taxonomically (e.g., Dalrymple 1979; Patchell and Shine 1986a). There have been no broad-based, rigorous studies that compare the distribution of features of the kinetic apparatus with phylogeny, behavior, size, or diet. Thus, what has been perceived as the central feature of the lizard feeding apparatus, the kinetic mechanism, remains incompletely examined.

Diet and Dentition. A number of papers have attempted to relate lizard dental morphology and diet. Hotton (1955) examines the relation of dentition to diet in North American iguanids. He particularly aims for comparisons where dietary differences, with their associated dental differences, occur within taxonomic boundaries or where dietary and dental similarities transgress taxonomic boundaries.

Hotton defines five dental types that largely relate to obtaining rather than to processing food. For example, the bladelike teeth of herbivores slice leaves from the plants; leaves are not masticated. Most iguanids are insectivorous. Hotton specifies a number of subcategories of insectivory that include degree of prey activity and weight of integument. He predicts that these functionally significant subcategories might be expected to sort different dental types. In many cases species possess similar dentitions, but are also closely related, and as Hotton points out, it is difficult to distinguish between phylogenetic and adaptive patterns. Some cases, however, cross taxonomic boundaries. *Callisaurus* and *Urosaurus* are not closely related, but both possess slender, cylindrical, sharp teeth. Their diets are likewise similar and distinct, consisting of the highest proportion of bees and wasps among the species examined. *Callisaurus* and *Urosaurus* are much more like each other than either is to its nearest relative. Hotton calls this a "striking convergence" and evidence for adaptation.

Molariform teeth provide the best examples of broad cross-taxonomic dental convergence in lizards (Cowles 1930; Dalrymple 1979; Krebs 1979; Lonnberg 1903; MacLean 1974; Rieppel and Labhardt 1979). Estes and Williams (1984) identify molariform teeth in members of the Iguanidae, Teiidae, Lacertidae, Scincidae, Anguidae, and Varanidae. However, they have difficulty in generalizing patterns of dental adaptation (fig. 4.3). For example, in some species such as *Chamaeleolis chamaeleonides* (Iguanidae) there is an ontogenetic shift in both diet and dentition, but in others such as *Tiliqua scincoides* (Scincidae), the teeth are fully molariform at hatching. Many animals that have molariform teeth are omnivorous rather than distinctly molluscivorous. Other species are known to consume significant amounts of molluscs but show no particular dental modifications from the primitive condition.

The relation between changes in diet and dentition through ontogeny has been studied by several authors with varying results (Capel-Williams and Pratten 1978; Dessem 1985; Montanucci 1968; Rieppel and Labhardt 1979). One of the most striking cases of dental specialization in lizards is

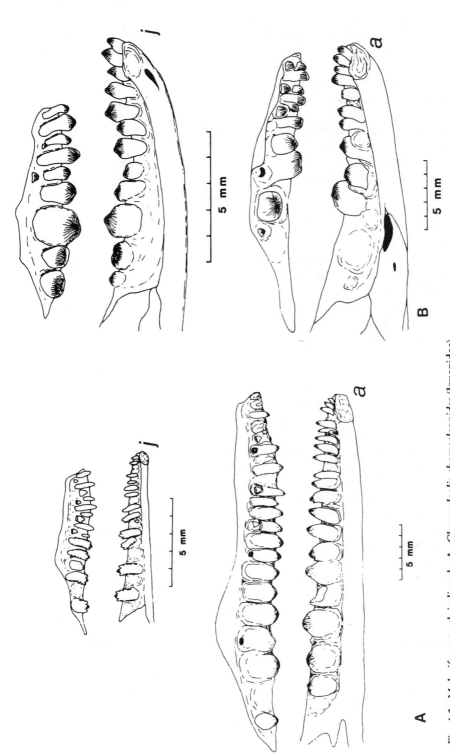

Fig. 4.3. Molariform teeth in lizards. A. *Chamaeleolis chamaeleonides* (Iguanidae). B. *Tiliqua scincoides* (Scincidae). In both cases the maxillary and mandibular tooth rows are shown in an adult (a) and a juvenile (j) individual (also indicated by changing scale). Note the striking ontogenetic shift in (A). Reprinted with permission from Estes and Williams (1984).

reported by Patchell and Shine (1986b) in *Lialis burtonis,* an Australian pygopodid lizard. *Lialis burtonis* is largely saurophagous, as opposed to its insectivorous relatives, *Pygopus lepidopodus* and *Delma inornata.* *L. burtonis* possesses hinged teeth, very similar to those found in snake species that also feed on hard-bodied prey (Savitzky 1981).

Evaluation and Summary. Lizards appear to be opportunistic, fairly generalistic feeders. It is, however, difficult to generalize about the relation between diet and the feeding apparatus in lizards. First, the relation between form and function has not been studied as broadly in lizards as in other groups. Second, the relation between form and function appears to be less exact in lizards than in the groups of terrestrial vertebrates discussed below. This latter point was discussed by Greene (1982), who provides numerous instances in which phenotypically generalized lizards consume the same food items as morphologically specialized lizards. In lizards few consistent interfamilial convergences in the trophic apparatus have been identified; instead it appears that many components of the feeding apparatus are conservative within specific phylogenetic groups. The pattern of phylogenetic uniformity appears to apply to a number of aspects of the trophic system, including the tongue and hyoid apparatus (Schwenk 1984, 1988; Smith 1984, 1986), teeth (Edmund 1969), cranial musculature (Gomes 1974; Haas 1973; Lakjer 1926), and many aspects of the kinetic apparatus. The absence of distinct patterns of interfamilial convergences in the trophic apparatus is in striking contrast to numerous convergences in general body form.

A number of alternative hypotheses might account for this pattern. First, the common hypotheses of the adaptive significance of skull features may not be correct, or general. For example, if active intracranial movement is not the functional basis for the basic skull pattern in lizards, then the proper functional questions have not yet been asked about the skull. Second, it may be that lizard feeding strategies are such that selection will not produce close tracking between the trophic apparatus and diet categories in the way it does in some other vertebrate groups. If lizards are for the most part opportunistic feeders, then a clear relation between a specific prey item and dentition would not be expected. Few studies that combine rigorous dietary information with careful morphological analysis exist for lizards. Such studies are required to address the issue of relative specialization (Greene 1982). Third, it may be that constraints operate on the lizard cranial system. If so, the components of the network of constraints have not been sufficiently identified. For example, it has been proposed that the existence of functional or mechanical constraints explains why herbivory in lizards is rare (Ostrom 1963; Sokol 1965; Szarski 1962). It has also been suggested that the cranial morphology in lizards is constrained by requirements of growth (e.g., Dalrymple 1979) or that dietary adaptations are constrained by body size (Pough 1973). However, with the exception of Pough's study these hypotheses have not been specific in their predictions, nor have they been tested by comparative data.

The Ophidian Feeding Apparatus

The most characteristic feature of the snake's skull is an amplification of the kinetic apparatus. The bones of the parietal-temporal segment are fused with the occipital segment, so that the braincase is solidly enclosed in bone and the metakinetic joint no longer exists. In contrast, the connection between the bones of the upper and lower jaws and the braincase are dramatically loosened (fig. 4.4). The upper temporal arcade has been lost,

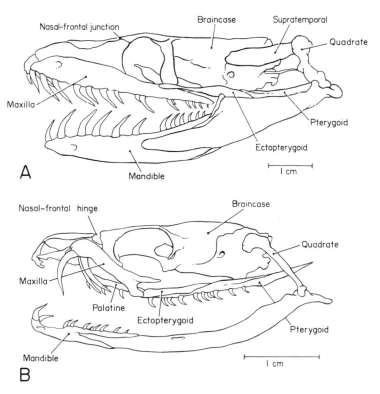

Fig. 4.4. Morphology of the cranial apparatus in two snakes. A. African rock python (*Python sebae,* Boidae). B. Green forest mamba (*Dendroaspis jamesoni,* Elapidae). Snakes are distinguished from lizards in that the braincase is a solid structure formed by the fusion of the occipital segment and dermal elements. The mesokinetic joint is solid, and secondary mobility develops at the nasal-frontal hinge. Further, the maxilla and pterygoid bars develop true, bilateral independent mobility. Redrawn from Parker and Grandison (1977).

the ectopterygoid and pterygoid bones lose their vertical and lateral supports, and the lower end of the quadrates are no longer anchored to the pterygoids. The maxillae are likewise loosely connected to the skull. In advanced snakes at least six jaw elements possess independent mobility: the two maxillary units, the two palato-pterygoid bars, and the two mandibles. The muscles necessary to move these units are hypertrophied and differentiated relative to lizards.

These modifications have at least two major functional consequences. First, independent movement and control of the tooth-bearing bones of the upper jaw relative to the braincase is possible, and second, the tips of the jaws, in particular the lower jaws, may be widely distended. While most other terrestrial amniotes use the tongue or thrusting movements of the head in space to ingest prey, snakes use independent movements of the bones of the upper and lower jaws and right and left sides to transport prey (Albright and Nelson 1959 a, b; Boltt and Ewer 1964; Cundall 1983; Cundall and Gans 1979; Dullemeijer 1959; Dullemeijer and Povel 1972; Gans 1952; Frazzetta 1966; Kardong 1974, 1977, 1979; Pough 1983; Rieppel 1980). This is a highly derived condition that bears little relation to the lizard feeding system.

Origin of the Ophidian Feeding Apparatus. Gans (1961) argues that the origin of the snake feeding apparatus was brought about by the elongation of the body, presumably a result of locomotor or habitat adaptations. Elongation of the body reduced the ratio of body diameter to body mass. As a consequence, maximum gape, and therefore maximum food item size was reduced relative to mass. Gans argues that in order to compensate for the reduction in gape relative to body mass, snakes developed adaptations to increase gape and consume larger prey. This model suggests that the diversity of the snake skull involves specializations for catching, immobilizing, and ingesting specific, large prey items.

Savitsky (1980) hypothesizes that envenomation is a key adaptation of higher snakes. Early snake radiations were dominated by boid and aniliid snakes with limited or modest cranial mobility. These animals were largely "sit and wait" predators that immobilized prey either by biting and stunning or by constriction. Savitsky (1980) and also Ruben (1977a, b), argue that prey immobilization by constriction links the trophic and locomotor systems into a single complex. The linkage of the locomotor and feeding systems constrains the locomotor system, which limits the capacity for locomotor and thus habitat diversification. In the late Miocene in North America and Europe the primary boid fauna was replaced by colubroids. Savitsky postulates that this shift reflects the replacement of the slow-moving, heavy-bodied boids by a radiation of snakes characterized by rapid movement. He hypothesizes that the locomotor system was liberated as a result of the development of prey immobilization via venom delivery systems. The radiation of colubroid snakes was thus keyed by the uncoupling of the locomotor and feeding system.

Savitsky argues that front-fanged venom delivery systems in elapids and vipers evolved independently from primitive rear-fanged systems at least five times. This parallel evolution of specialized venom delivery systems occurred, according to Savitsky, because serous oral glands and thus the ability to envenomate prey are primitive in higher snakes (caenophidians). Thus, the adaptation of the ancestor (the acquisition of serous oral glands) has made a certain course of evolution (the development of venom injection systems) more likely. Savitsky's analysis places the evolution of snake diversity in a historical context, but it is not fully confirmed by the distribution of characters in extant snakes. The venom of only approximately 40 species of extant colubroids (out of approximately 1,400) has been shown to produce intoxication in mammals and significant envenomation is rare (Gans 1978). Furthermore, many colubroids are powerful constrictors (Ditmars 1907).

Greene (1983) summarizes dietary patterns in extant snakes in order to re-examine hypotheses that the snake trophic apparatus is adapted for feeding on large prey. He finds that there is little evidence that living primitive snakes eat prey that is particularly large relative to body weight or that snakes, particularly boids, are food specialists. Greene proposes that the initial dietary shift in early snakes involved consumption of elongate, heavy prey. Subsequent morphological change allowed diversification in terms of prey shape and taxonomy.

The Evolution of Coadapted Functional Complexes. Pough and Groves (1983) examine the functional complex involved in the consumption of relatively very large prey. This complex consists of a relatively short, stout body, a large head, fangs on rotating maxillae, and rectilinear locomotion. It has evolved a number of times independently within the vipers. These authors use comparative data to test three specific hypotheses: (1) that the body form in vipers is different from nonvipers, (2) that the distinctive features constitute a suite of characters that change in concert, and (3) that vipers are able to swallow bulky prey more readily than nonvipers. The first two hypotheses are confirmed in a morphological study that shows that vipers exceed nonvipers in stoutness of body, skull length, head width, mandible length, and skull circumference at the quadrates.

Vipers swallow prey of any size with fewer maxillary protractions than nonvipers and can swallow prey that is absolutely and relatively larger than prey swallowed by nonvipers (fig. 4.5). Pough and Groves note that nonvipers attempted and failed to swallow prey at 11-29% of body mass and that vipers failed at only 40-45%. Their comparative study dem-

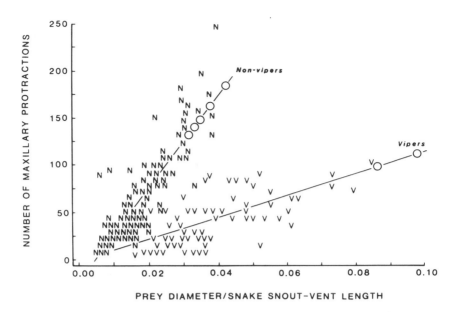

Fig. 4.5. The ability to ingest large prey in vipers and nonvipers. In the graph the relation between the number of maxillary protractions required to swallow prey and the relative size of the prey is diagrammed. N = nonvipers, V = vipers. Open circles indicate items that a snake tried and failed to swallow. Reprinted with permission from Pough and Groves (1983).

onstrates morphological and performance convergence. "Parallel, stepwise developments of the same suite of characters are seen among colubrids, viperines and crotalines. This parallelism strongly suggests a functional association among structural features that are as diverse as the circumference of the trunk and the length of the mandible" (p. 449).

Savitsky (1983) examines a number of character complexes involved with adaptations for fossoriality, piscivory, and durophagy in snakes. For example, at least two independent lineages of colubrids are predators on gastropod molluscs. In both, the exposed body is seized and the soft parts withdrawn from the shell by alternate mandibular retractions. Cranial modifications include long and slender teeth, often reduced in number, shortened pterygoid bones, development of serous glands on the lower, as opposed to upper, jaw, and a hypertrophied M. levator anguli oris. Savitsky argues that convergent evolution of character suites such as this "provide opportunities to test the likelihood of adaptationist explanations. Where shared, derived character states in demonstrably unrelated lineages correspond to shared attributes of natural history, adaptation becomes a parsimonious explanation" (p. 397).

Competing Demands. The conflicting demands imposed by the venom delivery and ingesting units of the skull have been investigated by several authors. Dullemeijer and Povel (1972) study rattlesnakes (*Crotalus*) and contrast the demands of the poisoning apparatus, which requires a precise kinematic pattern, with the construction for swallowing, which requires a highly mobile system. They state that this issue "presents a case of formation of a delicate structural balance to meet two contradictory demands in a part of the feeding construction" (p. 561).

Cundall (1983) also examines the problem of competing demands of swallowing and venom delivery. Cundall proposes that the head of advanced snakes displays a variety of prey-capture mechanisms, while maintaining a relatively conservative swallowing (prey-ingestion) mechanism. He tests this hypothesis with comparative electromyographic and cinematographic studies of four species, *Elaphe obsoleta, Nerodia fasciata, Heterodon platyrhinos,* and *Agkistrodon piscivorous* (fig. 4.6). These species differ both in prey-capture strategies and in cranial morphology. Only *Agkistrodon* possesses an elaborate envenomating apparatus and highly toxic venom. *Elaphe* constricts endothermic prey; *Nerodia* and *Heterodon* usually consume prey alive.

Cundall shows that the movements of the palato-pterygoid bar and mandible are conservative, while the movements of the maxilla are variable. Similarly, some craniofacial muscles have retained conservative patterns of activity and others have not. There is little variation in mandibular adductor or pterygoideus muscle activity. Cundall explains this with a reexamination of prey ingestion. In snakes, prey ingestion is largely a matter of advancing the palato-pterygoid bars, with the mandible serving primarily to keep the prey against the roof of the mouth. The prey is not actively retracted relative to the braincase; rather the braincase is advanced over the prey. The snake therefore employs little energy beyond that necessary to move the braincase. The maxilla, on the other hand, plays only a minor role in prey ingestion in all of the specimens examined, or in other species studied by other workers (e.g., Kardong 1979, 1980). Instead, the maxilla appears to be involved in prey capture, even in species without specialized venom injection systems. Thus, even in relatively unspecialized colubrids, the prey-capture and ingestion mechanisms are to some extent functionally and structurally separate. Cundall suggests that because of the independence of the maxilla and palato-pterygoid units in advanced snakes there is not a conflict between requirements for prey capture and ingestion.

Evaluation and Summary. A number of features characterize snakes: a highly specialized body form and locomotor apparatus and a derived cranial apparatus, including mechanical independence of up to six jaw units. The behavioral key to the snake feeding system typically has been thought

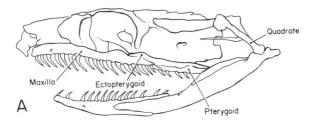

A

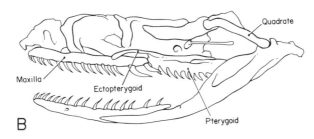

B

Fig. 4.6. Cranial
morphology of the four
snakes studied by
Cundall. Note the
increasing specialization
of the maxilla for
venom injection. A.
Elaphe obsoleta
(Colubridae). B.
Nerodia fasciata
(Colubridae). C.
Heterodon platyrhinos
(Colubridae). D.
*Agkistrodon
piscivorous* (Viperidae).
Redrawn from Cundall
(1983).

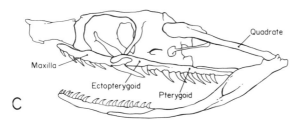

C

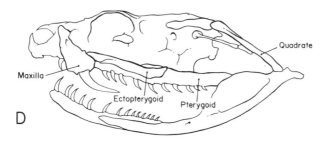

D

to involve specializations for feeding on large and specific food items. While this may not be an accurate generalization for all snakes (Greene 1983), a number of studies show remarkable specificity in prey choice (Gans 1983). In some cases this food preference appears to be genetic, and intraspecific polymorphisms in food choice have been identified (Arnold 1977, 1981a, b; Burghardt 1970).

The snake trophic apparatus is largely responsible for ingesting whole packets of food. Food is not mechanically prepared, broken down, or separated. In advanced snakes the trophic apparatus acquires a second specialization—envenomation. Envenomation may have evolved in order to begin the process of chemical preparation of the prey (Gans 1978; Kochva et al. 1983). While on the surface this dual role may appear to present a problem of competing demands, Cundall's work shows that the ingestion and envenomation units are separate in all advanced snakes.

Snakes appear to be a potential case for tests of the "decoupling hypothesis," as a number of elements of the skull are mechanically independent (Lauder 1981; Liem 1973; Vermeij 1973). This hypothesis predicts that "primitive members of a morphologically diverse monophyletic lineage possess functional, structural or morphogenetic networks which have a greater number of independent elements as compared to similar networks in closely related but less morphologically diverse monophyletic lineages" (Lauder 1981, 437). In the evolution of the snake feeding apparatus two separate uncoupling events have occurred. The first involves the decoupling of the upper jaws from the cranium and of the right and left halves of both the upper and lower jaws, leading to six potentially independent mechanical units. This adaptation is present in henophidians (e.g., boids) as well as caenophidians (e.g., colubroids) and therefore does not correlate with the diversification of colubroids. The second innovation is the independence of the maxillary and the pterygoid portions of the upper jaw. This latter innovation is present in all caenophidians and might supply an explanation for the explosive radiation of the advanced snakes. Most studies of the function of the maxillae in caenophidians are of the few species that possess specializations for envenomation. Few compare the use of the maxillae in less specialized colubrids and boids. To confirm the hypothesis that the decoupling of the maxillary and pterygoid bones has led to diversification within caenophidians would require that variation in the specialization of the maxilla correlate with the taxonomic diversification. An alternative but similar explanation for the diversification of the colubroids proposes that the liberation of the locomotor apparatus from the constraints of constriction has allowed locomotor and habitat diversification. Again, this hypothesis could be more completely tested by mapping the morphological innovations against taxonomic diversity.

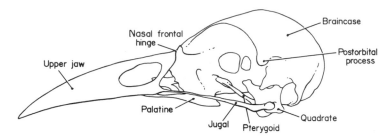

Fig. 4.7. The cranial apparatus of a crow (*Corvus*). As in snakes, birds possess a solid braincase, consisting of fused dermal and neurocranial elements. Mobility is present at the nasal frontal hinge, and at the quadrate. Movements of the quadrate are translated to the upper jaw via the jugal bone. Redrawn from Bock (1964).

The Feeding Apparatus of Birds

The bird skull, like the skull in snakes and lizards, includes regions of intracranial mobility. Like snakes, but unlike lizards, it is well established that intracranial movements are an integral part of feeding behavior. However, with the exception of the detailed studies by Zweers (1974, 1982), there have been few experimental studies on the kinematics and activity patterns of the muscles and bones of the avian skull.

The basic pattern of the avian skull has been summarized by Bock (1964), who presents a detailed mechanical analysis, and Buhler (1981) and Zusi (1993) who present reviews of the functional diversity. Avian kinesis involves anterior sliding of a palatal unit, composed of the palato-vomero complex and jugal, pterygoid, and quadrate bones, relative to a solid braincase (fig. 4.7). Bending between the upper jaw and skull occurs either between the frontal and nasal bones (prokinesis) or within the nasal bone (rhynchokinesis). Anterior movement of this unit may be produced by either anterior rotation of the quadrate induced by movements of the lower bill, or activity of the Mm. protractor ptyergoidei and quadrati. Movements of the upper and lower bills may be coupled or uncoupled and the degree to which the upper and lower bills are obligately coupled appears to vary (Zusi 1967). In both cases, elevation of the upper bill may be independent of depression of the lower bill. Additional mechanical analyses include Bock (1966), Bock and Kummer (1968), Bock and Morioka (1971), Lederer (1975), and Simonetta (1960).

Bock (1964) suggests six potential biological roles of the kinetic, and in particular coupled kinetic, mechanism. These include: (1) passive maintenance of the mandible in the closed position, (2) a mechanism to increase the force of bill opening in "gapers," (3) maintenance of a primary visual axis of orientation, (4) faster bill closing, because both bills close simultaneously, (5) a shock-absorption mechanism, or (6) increased areas for attachment of jaw muscles. Both Zusi (1967) and Beecher (1962) argue that the fundamental advantage of the kinetic apparatus in birds is in the potential diversity and versatility of the jaws as a manipulatory tool. This latter hypothesis appears to be endorsed by much of the behavioral and functional morphological data.

One of the major mechanical constraints operating on the avian skull is the necessity for light construction due to the requirements of flight. Buhler (1981) illustrates this with the weights of four skulls of approximately equal breadth and length: *Caprimulgus* (bird) 0.45 g; *Gallinula* (bird) 0.85 g; *Rattus* (mammal) 3.2 g; and *Lacerta* (lizard) 3.7 g. Bock (1966) presents an analysis of the construction of the skull and some of the ways that force is transmitted despite the requirements of lightness.

Relation of Form and Function within Avian Families. Beecher has investigated the functional significance of the feeding apparatus in birds by surveying the form and function relation within radiations of specific families (1951, 1962, 1978). In a study of the adaptive radiation within the American blackbirds, the Icteridae, Beecher (1951) inspects the skeletal morphology, musculature, diet, and behavior in 38 genera. He hypothesizes that the primitive condition is similar to that of the cowbird, *Molothrus*. The diet of cowbirds consists of approximately 77% seeds. Like other seed eaters, cowbirds possess skulls with short beaks, a high angle between the beak and skull base, relatively limited kinetic ability, and large, highly pinnate muscles. Beecher documents the changes that have occurred within the family that correlate with dietary and behavioral differences (fig. 4.8). For example, as birds such as the blackbirds, *Euphagus,* consume a greater proportion of insects, bills are elongated and the amount of kinetic mobility and the angle between the beak and skull base increase. The size of the muscles is also reduced in insectivorous members of the Icteridae, but they remain pinnate. (They are parallel-fibered in many primitively insectivorous groups such as the Old World warblers; Beecher 1978.) Beecher speculates that the pinnate nature of muscles may be "too deep-seated genetically" to be lost readily. He notes, however, that the fibers insert with a low angle on the tendon and thus may mechanically mimic parallel-fibered muscles. He also identifies a number of other adaptations within the group. For example, grackles utilize a hard keel that projects downward from the palate and is used to saw hard materials with a back and forth movement. Accompanying this is a hypertrophy of the M. adductor mandibulae externus superficialis.

One major characteristic of the Icteridae is the gaping adaptation of three specific groups: first, the ground-feeding meadowlarks; second, fruit gapers such as orioles (which protrude the bill into fruits, gape, and then lap

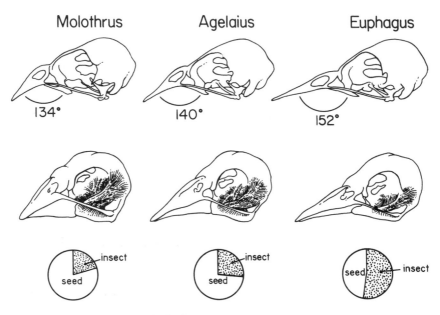

Fig. 4.8. Adaptations in the skull of individuals of the Icteridae. *Molothrus,* the cowbird, represents the primitive condition. *Agelaius* and *Euphagus* represent derived conditions, with increasingly insectivorous diets. The correlated changes in the angle of commissure, the jaw adductor musculature, and percentage of insects in the diet are diagrammed. Redrawn from Beecher (1951).

the pulp and juices); and third, powerful wood gapers. In all gapers upper-beak protractors hypertrophy as do the lower-beak depressor muscles. Thus the ability to open the jaws with power is increased relative to the primitive condition.

Beecher (1978) also examines the feeding adaptations of the starlings (family Sturnidae). Phylogenetic analysis is used to determine the most probable ancestor, an insectivorous species. From this ancestor Beecher details the changes in morphology with different behaviors. Starlings exhibit a diversity of form and function of the bill, but like the Icteridae, include a species, *Sturnus vulgaris,* with well-developed gaping adaptations. These adaptations include a "remarkably narrow" skull and a hypertrophy of the Mm. depressor mandibulae and protractor quadrati muscles.

Numerous additional studies on the form and function of the avian trophic apparatus exist. Many authors examine form in relation to behavior and diet. These include Bhattacharyya's (1987) study of Indian insectivorous birds, Burton's (1974b) study of the jaw and tongue in the tooth-billed pigeon, Owre's (1967) study of feeding and locomotion in the cormorant, and Zusi's (1962) study of the feeding adaptations of the skimmer. Other studies examine the variation in morphology in a closely related group given different behaviors (Bowman 1961, 1963; Burton 1974a, 1984; Jenkin 1957). Richards and Bock (1973), in a detailed study of the Hawaiian honeycreepers of the genus *Loxops,* describe a series of modifications of the beak and jaw muscles in relation to the manner of obtaining food. Other studies of form and function in a radiation of birds include Burt's (1930) and Spring's (1965) studies of North American woodpeckers, Burger's (1978) study of the feeding apparatus of four species of cormorants, and Brown and Bowers's (1985) and Feinsinger and Colwell's (1978) studies of hummingbirds.

Seed-Eating Birds. Numerous studies have focused on adaptations for seed eating in birds. Newton (1967) examines ecological aspects of a radiation of British seed-eating birds. The goldfinches and siskins have narrow beaks of different lengths and use their beaks to probe and manipulate ripe seed heads. They differ in the types of seed heads utilized. Greenfinches have the heaviest bills and crush hard fruiting bodies. Bullfinches also utilize closed seed heads, but instead of crushing the heads, they peel away portions of the seed head with their lighter, slightly recurved beaks. The chaffinch is the only species that feeds primarily on the ground; it takes the widest range of seed sizes, and possesses the second largest bill of those studied by Newton. It is the most common of all species. Newton's data show that the morphological and behavioral specializations of these finches largely relate to how the animals get their food from the plant.

Bock (1960) presents an analysis of the functional significance of the palatine process in seed-eating birds, and in the course of the analysis demonstrates alternate solutions to similar mechanical demands. The major modifications of this process appear to be associated with the functional demands of strengthening the skull against stresses induced by cracking seeds. Bock argues that this may be a particular problem in birds, because of the specializations for lightening the skull (Bock 1966; Buhler 1981). Two pathways for solving this problem are used by finches. In emberizine finches, the upper and lower jaws both retain independent mobility. Bock calls this the "nutcracker" method of cracking seeds. The cardinal represents the extreme of this type of seed eater: the adductor mandibulae and pterygoideus muscles are both hypertrophied, the beak is strong, but the upper jaw is not heavily buttressed. The alternative method is seen in cardueline finches, in which the upper jaw has lost its mobility and heavy buttressing exists between the upper jaw and skull. The adductor mandibulae muscles are also large, but the protractors and retractors of the upper jaw are reduced. Bock terms this method of cracking seeds the "vise" method. In both systems the upper beak is short, conical, and strongly recurved. "It must be emphasized that the important functional difference between the nutcracker and the vise methods of cracking seeds is not in terms of applying force on the seed, but in terms of protecting the braincase from the shocks associated with the breaking of the seed coat" (Bock 1960, 425). In the nutcracker apparatus stresses are isolated and absorbed in the jaw apparatus; in the vise morphology the stresses are distributed evenly through the braincase by a series of struts. Bock hypothesizes that the nutcracker method allows birds to retain upper-bill mobility and thus to consume both insects and seeds. Species utilizing the vise method such as the hawfinch may be limited to a diet of seeds. This case is a good example both of morphological responses to competing mechanical demands and of the existence of alternative adaptive pathways.

Summary and Evaluation. There are several general conclusions about the avian feeding apparatus. First, the bird feeding system, because of the independent mobility of the upper and lower bills, apparently allows tremendous diversity of function of the avian bill, in particular the ability for manipulation. Both Beecher (1962) and Zusi (1967) cite this versatility as one of the key innovations of birds. Zusi (1967) states that the true significance of the avian jaw lies not only in its feeding function, but also in preening, nest building, and defense. Beecher (1962) claims that "the unparalleled versatility of the bill as a tool stems from the achievement of this mobility or kinetism. It was a major adaptation as important to the whole class Aves as the origin of flight" (p. 10). Second, convergence of the significant design features is common. One example of this discussed above involves adaptations for gaping. Beecher (1951, 1962, 1978) was able to show that gaping adaptations have evolved convergently in two groups, the starlings and the blackbirds. This is particularly interesting because the primitive condition in the two is quite different: blackbirds are thought to have evolved from a seed eater with a short, recurved bill and heavy pinnate adductor muscles, and starlings from a warblerlike ancestor with a long, thin beak and thin jaw adductor muscles. Nevertheless, a similar suite of morphological characteristics defines the two derived taxa. Convergence between widely separated taxonomic groups is common, including finchlike adaptations and those for nectar feeding (references above). Third, these studies of the bird feeding apparatus show a distinct relation between the form of the feeding apparatus and the acquisition of food. Rarely is the avian trophic apparatus called upon to process food mechanically, instead, it obtains food in situ. The frequent pattern of relatively close tracking of the trophic apparatus to characters of where the food is in the environment rather than the intrinsic properties of the food itself has made birds a particularly fruitful group for ecological and ecomorphological studies that relate morphological characters and resource choice (e.g., Brown and Bowers 1985; Feinsinger and Colwell 1978; Herrera 1978; Hespenheide 1973; Hulsman 1981; Jackson 1985; Karr and James 1975; Wheelwright 1985).

The Mammalian Skull

The form of the mammalian trophic apparatus is distinguished from the ancestral condition by a number of features (e.g., Allin 1975; Barghusen 1968; Bramble 1978; Crompton and Hylander 1986; Crompton and Parker 1978). One is that in contrast to their ancestors and to the verte-brate groups just discussed, mammals are notable for the lack of kinetic joints within the skull. The most characteristic mammalian feeding adap-tation is mastication of food or intraoral processing of food. This latter adaptation is made possible by two major functional shifts from the an-cestral condition. The first is the development of teeth with complex mor-phology and precise occlusal patterns. Numerous workers have studied the functional significance of mammalian teeth on a broad scale (Crompton and Kielan-Jaworowska 1978; Lucas 1982; Lucas and Luke 1984; Rens-berger 1973, 1975, 1986; Rensberger et al. 1984). The second is the modi-fication of the primitive pattern of jaw muscles. Two distinct external adductor muscles, the masseter and temporalis, are present in mammals. The masseter and an internal adductor, the medial pterygoid, provide for mediolateral movements of the jaws. It is thought that during the evolution of mammals the directions of the jaw muscles have been modified from the primitive condition to better balance the reaction forces at the jaw joint (Bramble 1978; Crompton and Parker 1978; but see Gans et al. 1985; fig. 4.9). However, Crompton and Hylander (1986) discuss the fact that in

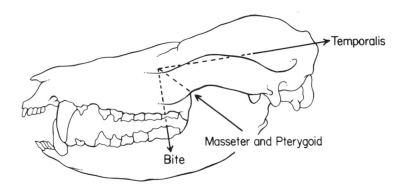

Fig. 4.9. The skull of the American opossum. In mammals, unlike the other groups discussed above, no intracranial joints are present. Jaw muscle forces are diagramed in lateral view. In this diagram the jaw muscle forces and the forces generated by the molar teeth meet so as to establish a triangle to prevent excessive forces from being generated at the jaw joint. Redrawn from Crompton and Parker (1978).

extant mammals during unilateral chewing and incisal biting, reaction forces at the jaw joint may be quite large.

Mastication and the extensive mechanical breakdown of food by the jaw apparatus distinguishes mammals from the other vertebrate groups examined thus far. The radiation of the mammalian trophic apparatus reflects a relatively tight correlation between the requirements for food breakdown and the form of the masticatory system. However, the mammalian system also is subject to a multiplicity of functional requirements.

Studies of the mammalian feeding system have included (1) analyses of the origin of the feeding system (e.g., Barghusen 1968; Bramble 1978; Crompton 1971; Crompton and Hylander 1986; Crompton and Parker 1978; Davis 1961), (2) experimental studies of bone-muscle systems (e.g., Crompton and Hiiemae 1970; Crompton et al. 1977; De Vree and Gans 1976; Gans 1985; Gorniak and Gans 1980; Herring 1976; Herring and Scapino 1973; Hiiemae 1978; Hylander 1979, 1984, 1985; Janis 1979; Kallen and Gans 1972; Oron and Crompton 1985; Weijs and Dantuma 1981), and (3) biomechanical modeling (e.g., Greaves 1978, 1980, 1982, 1983, 1985). Here, a few studies of the determinants of the form of the feeding system in mammals will be examined.

Maynard Smith and Savage Revisited. One of the early attempts to define broad organizing rules about the determinants of the masticatory system in mammals was a study of the form of the jaw and muscle system by Maynard Smith and Savage (1959; some of the major points are also found in Wolff-Exalto 1951). This study defines the major mechanical requirements and constraints imposed on the masticatory system in carnivores and herbivores by their respective diets (fig. 4.10). The major requirements for a carnivore include jaws with the capacity for fast closing, a reduction of lateral jaw movement so that precise shear of the carnassial can be maintained, and muscles with a major component of force directed posteriorly so as to resist the anteriorly directed forces of the struggling prey. The major features of the jaws of most carnivores meet these requirements. They possess relatively large temporalis muscles, and low mandibular condyles and high coronoid processes, which Maynard Smith and Savage suggest increase the moment arm of the temporalis. A hingelike glenoid fossa serves to reduce translation of the mandible and resist jaw dislocation. The food of herbivores imposes few externally applied forces on the jaw apparatus when compared to carnivores, and most herbivores do not possess morphology that would resist jaw dislocation. Instead, herbivores possess masticatory systems that emphasize lateral jaw movement in order to utilize the shearing facets of the teeth.

Maynard Smith and Savage suggest that the masseter and pterygoideus are the muscles primarily responsible for mediolateral jaw translation. In

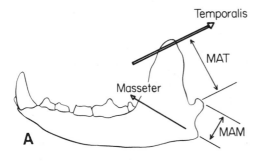

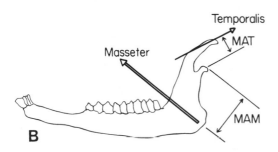

Fig. 4.10. The force vectors and moment arms of the masseter and temporalis muscles in (A) a mustelid carnivore (*Martes*) and (B) an ungulate herbivore (*Strepsiceros*). The relative sizes of the muscles are indicated by the relative thickness of the lines. Note the relative sizes of the moment arms of the temporalis (MAT) and masseter (MAM) muscles. Redrawn from Maynard Smith and Savage (1959).

herbivores the masseter and pterygoideus muscles are large, and their moment arm is increased by extension of the jaw condyles high above the occlusal plane. Maynard Smith and Savage's hypothesis of masticatory movements is supported by experimental data from the little brown bat (Kallen and Gans 1972), miniature pig (Herring and Scapino 1973), pygmy goat (De Vree and Gans 1976), and rabbit (Weijs and Dantuma 1981). In summary, the basic design differences in the jaws of herbivores and carnivores are due to (1) the requirements of specific lines of force transmission and jaw movement arising from the particular types of food and tooth shear, (2) requirements of reducing food-induced stresses, and (3) patterns of maximizing the leverage of particular muscle groups. The design of the jaws is necessarily a compromise between competing demands.

Many aspects of the Maynard Smith and Savage model have been refined by later workers (e.g., Turnbull 1970; Greaves 1978, 1983, 1985; Scapino 1972). Radinsky (1985) compares a series of fossil and extant ungulates and finds that an expanded angular process, reflecting an increase in the masseter muscle, evolved at least 12 times independently in ungulates. As Radinsky states, we are "surely dealing with a feature of adaptive significance." On the other hand, Radinsky finds no clear-cut pattern of raising the temporomandibular joint above the tooth row (also noted by Greaves 1974).

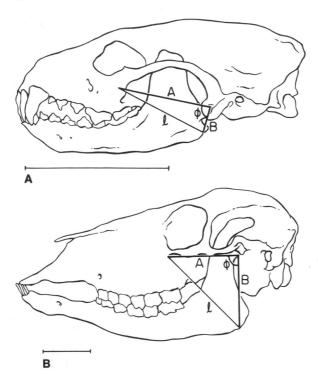

Fig. 4.11. Skulls of (A) a mustelid carnivore (*Martes pennanti*) and (B) an ungulate herbivore (*Tragelaphus buxtoni*). The factors important in the Herring and Herring model for the effect of the masseter muscle on gape are shown and include A, the distance between the jaw joint and the origin of the muscle; B, the distance between the joint and the insertion of the muscle; ϕ, the angle between the origin and the insertion; and 1, the fiber length of the muscle. Scale bars equal 5 cm. Skulls redrawn from Radinsky (1985).

One important mechanical aspect not examined in the Maynard Smith and Savage paper is the potential compromise between increasing the leverage of a masticatory muscle by moving it farther from the joint and the resulting restrictions of gape. Herring and Herring (1974) model the competing requirements of muscle position and gape and present quantitative hypotheses that may be tested by comparative data (see also Gans et al. 1985). They model the orientation of the superficial masseter relative to the amount of stretch for a given angle of mandibular rotation. In the model five parameters are important: (1) the distance between the jaw joint and the origin of the muscle, A; (2) the distance between the jaw joint and the insertion of the muscle, B; (3) the length of a fiber of the muscle, l; (4) the angle between the origin and insertion of the muscle, ϕ; and (5) the gape angle (fig. 4.11). The model predicts that animals requiring wide gape (i.e., carnivores) will retain a relatively high angle ϕ; if food is taken laterally, there will be little modification of the length of A or B, but the ratio of A to B will be high; if food is not taken laterally, then A and B will both lengthen. If gape is no longer of particular significance, as in herbivores, then mechanical advantage of the masseter will probably be improved, by lengthening A and B and decreasing ϕ. Herring and Herring test this model with comparative data and find that the above predictions are largely confirmed. Emerson and Radinsky (1980) apply this model to the temporalis muscle of saber-toothed cats and find that the predictions of the model help in providing an accurate mechanical basis for explaining many of the differences between saber-toothed cats and modern felids.

All the above mechanical models have a considerable advantage in that they elucidate major patterns of morphology and provide bases for broad comparative studies. However, because the approach is broad, potential problems in application arise. For example, as pointed out by Weijs (1980), most models of jaw mechanics are static and model only a single plane, while jaw movements are three-dimensional. Electromyographic studies have shown that muscular activity is complex and that asymmetric loading may be the rule in most mammals. Further, most analyses consider the adaptations of the jaw apparatus to transmit maximal forces. As Weijs points out, the most important movements may be the rapid and complicated movements that occur in mastication, which do not involve maximum force. Most studies are either rigorous, detailed studies of the function of the apparatus in a single animal or broad-based comparative studies that address evolutionary issues, but make large numbers of simplifying assumptions.

Cranial Form in Carnivores: Morphometric Approaches. Radinsky (1981a, b, 1982) approaches the function of cranial features in carnivores quantitatively. His analyses have consisted of measurements of features of functional significance, transformation to eliminate size effects, and then principle component analysis. In a comparison of felids, mustelids, canids, and viverrids, Radinsky (1981a) finds several major characteristics that separate the families (fig. 4.12). For example, factor 1 distinguishes mustelids and felids from canids. This factor is hypothesized to represent primarily features related to bite strength and to distinguish animals on the basis of diet. But when similar morphometric analyses are performed on additional carnivores—ursids, procyonids, and additional mustelids—the distinction between families is not as clear (Radinsky 1981b). The ursids and procyonids are particularly variable. Furthermore, this second study provides little evidence to support the hypothesis that high factor 1 loading reflects bite strength or that the differences between animals in factor 1 loading reflect correlations between bite strength and diet. For example, the panda, *Ailuropoda,* is not distinguished in this analysis from other ursids in the features related to bite strength, but is considered to possess general adaptations for strong jaws (Davis 1964).

This case illustrates the difficulties in establishing the functional basis of pattern as assessed by morphometric approaches. Radinsky (1981b) cites three explanations for the lack of correlation between factor 1 loading and bite strength in the additional species: (1) the hypothesis that

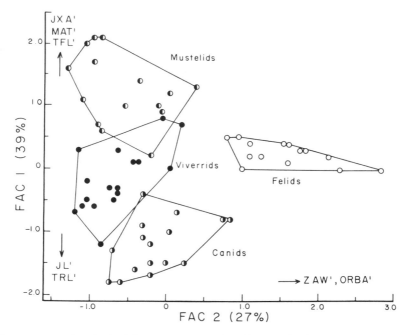

Fig. 4.12. Results of principle component analysis from Radinsky (1981a). Abbreviations for variables; JXA, jaw cross-sectional area; MAT, moment arm temporalis; TFL, temporal fossa length; JL, jaw length; TRL, tooth row length; ZAW, zygomatic arch width; ORBA, orbital area. Polygons enclose all species of a given family. Reproduced with permission from Radinsky (1981a).

factor 1 loading primarily reflects bite strength is too narrow, (2) the hypothesis that the primary biological role of bite strength is feeding is too narrow, or (3) a factor other than adaptation (i.e., constraint) may be significant in determining these aspects of skull form. Morphometric approaches alone cannot distinguish these hypotheses—detailed functional, behavioral, and comparative studies are necessary.

In a third paper, Radinsky (1982) applies the same measurements to fossil carnivores in an attempt to establish the origin of the major features of the various carnivore groups. Radinsky finds that the differences distinguishing modern viverrids, canids, felids, and mustelids are less pronounced in the Oligocene. He is not able to identify any key innovation characteristic of the Carnivora or any family within the order.

Werdelin (1986) compares Radinsky's results on placental carnivores with data for marsupial carnivores. Measurements similar to those made by Radinsky were made on members of the Dasyuroidea. Werdelin finds that despite a wide range of dietary habits, the Dasyuroidea, with the exception of *Sarcophilus,* are far more narrow in morphology than the

Carnivora. Further, Werdelin finds no significant convergence between placental and marsupial carnivores. "In terms of the morphological composition of the functioning skull, convergence due to similar ecologies is of very minor significance compared to the phylogenetic history of the taxa. At this phylogenetic distance, convergent similarity is apparently no more than skin deep" (p. 114). Werdelin (1983) studies the skull of cats, and discusses the effects of developmental constraints on the jaws of marsupial carnivores in a later paper (1987).

Primate Teeth and Jaws. The variation in mammalian teeth forms the basis of much of mammalian systematics, particularly of fossil forms. There have been a number of excellent analyses of the evolution and functional significance of mammalian teeth. Primate teeth provide a good example of a system in which the relation between form and diet has been thoroughly examined.

Kay has related the morphology of molar surfaces to different major dietary types in primates. Kay (1975) defines three general factors that might determine selection on tooth form in mammals: (1) body size—because of metabolic rate and body size relations, smaller mammals would be expected to prepare proportionately more food; (2) energy content of food—animals consuming food with low intrinsic energy would be expected to prepare proportionately more food per unit time; (3) food consistency—mechanical properties of food will affect the shape of food preparation surfaces. In addition to these general factors, tooth shape is influenced by its phylogenetic heritage. Because of this last factor, comparisons must be based on design features rather than specific morphological characters.

In a study of noncercopithecoid primates and tupaiids both bivariate and multivariate analyses separate molar morphology of frugivores from folivores and insectivores (Kay 1975). Folivores are separated from insectivores on the basis of body size. Further studies reveal that in extant Cercopithecidae folivorous species are separate from frugivorous species (Kay 1978). However, contrary to most expectations, linear or surface area measurements of teeth do not scale to metabolic rate. For example, in cercopithecines the relation between body mass and M2 surface area is not significantly different from isometry. Kay claims that this is also true for artiodactyls (thereby disputing Gould 1975).

While molar teeth are generally involved in only a single function—the mechanical preparation of food—the anterior dentition is involved in a variety of functions including scraping, prying, grooming, social displays, and food preparation. It would be expected that the tracking of incisor tooth morphology to diet would be more difficult to demonstrate. Hylander (1975) shows that within anthropoids and particularly the Cercopithe-

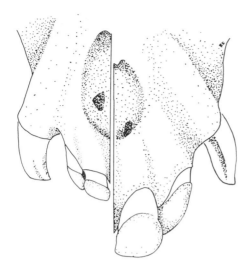

Fig. 4.13. Incisor size of *Erythrocebus patas* (left) and *Cercocebus albigena* (right) standardized for the breadth of the piriform aperture. This illustrates the variability in incisor size in cercopithecines. *Erythrocebus* is largely graminivorous, while *Cercocebus* eats very large quantities of fruit. Reprinted with permission from Kay and Hylander (1978).

cidae, incisor size is highly correlated with diet. The folivorous colobines have significantly smaller incisors than frugivorous cercopithecines. Even within cercopithecines, the more graminivorous species have smaller incisors than species that are frugivorous (fig. 4.13). Maier (1984) reaches similar conclusions about relative incisor size.

Kay and Hylander (1978) extend these studies broadly and compare folivorous primates and phalangeroids (Marsupialia). A number of the trends seen in primates, such as increased molar shearing surfaces in folivorous species relative to nonfolivorous species, variability in incisor morphology due to competing demands, and larger incisors in frugivores, are also observed in phalangeroid marsupials. This paper, which compares diverse and distantly related taxa, makes the important point that the "simple formula of tooth structure being related to tooth function is rendered inexact by the unique ancestry of each animal. Thus, species which eat foods requiring large amounts of shearing during mastication need not necessarily emphasize the same molar shearing blades" (pp. 173–174). However, all herbivores emphasize molar shearing blades.

Summary and Evaluation. Studies of mammalian dental form and function can serve as an excellent model for studying the basis for diversity of morphology in relation to diet. The developmental and genetic basis of dental morphology is well known. The specific relation between aspects of tooth morphology and performances has been modeled (e.g., Lucas and Luke 1984; Rensberger 1973, 1975), and in some cases tested (e.g., Kay and Sheine 1979; Sheine and Kay 1982). Further, primate ecology and diet have been studied by numerous workers so that the relevance of these data to natural behavior is established. Comparative data have been used to confirm the inference of an adaptive relation among form, performance, and fitness. Finally, the influence of phylogenetic patterning or constraint is recognized. The most important aspects of this latter factor is that the comparisons are of the design features (e.g., the relative development of shearing structures) rather than of specific morphological features. Folivorous Old and New World monkeys always have more shearing crests than their frugivorous relatives; however, all Old World monkeys have better developed shearing crests than all New World monkeys. Predictions of convergence do not require morphological identity. Comparison of design features not only allows comparison at the broadest level, but insures that the comparison is of the mechanically or functionally most significant traits.

The mammalian masticatory apparatus closely tracks diet in those species that masticate food. This tracking is reflected in dental morphology, cranial and jaw shape, and the masticatory muscles. While phylogenetic patterning is clearly present in all these features within a group, workers have again and again been able to define design features of functional significance that consistently correlate with particular diets. The iterative evolution of functional patterns strongly corroborates hypotheses of adaptation.

The issue of comparison of design features rather than morphology also arises in the comparison of metatherian and eutherian carnivores. One problem in interpreting results of morphometric comparisons among taxa as far removed as metatherian and eutherian carnivores is that it may not be possible to equate morphological similarity with functional similarity. Similar biomechanical ends may arise from different specific morphological configurations. For example, Werdelin (1986) shows that the shape of the temporal fossa differs between marsupials and placental carnivores, but he notes that nevertheless, similar functional ends may have been achieved. Thus, the negative results of morphometric comparisons may not necessarily refute the hypothesis that functional convergence or divergence exists. In studies of adaptation the comparison of design features, and not specific morphology, is most relevant in testing hypotheses.

One additional caution in interpreting the results of morphometric approaches is that while such approaches allow the quantitative assessment of hypotheses of morphological convergence or divergence, remove the effects of size, and allow study of a wide range of species, the significance of the patterns may be obscure. For example, Radinsky (1981a) notes the relative constancy of the carnassial position in eutherian carnivores. However, as discussed by Radinsky, it is impossible to resolve the two competing and perhaps diametrically opposed hypotheses to explain the consistency: mechanical optima maintained by selection or developmental or phylogenetic constraint resistant to selection.

DISCUSSION

Comparison of Diverse Taxa

Despite the attention paid to the function and morphology of the skull of individual terrestrial vertebrate groups, there are few comparisons of the skull across vertebrate classes. One reason is that it is difficult to make broad-based, cross-taxonomic comparisons. Very often, comparable data are not available. Perhaps for historical reasons, workers examining the different classes have tended to take different approaches to the study of form and function. There are numerous excellent studies of behavior, ecology, diet, and morphology in birds. There are fewer such studies for other groups. There are many detailed experimental (i.e., kinematic and electromyographic) studies of the feeding system in mammals and fewer in other terrestrial vertebrates. The mammalian skull has been analyzed with numerous broad-based or morphometric comparisons; this is not the case for the avian or reptilian skull.

The difficulty in constructing broad, cross-taxonomic rules of the determinants of the feeding apparatus, however, goes deeper than methodology. The trophic apparatus in each vertebrate group plays a fundamentally different biological role. This observation has two major implications. First, the expected relation between form and function will be different for different groups. For example, the functional significance of teeth is different in animals that masticate food and animals that do not. Therefore, predictions on the relation of tooth form to diet necessarily will be different in the two different groups. This difference will be reflected in the absence of specific morphological similarity, the absence of similarity in design features, and the absence of similar patterns of diversification. For example, the question of why there are not more reptilian herbivores generated a flurry of work, but was actually a question of why there are not more mammal-like herbivores. There are numerous lacertilian herbivores—but they do not develop large body size, ruminating chambers, or extensive dental batteries. This is not necessarily because of any intrinsic constraint (Ostrom 1963; Sokol 1965; Szarski 1962), but perhaps merely because the biological role of the trophic apparatus patterns the adaptations to food in a different way in mammals and lizards.

The second major implication of differences in the specific biological role of the trophic apparatus in each vertebrate group is that the way the trophic apparatus diversifies in response to dietary diversification will be different in each group. The mammalian trophic apparatus is specialized for processing food; much of the diversity of the mammalian skull reflects changes in the masticatory apparatus. Within mammals, numerous cross-taxonomic dental convergences have been identified. Birds, with a few exceptions, do relatively little processing or mechanical breakdown of food with their cranial apparatus, but instead often specialize the skull and bill for obtaining food in situ. The cranial apparatus in birds often tracks this latter function. Snakes may often specialize the skull for very specific prey items; lizards appear to be more opportunistic, taking anything of an appropriate size with little or no processing. The teeth must merely be able to grab, hold, and in some cases subdue a prey item. In pursuing questions about adaptation and constraint of the trophic apparatus, the predictions on diversity must reflect the fundamental function within that group. "All things being equal" cannot be assumed when comparing organisms from widely differing taxa. Different rules of performance, adaptation, and constraint operate in each of the groups.

The problem in constructing generalizations about the determinants of the form of the trophic apparatus is further complicated because even within each group notable exceptions can be found to any generalization. Landry (1970) and others have noted numerous examples within the Rodentia where diets between relatively closely related species vary widely, with little or no dentitional differences. For example, Landry compares *Dipodomys* and *Microdipodops* and claims that "no overt structural difference" indicates that individuals of the former species seldom eat animal material while those of the latter species are often insectivorous. Carlton (1973) claims that in many New World cricetine rodents the digestive tract rather than masticatory systems reflects diet. In mammalian myrmecophages the major functional requirement appears to be fast consumption of items rather than mastication. Food processing often occurs via specialized tongue and palate structures or in muscularized stomachs. With this adaptation there is apparently a release in the selection on teeth; many mammalian myrmecophages have reduced or extremely variable tooth numbers (Redford 1987). Smith and Redford (1990) show that as the nine-banded armadillo, *Dasypus novemcinctus*, expands its range into North America it consumes a wide range of prey despite its morphological specializations for ant-eating and its limited diet in its original range (fig. 4.14). Bhattacharyya (1987) shows that three species of Indian birds with fly-catching behaviors and very similar diets possess very different bill and muscle morphology. Some lizards appear relatively specialized for a given diet, while other taxa with the same diet may appear completely unspecialized (Greene 1982). It is thus difficult to generalize about the determi-

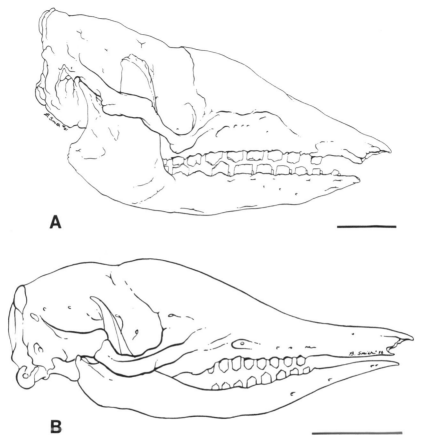

Fig. 4.14. The jaw apparatus of two genera of armadillos. A. *Euphractus sexcinctus.*
B. *Dasypus novemcinctus.* Note the reduced teeth, areas for jaw muscles, and moment
arms of the muscles in *Dasypus.* The condition in *Ephractus* is closer to the primitive
condition, and the reductions of the feeding apparatus in *Dasypus* are derived. These
derived morphological characteristics have evolved convergently in individuals
adapted for ant and termite eating from a number of mammalian orders. Scale bar in
both = 2 cm. Redrawn from Smith and Redford (1990).

nants of the form of the trophic apparatus within any single class, much
less across terrestrial vertebrates.

Finally, it is not easy to evaluate the significance of the differences
between groups. For example, it is meaningless to argue that mammals, by
virtue of their close tracking of the teeth to diet, have a better adapted
feeding apparatus than lizards. The alternative, that the lizard's feeding
apparatus is constrained, is no more satisfactory. The studies most suc-

cessful at demonstrating adaptation or constraint are those that have limited themselves to examining the bases of diversity within a group where the biological role of the feeding apparatus and the phylogenetic relations are known.

Adaptation and Constraint

One of the goals of this chapter was to discuss the relative contributions of adaptation and constraint in determining the form of the trophic apparatus. I have reviewed many representative papers on the adaptation of the feeding apparatus. Most studies place their analysis in a comparative or phylogenetic context, recognize the existence of limits to evolution, discuss multiple determinants of form, and seek to explain observed variability. These studies do not seek to demonstrate perfection. Admittedly, most fall short of some methodogical ideal. Most recognize the diversity of influences on form but few discuss these diverse influences in depth. Heritable variation and independence (in a genetic and epigenetic sense) of the features under consideration is assumed, generally with little supporting data. And virtually all merely infer, but do not demonstrate directly, a relation between morphology and performance or between performance and fitness. However, the generalization that most studies of morphological adaptation are Panglossian scenarios (Gould and Lewontin 1979) is simply incorrect.

Most morphologists perform their analyses with consideration of constraints due to mechanical limits, competing demands, and phylogenetic heritage. "A comparative anatomist is a scientist who believes that, notwithstanding what a species may have become, it can never escape from what it has been" (Beecher 1978). If constraints are not directly addressed it is largely because the focus of studies is the diversity that exists rather than morphologies that do not.

In the introduction, four categories of constraint were defined. One of the reasons constraint has proven to be a relatively nebulous explanation is that the different types of constraint are distinct in the levels on which they act, the types of processes they effect, and the way in which hypotheses of effect can be tested. At least two, physical (or mechanical) constraints and selective (or compromise) constraints, operate firmly within the bounds of typical adaptational studies. The operation of these constraints does not rely on particular biases in variation, but on the result of natural selection. Many scaling and allometric relations are of this type. These constraints operate not in opposition or in addition to the processes of adaptation via natural selection, but precisely because of these processes.

On the other hand, developmental and phylogenetic constraints are thought primarily to influence evolution largely in the production of biases in variation upon which selection may act. These constraints may therefore provide a directionality in evolution at a hierarchical level that is different from adaptation via natural selection (Alberch 1980). These biases may be fundamental (e.g., some patterns cannot be generated) or happenstance (e.g., one sort of variation is more likely to occur than another). The consequences of these extremes and the way in which these hypotheses are constructed and tested are different. In the former case, where it is hypothesized that some sorts of variation will not be produced because of the mechanisms of development, these mechanisms must be precisely understood and the hypotheses be based and tested within these mechanisms. A single exception falsifies the hypothesis. In the latter case, the hypothesis consists of "this is more likely than that to happen." It can be corroborated, but not falsified. How strongly it can be corroborated depends on the strength of the "more likely" statement. Such hypotheses of constraint are in fact very difficult to test. However, without specific hypotheses and explicit tests of the processes of constraint, constraint as an explanation is subject to the same criticism applied to rampant "adaptationism": untestable predictions, ad hoc hypotheses, and post hoc explanations.

Maynard Smith et al. (1985) discuss the use of the comparative method to demonstrate the operation of a developmental constraint: "More promising yet are comparative studies of two different taxa whose members have been exposed to a similar range of ecological conditions. Should one taxon show variants of a kind not shown by the other, it would be likely that the latter taxon was subject to some degree of developmental constraint" (p. 277). The degree to which such a test would be convincing would depend on the taxa compared and the form of the hypothesis of constraint. The mere observation that one taxon possesses variation absent in another is not sufficient evidence of constraint.

In the current context, the biological role of the trophic apparatus differs in the various groups of vertebrates discussed, and these differences influence the course of specialization to food type. Patterns of adaptation vary in different groups not only because of potential constraints, but because of different adaptive regimes. There is no reason to believe that carnivory, herbivory, frugivory, or insectivory is the same for snakes, birds, mammals, and lizards. In fact, it is probable that even within a vertebrate class different patterns exist. For example, insectivory generates very different "adaptive strategies" in large- and small-bodied mammals. In this case the comparative tests suggested by Maynard Smith et al. are not sufficient because to observe "variants of a kind not shown by the other" in one taxon and attribute the pattern to constraint may be an explanation for a phenomenon that does not exist. Different patterns of variation are to be expected. If constraint is proposed as an explanation for lack of any kind of expected variation, the concept loses its power. Without a more rigorous and narrow definition of constraint, be it phylogenetic, developmental, or mechanical, constraint takes on the role of being everything not demonstrably adaptive. This weakens the explanatory power and impact of an extremely significant concept.

Form is not determined by either adaptation or constraint. As is increasingly recognized, they are two sides of the same process. An adaptation may produce certain kinds of patterning in descendants. In some cases this patterning may lead to a process that actively constrains certain pathways in its descendants; in some cases it is a mere pattern just because evolution is happenstance. Sometimes this patterning may lead to specific new adaptive and selective regimes so that adaptive evolution in response to the same ecological conditions may take very different pathways in different organisms. The alternatives become particularly complex when taxa at very high levels are compared. Most biologists recognize the interaction of constraint and adaptation in a general sense, although few discuss this interaction specifically and rigorously. Such specific and rigorous studies are increasingly appearing and will eventually allow a thorough understanding of the interacting influences of adaptation and constraint in the determination of form.

ACKNOWLEDGMENTS

I thank C. T. Clark, D. Cundall, C. Gans, W. L. Hylander, W. M. Kier, D. McClearn, D. A. Pabst, A. D. Yoder, and the editors of the volume for comments on earlier drafts of this manuscript; B. Smith for drawing figures 1, 3, 7–11, and 14; and K. MacKay for general research assistance. The National Institute of Dental Research grant DEO 7351-03 provided support during the preparation of this review.

REFERENCES

Alberch, P. 1980. Ontogenesis and morphological diversification. American Zoologist 20: 653–667.

Albright, R. G., and E. M. Nelson. 1959a. Cranial kinetics of the generalized colubrid snake *Elaphe obsoleta quadrivittata*. I. Descriptive morphology. Journal of Morphology 105: 193–240.

———. 1959b. Cranial kinetics of the generalized colubrid snake *Elaphe obsoleta quadrivittata*. II. Functional morphology. Journal of Morphology 105: 241–292.

Alexander, R. McN. 1985. The ideal and the feasible: Physical constraints on evolution. Biological Journal of the Linnean Society 26: 345–358.

Alexander, R. McN., and A. G. Sinclair. 1987. Estimates of forces exerted by the jaw muscles of some reptiles. Journal of Zoology, London 213: 107–115.

Allin, E. F. 1975. Evolution of the mammalian middle ear. Journal of Morphology 147: 403–438.

Arnold, S. J. 1977. Polymorphism and geographic variation in the feeding behavior of the garter snake, *Thamnophis elegans*. Science 197: 676–678.

———. 1981a. Behavioral variation in natural populations. I. Phenotypic, genetic, and environmental correlations between chemoreceptive responses to prey in the garter snake, *Thamnophis elegans*. Evolution 35: 489–509.

———. 1981b. Behavioral variation in natural populations. II. The inheritance of a feeding response in crosses between geographic races of the garter snake, *Thamnophis elegans*. Evolution 35: 510–515.

———. 1983. Morphology, performance, and fitness. American Zoologist 23: 347–361.

Barghusen, H. R. 1968. The lower jaw of cynodonts (Reptilia, Therapsida) and the evolutionary origin of mammal-like jaw musculature. Postilla 116: 1–49.

Beecher, W. J. 1951. Adaptations for food-getting in the American Blackbirds. Auk 68: 411–441.

———. 1962. The biomechanics of the bird skull. Bulletin of the Chicago Academy of Science 11: 10–33.

———. 1978. Feeding adaptations and evolution in the starlings. Bulletin of the Chicago Academy of Science 11: 268–297.

Bhattacharyya, B. N. 1987. On the structural adaptations of the bill, skull-elements, tongue, and hyoid of some Indian insect-eating birds. Gegenbaurs Morphologisches Jahrbuch 133: 311–351.

Bock, W. J. 1960. The palatine process of the premaxilla in the Passeres. Bulletin of the Museum of Comparative Zoology 122: 361–488.

———. 1964. Kinetics of the avian skull. Journal of Morphology 114: 1–41.

———. 1966. An approach to the functional analysis of bill shape. Auk 83: 10–51.

Bock, W. J., and B. Kummer. 1968. The avian mandible as a structural girder. Journal of Biomechanics 1: 89–96.

Bock, W. J., and H. Morioka. 1971. Morphology and evolution of the ectethmoid-mandibular articulation in the Meliphagidae (Aves). Journal of Morphology 135: 13–50.

Boltt, R. E., and R. F. Ewer. 1964. The functional anatomy of the head of the puff adder, *Bitis arietans*. Journal of Morphology 113: 83–106.

Bowman, R. I. 1961. Morphological differentiation and adaptation in the Galapagos finches. University of California Publications in Zoology 58: 1–302.

———. 1963. Evolutionary patterns in Darwin's finches. Occasional Papers of the California Academy of Science 44: 107–140.

Bradley, O. C. 1903. The muscles of mastication and movements of the skull in Lacertilia. Zoologische Jahrbücher, Anatomie 18: 475–486.

Bramble, D. M. 1978. Origin of the mammalian feeding complex: Models and mechanisms. Paleobiology 4: 271–301.

Brown, J. H., and M. A. Bowers. 1985. Community organization in hummingbirds: Relationships between morphology and ecology. Auk 102: 251–269.

Buhler, P. 1981. Functional anatomy of the avian jaw apparatus. In *Form and*

Function in Birds, vol. 2, A. S. King and J. McLelland, eds. New York: Academic Press, pp. 439–468.

Burger, A. E. 1978. Functional anatomy of the feeding apparatus of four South African cormorants. Zoologica africana 13: 81–102.

Burghardt, G. M. 1970. Chemical perception in reptiles. In *Communication by Chemical Signals,* J. W. Johnston, D. G. Moulton, and A. Turk, eds. New York: Appleton-Century Crofts, pp. 241–308.

Burt, W. H. 1930. Adaptive modifications in the woodpeckers. University of California Publications in Zoology 32: 455–524.

Burton, P. J. K. 1974a. *Feeding and the Feeding Apparatus in Waders: A Study of Anatomy and Adaptations in the Charadrii.* London: British Museum (Natural History).

———. 1974b. Jaw and tongue features in Psittaciformes and other orders with special reference to the anatomy of the tooth-billed pigeon (*Didunculus strigirostris*). Journal of Zoology, London 174: 255–276.

———. 1984. Anatomy and evolution of the feeding apparatus in the avian orders Coraciiformes and Piciformes. Bulletin of the British Museum (Natural History) 47: 331–443.

Capel-Williams, G., and D. Pratten. 1978. The diet of adult and juvenile *Agama bibroni* (Reptilia: Lacertae) and a study of the jaw mechanisms in the two age groups. Journal of Zoology, London 185: 309–318.

Carlton, M. D. 1973. A survey of gross stomach morphology in New World Cricetinae (Rodentia, Muroidea), with comments on functional interpretations. Miscellaneous Publications of the Museum of Zoology, University of Michigan 146: 1–43.

Carroll, R. L. 1976. The origin of lizards. In *Problems in Vertebrate Evolution* (Linnean Society Symposium Series no. 4), S. M. Andrews, R. S. Miles, and A. D. Walker, eds. London: Academic Press, pp. 359–396.

Clutton-Brock, T. H., and P. H. Harvey. 1979. Comparison and adaptation. Proceedings of the Royal Society of London B 205: 547–565.

Condon, K. 1987. A kinematic analysis of mesokinesis in the Nile monitor (*Varanus niloticus*). Journal of Experimental Biology 47: 73–87.

Cowles, R. B. 1930. The life history of *Varanus niloticus* (Linnaeus) as observed in Natal South Africa. Journal of Entomology and Zoology 22: 1–31.

Crompton, A. W. 1971. The origin of the tribosphenic molar. In *Early Mammals,* D. M. Kermack and K. A. Kermack, eds. Zoological Journal of the Linnean Society (suppl. 1). London: Academic Press, pp. 65–87.

Crompton, A. W., and K. Hiiemae. 1970. Molar occlusion and mandibular movements during occlusion in the American opossum, *Didelphis marsupialis.* Zoological Journal of the Linnean Society 49: 21–47.

Crompton, A. W., and W. L. Hylander. 1986. Changes in mandibular function following the acquisition of a dentary-squamosal jaw articulation. In *The Ecology and Biology of Mammal-like Reptiles,* N. Hotton, P. MacLean, J. Roth, and E. Roth, eds. Washington, D.C.: Smithsonian Institution Press, pp. 263–287.

Crompton, A. W., and Z. Kielan-Jaworowska. 1978. Molar structure and occlusion in Cretaceous therian mammals. In *Development, Function, and Evolution of Teeth,* P. M. Butler and K. A. Joyse, eds. New York: Academic Press, pp. 249–287.

Crompton, A. W., and P. Parker. 1978. Evolution of the mammalian masticatory apparatus. American Scientist 66: 192–201.

Crompton, A. W., A. J. Thexton, P. Parker, and K. Hiiemae. 1977. The activity of the jaw and hyoid musculature in the Virginian opossum, *Didelphis virginiana.* In *The Biology of Marsupials,* B. Stonehouse and D. Gilmore, eds. New York: Macmillan Press, pp. 287–305.

Cundall, D. 1983. Activity of head muscles during feeding by snakes: A comparative study. American Zoologist 23: 383–396.

Cundall, D., and Gans, C. 1979. Feeding in water snakes: An electromyographic study. Journal of Experimental Zoology 209: 189–208.

Dalrymple, G. H. 1979. On the jaw mechanism of the snail-crushing lizards, *Dracaena* Daudin 1802 (Reptilia, Lacertilia, Teiidae). Journal of Herpetology 13: 303–311.

Davis, D. D. 1961. Origin of the mammalian feeding mechanism. American Zoologist 1: 229–234.

———. 1964. The Giant Panda: A morphological study of evolutionary mechanisms. Fieldiana: Zoology, Memoirs 3: 5–339.

Dessem, D. 1985. Ontogenetic changes in the dentition and diet of *Tupinambis* (Lacertilia: Teiidae). Copeia: 245–247.

De Vree, F., and C. Gans 1976. Mastication in pygmy goats (*Capra hircus*). Annales de la Société royale zoologique de Belgique 105: 255–306.

Ditmars, R. L. 1907. *The Reptile Book.* New York: Doubleday, Page and Co.

Dullemeijer, P. 1959. A comparative functional-anatomical study of the heads of some Viperidae. Gegenbaurs Morphologisches Jahrbuch 99: 881–985.

———. 1968. Some methodology problems in a holistic approach to functional morphology. Acta biotheoretica 18: 203–214.

———. 1974. *Concepts and Approaches in Animal Morphology.* Assen, The Netherlands: Van Gorcum and Co.

Dullemeijer, P., and C. D. N. Barel. 1976. Functional morphology and evolution. In *Major Patterns in Vertebrate Evolution,* M. K. Hecht, P. C. Goody, and B. M. Hecht, eds. New York: Plenum Press, pp. 83–117.

Dullemeijer, P., and G. D. E. Povel. 1972. The construction for feeding in rattlesnakes. Zoologische mededelingen 47: 561–578.

Edmund, A. G. 1969. Dentition. In *Biology of the Reptilia,* vol. 1, C. Gans, A. d'A. Bellairs, T. S. Parsons, eds. New York: Academic Press, pp. 117–200.

Emerson, S. B., and L. Radinsky. 1980. Functional analysis of sabertooth cranial morphology. Paleobiology 6: 295–312.

Estes, R., and E. E. Williams. 1984. Ontogenetic variation in the molariform teeth of lizards. Journal of Vertebrate Paleontology 4: 96–107.

Feinsinger, P., and R. K. Colwell. 1978. Community organization among neotropical nectar-feeding birds. American Zoologist 18: 779–795.

Frazzetta, T. H. 1962. A functional consideration of cranial kinesis in lizards. Journal of Morphology 111: 287–319.

————. 1966. Studies on the morphology and function of the skull in the Boidae (Serpentes). Part II. Morphology and function of the jaw apparatus in *Python sebae* and *Python molurus*. Journal of Morphology 118: 217–296.

————. 1983. Adaptation and function of cranial kinesis in reptiles: A time-motion analysis of feeding in alligator lizards. In *Advances in Herpetology and Evolutionary Biology*, A. Rhodin and K. Miyata, eds. Cambridge: Museum of Comparative Zoology, Harvard University, pp. 222–244.

————. 1986. The origin of amphikinesis in lizards: A problem in functional morphology and the evolution of adaptive systems. In *Evolutionary Biology*, vol. 20, M. K. Hecht, B. Wallace, and G. T. Prance, eds. New York: Plenum Publishing, pp. 419–461.

Gans, C. 1952. The functional morphology of the egg-eating adaptations in the snake genus *Dasypeltis*. Zoologica 37 (4): 209–244.

————. 1961. The feeding mechanism of snakes and its possible evolution. American Zoologist 1: 217–227.

————. 1968. Relative success of divergent pathways in amphisbaenian specialization. American Naturalist 102: 345–362.

————. 1974. *Biomechanics: An Approach to Vertebrate Biology*. Philadelphia: J. B. Lippincott, Co.

————. 1978. Reptilian venoms: Some evolutionary considerations. In *Biology of the Reptilia*, vol 8, C. Gans and K. A. Gans, eds. New York: Academic Press, pp. 1–42.

————. 1983. Snake feeding strategies and adaptations—conclusions and prognosis. American Zoologist 23: 455–460.

————. 1985. Differences and similarities: Comparative methods in mastication. American Zoologist 25: 291–301.

————. 1988. Adaptation and the form-function relation. American Zoologist 28: 681–697.

Gans, C., and F. De Vree. 1987. Kinetic movements in the skull of adult *Trachydosaurus rugosus*. Anatomia, Histologia, Embryologia 16: 206–209.

Gans, C., F. De Vree, and D. Carrier. 1985. Usage pattern of the complex masticatory muscles in the shingleback lizard, *Trachydosaurus rugosus:* A model for muscle placement. American Journal of Anatomy 173: 219–240.

Gomes, N. 1974. Anatomie comparée de la musculature trigéminale des lacertiliens. Mémoires du Muséum national d'histoire naturelle, ser. A, Zoologie 90: 1–107.

Gomes, N., and J. P. Gasc. 1973. Étude biomécanique du movement de fermeture de la mandibule chez *Ophisaurus apodus*. Papeis avulsos de zoologia 27: 1–25.

Gorniak, G. C., and C. Gans. 1980. Quantitative assay of electromyograms during mastication in domestic cats (*Felis catus*). Journal of Morphology 163: 253–281.

Gould, S. J. 1975. On the scaling of tooth size in mammals. American Zoologist 15: 351–362.

————. 1980. The evolutionary biology of constraint. Daedalus 109: 39–52.

Gould, S. J., and Lewontin, R. C. 1979. The spandrels of San Marco and the

Panglossian paradigm: A critique of the adaptationist programme. Proceedings of the Royal Society of London B 205: 581–598.

Greaves, W. S. 1974. Functional implications of mammalian jaw joint position. Forma et Functio 7: 363–376.

———. 1978. The jaw lever system in ungulates: A new model. Journal of Zoology, London 184: 271–285.

———. 1980. The mammalian jaw mechanism—The high glenoid cavity. American Naturalist 116: 432–440.

———. 1982. A mechanical limitation on the position of the jaw muscles of mammals: The one third rule. Journal of Mammalogy 63: 261–266.

———. 1983. A functional analysis of carnassial biting. Biological Journal of the Linnean Society 20: 353–363.

———. 1985. The generalized carnivore jaw. Zoological Journal of the Linnean Society 85: 267–274.

Greene, H. W. 1982. Dietary and phenotypic diversity in lizards: Why are some organisms specialized? In Environmental Adaptation and Evolution, D. Mossakowski and G. Roth, eds. Stuttgart: Gustav Fischer, pp. 107–128.

———. 1983. Dietary correlates of the origin and radiation of snakes. American Zoologist 23: 431–441.

———. 1986. Diet and arboreality in the emerald monitor, Varanus prasinus, with comments on the study of adaptation. Fieldiana: Zoology 31: 1–12.

Haas, G. 1973. Muscles of the jaws and associated structures in the Rhynchocephalia and Squamata. In Biology of the Reptilia, vol. 4, C. Gans and T. Parsons, eds. New York: Academic Press, pp. 285–490.

Herrera, C. M. 1978. Individual dietary differences associated with morphological variation in robins Erithacus rubecula. Ibis 120: 542–545.

Herring, S. W. 1976. The dynamics of mastication in pigs. Archives of Oral Biology 21: 473–480.

Herring, S. W., and S. E. Herring. 1974. The superficial masseter and gape in mammals. American Naturalist 108: 561–576.

Herring, S. W., and R. P. Scapino. 1973. Physiology of feeding in miniature pigs. Journal of Morphology 141: 427–460.

Hespenheide, H. A. 1973. Ecological inferences from morphological data. Annual review of Ecology and Systematics 4: 213–229.

Hiiemae, K. M. 1978. Mammalian mastication: A review of the activity of the jaw muscles and the movements they produce in chewing. In Development, Function, and Evolution of Teeth, P. M. Butler and K. A. Joyse, eds. New York: Academic Press, pp. 359–398.

Hofer, H. 1960. Vergleichende untersuchugen am Schadel von Tupinambis und Varanus mit Besonderer Berucksichtigung ihrer Kinetik. Gegenbaurs Morphologisches Jahrbuch 100: 706–746.

Hotton, N. 1955. A survey of adaptive relationships of dentition to diet in the North American Iguanidae. American Midland Naturalist 53: 88–114.

Hulsman, K. 1981. Width of gape as a determinant of size of prey eaten by terns. Emu 81: 29–32.

Hylander. W. L. 1975. Incisor size and diet in anthropoids with special reference to Cercopithecidae. Science 189: 1095–1098.

————. 1979. The functional significance of Primate mandibular form. Journal of Morphology 160: 223–240.

————. 1984. Stress and strain in the mandibular symphysis of primates: A test of competing hypotheses. American Journal of Physical Anthropology 64: 1–46.

————. 1985. Mandibular function and biomechanical stress and scaling. American Zoologist 25: 315–330.

Impey, O. R. 1967. Functional aspects of cranial kinetism in the Lacertilia. Ph.D. diss. Oxford University.

Iordansky, N. N. 1966. Cranial kinesis in lizards: Contribution to the problem of the adaptive significance of skull kinesis. Zoologicheskii zhurnal 45: 1398–1410. Translation through Smithsonian Herpetological Information services.

————. 1970. Structure and biomechanical analysis of functions of the jaw muscles in the lizards. Anatomical Anzeiger 127: 383–413.

Jackson, H. D. 1985. Mouth size in *Macrodipteryx* and other African nightjars. Bulletin of the British Ornithological Club 105: 51–54.

Janis, C. M. 1979. Mastication in the hyrax and its relevance to ungulate dental evolution. Paleobiology 5: 50–59.

Jenkin, P. M. 1957. The filter-feeding and food of flamingoes (Phoenicopteri). Philosophical Transactions of the Royal Society of London B 240: 401–493.

Kallen, F. C., and C. Gans. 1972. Mastication in the little brown bat, *Myotis lucifugus*. Journal of Morphology 136: 385–420.

Kardong, K. V. 1974. Kinesis of the jaw apparatus during the strike in the cottonmouth snake, *Agkistrodon piscivorus*. Forma et Functio 7: 327–354.

————. 1977. Kinesis of the jaw apparatus during swallowing in the cottonmouth snake, *Agkistrodon piscivorus*. Copeia: 338–348.

————. 1979. "Protovipers" and the evolution of snake fangs. Evolution 33: 433–443.

————. 1980. Evolutionary patterns in advanced snakes. American Zoologist 20: 269–282.

Karr, J. R., and F. C. James. 1975. Ecomorphological configurations and convergent evolution. In *Ecology and Evolution of Communities*, M. L. Cody and J. M. Diamond, eds. Cambridge, Mass.: Belknap Press, pp. 258–291.

Kay, R. F. 1975. The functional adaptations of primate molar teeth. American Journal of Physical Anthropology 43: 195–216.

————. 1978. Molar structure and diet in extant Cercopithecidae. In *Development, Function, and Evolution of Teeth*, P. M. Butler and K. A. Joyse, eds. New York: Academic Press, pp. 309–339.

————. 1984. On the use of anatomical features to infer foraging behavior in extinct primates. In *Adaptations for Foraging in Nonhuman Primates*, R. S. Rodman and J. Cant, eds. New York: Columbia University Press, pp. 21–53.

Kay, R. F., and M. Cartmill. 1977. Cranial morphology and adaptations of *Palaechthon nacimienti* and other paromomyidae (Plesiadapoidea, ? Primates), with a description of a new genus and species. Journal of Human Evolution 6: 19–53.

Kay, R. F., and W. L. Hylander. 1978. The dental structure of mammalian folivores with special reference to Primates and Phalangeroidea. In *The Ecology of Ar-*

boreal Folivores, G. Montgomery, ed. Washington, D.C.: Smithsonian Institution Press, pp. 173–191.

Kay, R. F., and W. S. Sheine. 1979. On the relationship between chitin particle size and digestibility in the primate *Galago senegalensis.* American Journal of Physical Anthropology 50: 301–308.

Kochva, E., O. Nakar, and M. Ovadia. 1983. Venom toxins: Plausible evolution from digestive enzymes. American Zoologist 23: 427–430.

Krebs, U. 1979. Der Dumeril-Waran (*Varanus dumerilii*): Ein spezialisierter Krabbenfresser? (Reptilia, Sauria, Varanidae). Salamandra 15: 146–157.

Lakjer, T. 1926. *Studien uber die Trigeminus versorgte Kaumuskulatur der Sauropsiden.* Kopenhagen: C. A. Rietzel.

Landry, S. O. 1970. The Rodentia as omnivores. Quarterly Review of Biology 45: 351–372.

Lauder, G. B. 1981. Form and function: Structural analysis in evolutionary morphology. Paleobiology 7: 430–442.

Lederer, R. J. 1975. Bill size, food size, and jaw forces of insectivorous birds. Auk 92: 385–387.

Liem, K. F. 1973. Evolutionary strategies and morphological innovations: Cichlid pharyngeal jaws. Systematic Zoology 22: 425–441.

————. 1978. Modulatory multiplicity in the functional repertoire of the feeding mechanism in cichlid fishes. Journal of Morphology 158: 323–360.

Lombard, R. E., and D. B. Wake. 1976. Tongue evolution in lungless salamanders, Family Plethodontidae. I. Introduction, theory, and a general model of dynamics. Journal of Morphology 148: 265–286.

————. 1977. Tongue evolution in the lungless salamanders, Family Plethodontidae. II. Function and evolutionary diversity. Journal of Morphology 153: 39–80.

Lonnberg, E. 1903. On the adaptations to molluscivorous diet in *Varanus niloticus.* Arkiv für Zoologi 1: 67–83.

Lucas, P. W., and D. A. Luke 1984. Chewing it over: Basic principles of food breakdown. In *Food Acquisition and Processing in Primates,* D. A. Chivers, B. A. Wood, and A. Bilsborough, eds. New York: Plenum Press, pp. 283–301.

MacLean, W. P. 1974. Feeding and locomotor mechanisms of teiid lizards: Functional morphology and evolution. Papeis avulsos de zoologia 27: 179–213.

Maier, W. 1984. Tooth morphology and dietary specialization. In *Food Acquisition and Processing in Primates,* D. A. Chivers, B. A. Woods, and A. Bilsborough, eds. New York: Plenum Press, pp. 303–330.

Maynard Smith, J., R. Burian, S. Kauffman, P. Alberch, J. Campbell, B. Goodwin, R. Lande, D. Raup, and L. Wolpert. 1985. Developmental constraints and evolution. Quarterly Review of Biology 60: 265–287.

Maynard Smith, J., and R. J. G. Savage. 1959. The mechanics of mammalian jaws. School Science Review, London 141: 289–301.

Mayr, E. 1983. How to carry out the adaptationist program? American Naturalist 121: 324–334.

Montanucci, R. R. 1968. Comparative dentition in four iguanid lizards. Herpetologica 24: 305–315.

Newton, I. 1967. The adaptive radiation and feeding ecology of some British finches. Ibis 109: 33–98.

Novacek, M. 1993. Patterns of diversity in the mammalian skull. In *The Vertebrate Skull*, vol. 2, J. Hanken and B. K. Hall, eds. Chicago: University of Chicago Press.

Oron, U., and A. W. Crompton. 1985. A cineradiographic and electromyographic study of mastication in *Tenrec ecaudatus*. Journal of Morphology 185: 155–182.

Ostrom, J. H. 1963. Further comments on herbivorous lizards. Evolution 17: 368–369.

Owre, O. T. 1967. Adaptations for locomotion and feeding in the anhinga and the double-crested cormorant. Ornithological Monographs 6: 1–138.

Parker, H. W., and A. G. C. Grandison. 1977. *Snakes*. Ithaca, N.Y.: Cornell University Press.

Patchell, F. C., and R. Shine. 1986a. Feeding mechanisms in pygopodid lizards: How can *Lialis* swallow such large prey? Journal of Herpetology 20: 59–64.

———. 1986b. Hinged teeth for hard-bodied prey: A case of convergent evolution between snakes and legless lizards. Journal of Zoology, London 208: 269–275.

Pough, F. H. 1973. Lizard energetics and diet. Ecology 54: 837–844.

———. 1983. Feeding mechanisms, body size, and the ecology and evolution of snakes. American Zoologist 23: 339–342.

Pough, F. H., and J. D. Groves. 1983. Specialization of the body form and food habits of snakes. American Zoologist 23: 443–454.

Radinsky, L. B. 1981a. Evolution of skull shape in carnivores. 1. Representative modern carnivores. Biological Journal of the Linnean Society 15: 369–388.

———. 1981b. Evolution of skull shape in carnivores. 2. Additional modern carnivores. Biological Journal of the Linnean Society 16: 337–355.

———. 1982. Evolution of skull shape in carnivores. 3. The origin and early radiation of the modern carnivore families. Paleobiology 8: 177–195.

———. 1985. Patterns in the evolution of ungulate jaw shape. American Zoologist 25: 303–314.

Redford, K. H. 1987. Ants and termites as food: Patterns of mammalian myrmecophagy. Current Mammalogy 1: 349–399.

Rensberger, J. M. 1973. An occlusion model for mastication and dental wear in herbivorous mammals. Journal of Paleontology 47: 515–528.

———. 1975. Function in the cheek tooth evolution of some hypsodont geomyoid rodents. Journal of Paleontology 49: 10–22.

———. 1986. Early chewing mechanisms in mammalian herbivores. Paleobiology 12: 474–494.

Rensberger, J. M., A. Forsten, and M. Fortelius. 1984. Functional evolution of the cheek tooth pattern and chewing direction in Tertiary horses. Paleobiology 10: 439–452.

Richards, L. P., and W. J. Bock. 1973. Functional anatomy and the adaptive evolution of the feeding apparatus in the Hawaiian honeycreeper genus *Loxops* (Drepanididae). Ornithological Monographs 15: 1–173.

Rieppel, O. 1978a. The phylogeny of cranial kinesis in lower vertebrates, with special reference to the Lacertilia. Neues Jahrbuch für Geologie und Palaeontologie 156: 353–370.

———. 1978b. Streptostyly and muscle function in lizards. Experientia 34: 776–777.

———. 1979. A functional interpretation of the varanid dentition (Reptilia, Lacertilia, Varanidae). Gegenbaurs Morphologisches Jahrbuch 125: 797–817.

———. 1980. The evolution of the ophidian feeding system. Zoologische Jahrbücher 103: 551–564.

———. 1993. Patterns of diversity in the reptilian skull. In The Skull, vol. 2, J. Hanken and B. K. Hall, eds. Chicago: University of Chicago Press.

Rieppel, O., and L. Labhardt. 1979. Mandibular mechanics in Varanus niloticus (Reptilia: Lacertilia). Herpetologica 35: 158–163.

Robinson, P. L. 1967. The evolution of the Lacertilia: Problèmes actuels de paleontologie (évolution des vertébrés). CNRS, Paris: 395–407.

———. 1973. A problematic reptile from the British upper Trias. Journal of the Geological Society, London 129: 457–479.

Romer, A. S. 1956. Osteology of the Reptiles. Chicago: University of Chicago Press.

Ruben J. A. 1977a. Morphological correlates of predatory modes in coachwhip (Masticophis flagellum) and rosy boa (Lichanura roseofusca). Herpetologica 33: 1–6.

———. 1977b. Some correlates of cranial and cervical morphology with predatory modes in snakes. Journal of Morphology 152: 89–100.

Savitzky, A. H. 1980. The role of venom delivery strategies in snake evolution. Evolution 34: 1194–1204.

———. 1981. Hinged teeth in snakes: An adaptation for swallowing hard-bodied prey. Science 212: 346–348.

———. 1983. Coadapted character complexes among snakes: Fossoriality, piscivory, and durophagy. American Zoologist 23: 397–409.

Scapino, R. P. 1972. Adaptive radiation of mammalian jaws. In Morphology of the Maxillo-Mandibular Apparatus, G. H. Schumacher, ed. Leipzig: G. Thieme, for the International Congress of Anatomy, pp. 33–39.

Schwenk, K. 1984. Evolutionary morphology of the lepidosaur tongue. Ph.D. diss. Berkeley: University of California, 174 pp.

———. 1988. Comparative morphology of the lepidosaur tongue and its relevance to squamate phylogeny. In The Phylogenetic Relationships of the Lizard Families: Essays Commemorating Charles L. Camp, R. Estes and G. Pregill, eds. Palo Alto: Stanford University Press, pp. 569–598.

Sheine, W. S., and R. F. Kay. 1982. A model for comparison of masticatory effectiveness in primates. Journal of Morphology 172: 139–149.

Simonetta, A. M. 1960. On the mechanical implications of the avian skull and their bearing on the evolution and classification of birds. Quarterly Review of Biology 35: 206–220.

Smith, K. K. 1980a. The functional morphology of feeding in lizards. Ph.D. diss., Harvard University.

———. 1980b. Mechanical significance of streptostyly in lizards. Nature 283: 778–779.

———. 1982. An electromyographic study of the function of the jaw adducting muscles in *Varanus exanthematicus*. Journal of Morphology 173: 137–158.

———. 1984. The use of the tongue and hyoid apparatus during feeding in lizards (*Ctenosaura similis* and *Tupinambis nigropunctatus*). Journal of Zoology, London 202: 115–143.

———. 1986. Morphology and function of the tongue and hyoid apparatus in *Varanus* (Varanidae, Lacertilia). Journal of Morphology 187: 261–287.

———. 1992. The evolution of the mammalian pharynx. Zoological Journal of the Linnean Society 104: 313–349.

Smith, K. K., and W. L. Hylander. 1985. Strain gage measurement of mesokinetic movement in *Varanus exanthematicus*. Journal of Experimental Biology 114: 53–70.

Smith, K. K., and K. H. Redford. 1990. The anatomy and function of the feeding apparatus in two armadillos (Dasypodidae): Anatomy is not destiny. Journal of Zoology, London 222: 27–47.

Sokol, O. M. 1965. Herbivory in lizards. Evolution 21: 192–194.

Spring, L. W. 1965. Climbing and pecking adaptations in some North American woodpeckers. Condor 67: 457–488.

Szarski, H. 1962. Some remarks on herbivorous lizards. Evolution 16: 529.

Throckmorton, G. S. 1976. Oral food processing in two herbivorous lizards, *Iguana iguana* and *Uromastix aegyptius*. Journal of Morphology 148: 363–390.

Throckmorton, G. S., and L. K. Clarke. 1981. Intracranial joint movements in the agamid lizard *Amphibolurus barbatus*. Journal of Experimental Zoology 216: 25–35.

Turnbull, W. D. 1970. Mammalian masticatory apparatus. Field Museum of Natural History, Fieldiana: Geology 18: 149–356.

Vermeij, G. J. 1973. Adaptation, versatility, and evolution. Systematic Zoology 22: 466–477.

Versluys, J. 1910. Streptostyly bei Dinosaurien, nebst Bemekungen uber die verwandschaft der Vogel und Dinosaurier. Zoologische Jahrbücher, Anatomie 30: 177–260.

———. 1912. Das Streptostylie-problem und die Berwegungen im Schadel bei Sauropsiden. Zoologische Jahrbücher 15 (suppl.): 545–714.

Weijs, W. 1980. Biomechanical models and the analysis of form: A study of the mammalian masticatory apparatus. American Zoologist 20: 707–719.

Weijs, W., and R. Dantuma. 1981. Functional anatomy of the masticatory apparatus in the rabbit (*Oryctolagus cuniculus* L.). Netherlands Journal of Zoology 31: 99–147.

Werdelin, L. 1983. Morphological patterns in the skulls of cats. Biological Journal of the Linnean Society 19: 375–391.

———. 1986. Comparison of skull shape in marsupial and placental carnivores. Australian Journal of Zoology 34: 109–117.

———. 1987. Jaw geometry and molar morphology in marsupial carnivores:

Analysis of a constraint and its macroevolutionary consequences. Paleobiology 13: 342–350.

Wheelwright, N. T. 1985. Fruit size, gape width, and the diets of fruit-eating birds. Ecology 66: 808–818.

Wolff-Exalto, A. de. 1951. On differences in the lower jaw of animalivorous and herbivorous mammals. Proceedings of Koninklijke Nederlandse Akademie van Wentenschappen, ser. C 54: 237–246; 405–410.

Zusi, R. 1962. Structural adaptations of the head and neck in the black skimmer *Rynchops nigra*. Publications of the Nuttall Ornithological Club 3: 1–101.

———. 1967. The role of the depressor mandibulae muscle in kinesis of the avian skull. Proceedings of the United States National Museum 123: 1–28.

———. 1993. Patterns of diversity in the avian skull. In *The Vertebrate Skull*, vol. 2, J. Hanken and B. K. Hall, eds. Chicago: University of Chicago Press.

Zweers, G. A. 1974. Structure, movement, and myography of the feeding apparatus of the mallard (*Anas platyrhynchos*): A study in functional anatomy. Netherlands Journal of Zoology 24: 323–467.

———. 1982. The feeding system of the pigeon (*Columba livia* L.). Advances in Anatomy, Embryology, and Cell Biology 73: 1–104.

5

The Skull as a Locomotor Organ

MARVALEE H. WAKE

THE CONCEPT OF THE SKULL as a locomotor organ is, at best, merely an allusion in most studies of vertebrate locomotion. When mentioned, it is usually in the context of aberrant digging modes or as a correlate of fossoriality, and even those locomotor patterns usually utilize undulatory body locomotion or limb movements as effectors. Yet, there are at least anecdotal reports of some members of all vertebrate classes using their heads as the primary effectors of locomotion, and in ways other than burrowing.

There are three broad areas of skull use in locomotion: (1) the skull as a tool, perhaps involved in locomotion or other activities, but for which movement is initiated and controlled by other parts of the body; (2) the skull, or head, as the bearer of the special sensory organs, other receptors, their neural pathways, and their organizing and integrating center, the brain; and (3) the head as a primary effector of locomotion.

First, the skull is a tool in many situations. It is a wedge driven in burrowing, a shovel to move rocks or sand during nest-building, a feeding probe, a sensory probe, and a tool for molding the form of burrows and similar structures—and these are but a few examples. Further, skull structures may also serve as holdfast organs. Two examples are sucking devices (some discussed herein) and the opercular spines of the dreaded candiru, an Amazonian catfish that follows water currents generated by the gills, and anchors with its spines in the gill cavities of other catfishes which it parasitizes. It occasionally follows urinary water currents, and lodges in the urethras of unprotected persons (Norman 1931). However, for all such examples, locomotion per se is driven by other parts of the body, and skull involvement is often part of an activity differently directed but effected in part by locomotor mechanics. Secondly, that product of cephalization, the head, with its concentration of sensory components, is certainly important to locomotion, but as a mediator, not as an effector in the context I will emphasize. I will consider some of the modifications of sensory structures

197

that appear to be correlated with use of the skull in locomotion in order to try to distinguish nonmotor adaptations for fossoriality from those for locomotion per se. To provide consistency, I will limit consideration of the skull as a locomotor organ to the use of the skull, or components of it, and its associated musculature and integument, as the primary initiator and/or maintainer of locomotion, i.e., the active effector. The central theme, then, of this chapter is an examination of the structure and function of skulls as applied to a diversity of kinds of locomotion.

The concept of the skull as a locomotor organ raises several questions. Are modifications of the skull of species in which it is a primary effector of locomotion correlated with any measures of increased effectiveness of locomotion? Are modifications apparently used in locomotion the products of selection primarily for locomotor efficiency, or are they correlates of a fossorial way of life that were later co-opted for locomotion in such habitats? Why are certain members of each vertebrate group that lack skull modifications apparently as effective in skull-directed locomotion as those that have apparent "adaptations" for such locomotion? What are the mechanics of skull-initiated locomotion in various groups? What is the effect of the air, water, or terrestrial medium on such modes of locomotion? Are there any generalizations that seem to obtain for the diverse vertebrates that use the skull as a locomotor organ?

A search of the literature reveals—not much. Most of the reports of skull/head use in locomotion are short and anecdotal. There are few complete observational studies, fewer that correlate morphology with activity, still fewer functional or physiological studies, and fewer yet quantitative analyses of the use of the head in locomotion. At one level, however, the reason for this paucity is clear—most of these animals burrow, so they disappear from sight during most of the action. At another, the few rigorous studies available utilize techniques that could be applied with little modification to other organisms. This would allow studies of the head in locomotion within lineages, among taxa with apparently similar adaptations, and broadly among vertebrates in different habitats. Such studies are requisite to understanding diversity and similarity of locomotor function, and therefore would provide a perspective on the nature of adaptation, and its absence, in locomotor patterns.

I take a case-study approach to examination of the skull as a locomotor organ, citing examples of both the anecdotal and the more extensively functional approaches. The examples are specifically chosen, in order to focus on problems rather than to list taxa; they are not an exhaustive survey. I present these in a broadly phylogenetic framework by major groups, so that within-group as well as broader comparisons can be made. I consider structure-function correlations, but the limited data available reveal the need for more extensive investigations of these questions. Finally, I suggest research areas and problem-oriented approaches to skull morphology that would provide insight into structure-function relationships and patterns of evolution.

USE OF THE HEAD FOR LOCOMOTION BY AQUATIC ANIMALS

The head, or parts of it, initiates or maintains locomotion in a diversity of aquatic situations. These include burrowing in the substrate, travel by use of suckers, and jet propulsion.

Burrowing

Burrowing is the most common of these behaviors. A phylogenetic and functional comparison is provided by examination of burrowing in bony fishes; in cyclostomes; in cephalochordates, the vertebrate sister-group; and in the probable sister-group of chordates, the hemichordates. I shall consider these in reverse order, beginning with hemichordates, in order to draw some functional correlates with vertebrates.

Hemichordates do not have a skull, and questionably have a head. However, they combine a number of "invertebrate" features of anatomy (basically a nerve net and a fluid skeleton) with some chordate features (the nerve net sequestered in part in a dorsal nerve cord in the proboscis, collar, and trunk and a ventral cord in the trunk, an anterior "mouth" and gills; i.e., primitive cephalization). The anterior proboscis functions in feeding and is the primary locomotor organ. I consider it at least analogous to a specialized part of a head, and its fluid skeleton analogous to skull components. Burrowing has been described by Ritter (1902) and Knight-Jones (1952) and others in *Saccoglossus* and *Ptychodera,* all summarized in Trueman and Ansell (1969). The proboscis tip is placed on the sand substrate, and ciliary action pulls a stream of sand over the proboscis to form a cavity in the sand. The proboscis then elongates, and the trunk and collar form an anchor at the substrate surface. The longitudinal muscles of the proboscis then contract, forming a traveling bulge that acts as a terminal anchor. The proboscis thrusts forward again before the peristaltic longitudinal wave reaches the base of the proboscis, and up to three bulges have been noted on the proboscis. The bulges are thought to act as holdfasts so that the body is drawn into the substrate. After a succession of penetrative thrusts, undulatory body movements alternate with thrusts of the proboscis to drive the animal into the substrate. This "retrograde wave" motion is considered similar to that of earthworms by Trueman and Ansell (1969), and is markedly similar to the pattern of burrowing seen in uropeltid snakes. The animals form burrows in which the proboscis can be exposed to the water current, often through a second burrow opening.

In a largely ecological study of the responses of the cephalochordate *Branchiostoma* (amphioxus) to substrate conditions, salinity gradients, and temperature, Webb and Hill (1958) also reported on burrowing behavior. They performed rigorous experiments in the laboratory to assess burrowing behavior in substrates of different particle sizes and structured with and without organic growth. Young larvae are bottom dwellers, later larvae are planktonic, and metamorphs and adults are relatively sedentary burrowers. Webb and Hill noted that different positions are taken on different substrates, and at different ages. They concluded that amphioxus select particle sizes in which they can stay buried as long as possible, and in which a good water flow among particles can be maintained, to meet both feeding and metabolic demand. Therefore, adults prefer mixed or coarse sand; young larvae can tolerate mud better than adults. Amphioxus, like hemichordates, assume a position in finer substances so that the oral region emerges from the burrow into the water current. Webb and Hill reviewed the debate whether amphioxus burrow head or tail first, and concluded, based on the literature and especially their own observations, that head-first burrowing is virtually always the case. However, Webb (1973) determined from high-speed cine analysis that amphioxus can swim and burrow either head or tail first, and that undulatory movement is generated at whichever is the leading end. Webb carefully analyzed the role of the notochord in controlling differential rigidity and flexion of the body axis to produce undulatory amplitude. It is clear that both swimming and burrowing are responses to stimuli. Webb and Hill (1958) suggested that burrowing is due to a tactile response, and since they thought burrowing to be head-first, they indicate that the head, in a sense, initiates burrowing locomotion because it effects an anterior contact with the substrate. On the other hand, Webb (1973) considered locomotion to be a response to light. Light is sensed by the eye cups of Hesse, located in pairs in the nerve cord. These are largely anterior in larvae, but at metamorphosis increase in number and occur the entire length of the nerve cord. In adults there are large numbers of eye cups anteriorly, a lesser concentration in the tail, and few in midbody. Webb suggests that the concentrations of light-sensitive organs are important in initiating activity at either end of the animal, and that therefore larvae may not be capable of tail-first locomotion.

Cyclostomes, both hagfish and lampreys, burrow. However, it seems apparent from diverse reports (Foss 1963, 1968; Strahan 1963) that hagfish use only undulatory body movement to drive the positioned head into the substrate. The head may serve as a wedge, but its active function is feeding, not locomotion. Among lampreys, burrowing is more complex (Hubbs and Potter 1971). The larvae of most species burrow; among adults burrowing behavior is "slight" in the families Petromyzontidae and Geotriidae, and "marked" in Mordaciidae. In some larvae, stages of development are characterized by initiation of burrowing and the acquisition of lateral eyespots (Piavis 1971). Piavis reported that prolarvae burrow by the action of both tail and head. The head moves side to side in the substrate to open a cavity; the tail generates the propulsive force. Among adults, especially *Mordacia,* burrowing is a response to light. *Mordacia* has strongly dorso-lateral eyes, thought to be correlated with burrowing. Hardisty and Potter (1971) reported that burrowing is initiated by whipping the tail, which drives the head vertically into the substrate. The head is an effector in a somewhat limited way because the oral hood probes for a flexible route of penetration, and the flared oral hood is used as an anchor as the body muscular contractions pull the animal into the substrate. A skull element, the annular cartilage, supports the oral hood, so, by inference, the skull is indeed involved in locomotion (Sawyer 1959). As do hemichordates, lampreys position themselves in burrows so that the snout emerges into the water.

I found no reports of chondrichthyans using the skull as a locomotor effector. The head in some sharks does probe the substrate for feeding, but it does not seem to be involved in locomotion per se. A few sharks, and many skates and rays, burrow, or cover themselves in the substrate, but by use of undulatory body locomotion or, in the case of skates and rays, by using the pectoral fins to throw sand and/or mud over the body.

Osteichthyans use their heads and associated skull elements in several modes of locomotion. Some are lineage-specific; some occur repeatedly in diverse, unrelated lineages. Burrowing, jet propulsion, and climbing all are reported among bony fish (Lindsey 1978); in some, use of the skull, or its derivatives and attachments, is involved in active locomotion. A number of fishes burrow, but most use undulatory or anguilliform body muscular contraction to drive the head and body into the substrate (many eels and other members of a few but diverse teleost taxa: Breder 1926; *Protopterus dolli:* Brien et al. 1959), or throw sand over themselves by undulatory movement of fins (e.g., flatfish). Nikolsky (1963) reported that many benthic-feeding fish penetrate the substrate by ejecting water from the buccal cavity, but he did not give any specific examples. Greenwood (1986) reported that the dipnoan *Protopterus annectens,* when greater than 40 mm in length, burrows into soft submerged mud (fide Johnels and Svensson 1954) by biting its way into the substrate, and expelling mouthfuls of mud and water through its branchial openings. He comments that body movement may contribute to burrowing. The animal turns 180 degrees with its snout upward; in doing so it widens the base of the vertical-to-tangential burrow to two times its body width. The fish goes to the mouth of the tube to breathe until the water table falls below the fish's snout level, whence it begins its seven- to eight-month estivation. The final depth of the burrow is 30 to 250 mm below the mud-water interface and is positively correlated with body length. I infer, therefore, that teeth, jaws and their musculature, and the branchial components are essential to burrowing in *P. annectens,* though there has been no evaluative description of their function. There is no information about the way that *P. aethiopicus* burrows (Greenwood 1986); as noted above, *P. dolli* does not use its head, so to speak, in burrowing; there is no information how breeding, in contrast to estivating, burrows are constructed. Kerr (1900) reported that *Lepidosiren* estivates in mud-mucus burrows, but he did not consider burrow construction. Kemp (1986) indicates that *Neoceratodus* does not really burrow, but embeds in damp leaves, water weeds, and mud in dried ponds. She states that *Neoceratodus* is "vastly inferior" to *P. annectens* in its ability to withstand desiccation.

Several cyprinodonts, among other teleosts (gobies, blennies, etc.), are known to burrow. An ancedotal account of burrowing in a cyprinodont involves the plains killifish, *Fundulus kansae.* Minckley and Klaassen (1969) report that killifish use shallow water sediments for refuge. They dive head-first at an angle of 45 degrees or less. Burrowing is primarily effected by undulatory body propulsion or by body contractions that throw sand. However, sand is also expelled from the mouth and settles over the fish. As is common among aquatic burrowers, the mouth and eyes are exposed at the burrow surface.

The effects of particle size of the substrate, use of the anterior end of the body coupled with undulatory body locomotion, and final position in the burrow are somewhat similar for all of the aquatic/burrowing taxa considered. Ecological as well as morphological constraints profoundly influence burrowing behaviors, effecting convergent patterns of locomotion in distantly related taxa.

A number of aquatic amphibians, reptiles, birds, and mammals use their heads to poke about the substrate, usually in search of food. Some also plow into the substrate by undulatory body locomotion and are therefore covered and inconspicuous. Others follow channels among rocks and submerged plants for cover. However, I know of no records of any that actively burrow, except for caecilians (see below).

Jet Propulsion

Jet propulsion as a mode of locomotion among teleosts is controversial. Breder (1926) described it as the force of water expelled from the gill orifices that "of necessity must be of some aid in sending them forward," that is, propellant due to reaction energy. He commented that force and its importance in locomotion vary greatly among taxa. Breder cited the standard streamline propulsion ship's model as his analog for evaluation of propulsion in fish. He also suggested that the exhaled water would form a sheath around the fish to reduce frictional drag, also in accord with the ship model. He gave examples of teleosts and sharks of diverse speeds that use jet propulsion. Breder suggested that the branchiostegal rays and other compressible parts of the head, with the strong adductor mandibulae, make water ejection of considerable velocity possible. He did not quantify his study, however, and his conclusions are inferential.

Bainbridge (1983) dismissed exhaled water alone as of any significance as an active propellant, but suggested that drag reduction merited further examination. Gradwell (1971b) examined jet propulsion in banjo catfish (*Agmus* and *Bunocephalus*). He quantified thrust distance and cyclicity of water expulsion from opercular valves, concluding that the "posteroventral expulsion of jets of water from the opercular cavities" effected "progression . . . by forward lunges during opercular expiration," and that such propulsion is independent of that of undulation of fins and body. He noted that thrust velocity may be increased by the additive effect of tail propulsion. Clearly, a study to analyze locomotor effects separate from those of feeding or respiration is needed to resolve this issue.

Climbing and "Hitching" with Suckers

A particular modification of fishes in several lineages, mostly forms that inhabit swiftly moving streams, is the development of "suckers" or adhesive devices. They are usually used in two ways: as holdfasts against water flow, and as positioners for algal scraping during feeding. Benjamin (1986) notes that fish adhesive organs are of three functional sorts: means of increasing friction, vacuum-producing suckers, and organs that lower hydrostatic pressure and increase the coefficient of friction. He comments that frictional devices are usually ventral—on the thorax, abdomen, or the paired fins. In some cases a sucker develops near the mouth, and in a few taxa it surrounds the mouth. Given these general functions, the sucker is not obviously an active locomotor agent, movement being effected by body and fin activity when suction is released. However, there are numerous reports in the aquarium literature of fishes using their suckers to climb the walls of tanks without any other means of propulsion. Few have been documented functionally. One of the most interesting sets of observations is that of R. D. O. Johnson, a mining engineer working in Colombia at the turn of the century. He reported (1912) that *Arges* (now *Astroblepus*) *marmoratus,* a loricariid catfish living in torrential streams, is a very poor swimmer, but that it has a unique mode of locomotion. It has a flat sucker mouth surrounded by a rubberlike flap, and a triangular bony plate in the abdomen to which the pelvic fins attach. The rays of the fins bear sharp, posteriorly directed denticles. Paired protractor ischii muscles can move the ventral plate a distance of about one-sixth the length of the fish. These muscles originate on the posterior sides of the plate and insert on "the bony arch just below the gill openings." A posterior pair of muscles extends from the center of the posterior edge of the plate to the anal fin and presumably is a retractor of the plate.

By alternate action of the sucking mouth and the friction plate, the fish creeps against strong currents. Johnson was most impressed to see the fish climb the walls of a 22-foot pothole from which he had diverted a mountain stream. The fish found a thin trickle of water from the dam above the hole, and, in it, traversed the nearly vertical, and in one region inwardly inclined, wall in approximately half an hour. They would hitch upward rapidly for a foot or so, then rest for a minute, repeating this activity until they were out of the hole and into a flowing stream. Johnson observed that they would not swim up a falls, but needed a rock substrate. Alexander (1965) featured this fish in his discussion of the structure and function of catfish as an example of a member of a primitive group within a lineage that has evolved a unique structure-function complex.

Gyrinocheilids are among the cypriniform taxa of Southeast Asian aquarium fish that may use the oral sucker in locomotion, though the sucker is mainly involved in increasing the coefficient of friction for adhesion during feeding on encrusted algae. Benjamin (1986) presents an exquisite investigation of the morphology of the sucker in *Gyrinocheilus aymonieri* and considers the functional implications of the morphology. He found that the expanded fleshy lips (fig. 5.1A, B) are supported by flexible chondroid tissues. They allow the sucker to evert during attachment and are associated with the maxillae, premaxillae, and dentaries. Two horny scraping blades that bear rows of hooks lie inside the lips (fig. 5.1C). The anterior margin of the sucker isolates the chamber of the sucker from the buccal and pharyngeal cavities when the mouth is closed. Benjamin suggests that a true vacuum is formed, and that water need not be taken into the mouth for long periods. Benjamin postulates a model for sucker action that emphasizes the quantity and elasticity of the chondroid, the close apposition of the oral valve to the *inner* surface of the mandible (in contrast to several other fish with oral suckers), the invaginations of the lower lip, and the negative buoyancy of the fish. He suggests that myological organization and sequence of actions in *Gyrinocheilus* are similar to that of catostomids, and used primarily in feeding. He indicates that further comparative work on the electromyography of the system and analysis of the chondroid material and the keratinization of the rasps (both interesting problems in the evolution of morphology in vertebrates) would shed more light on the functional morphology of suckers.

Some anuran tadpoles also use oral suckers as holdfasts, for feeding and for locomotion. The use of suckers in mountain streams and the relative similarity of their structure in both fish and amphibians was noted by Annandale and Hora (1922) in their study of "parallel evolution" in Indian streams. They considered the structures to be mere holdfasts and

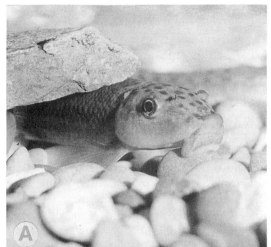

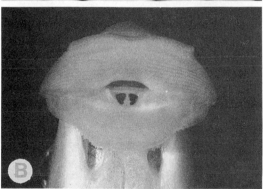

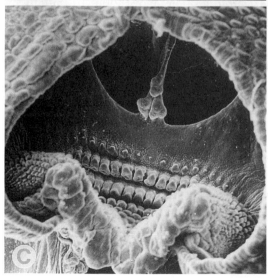

Fig. 5.1. Morphology of a teleost sucker (From Benjamin 1986). A. *Gyrinocheilus aymonieri*. B. The sucker. C. Scanning electron microscopy of the rasp of the sucker.

feeding devices, however. Two studies examine the myology and histology of tadpole suctorial discs, and suggest activity that one could infer might produce locomotion if suction and release were activated sequentially. Noble (1929) described sucker morphology of an *Amolops* (*Staurois*). The sucker is posterior to the buccal area and has a large connective tissue pad. The pad is connected to quadrate, hyoid, and maxilla by ligaments. Action is effected by paired bicipital subbranchial muscles that originate on lateral connective tissue sheets and insert on the ventral surface of the disc, and by stout rectus abdominis muscles that insert on the posterior margins of the pad. The posterior wall of the pericardium is attached to the pad. Smooth muscle fibers and collagenous fibers that form ligaments attach to the otic capsule and the sheath over the dorsal musculature. Noble suggested that suction is formed by contraction of the ventral musculature to lift the pad and form a vacuum. The posterior pad has numerous small denticles that further increase friction for adhesion. Wassersug (personal communication) hypothesizes that since the body is flexed by the recti as part of the suction-forming action, release of suction and of rectus contraction might provide recoil that would effect forward locomotion. He suggests that the *Otophryne* tadpole, with a similar morphology (Wassersug and Pyburn 1987) might also use its disc and therefore the skull in locomotion.

One case of a tadpole oral sucker used in locomotion is particularly well documented. Gaige (1920) and Altig and Brodie (1972) described forward locomotion in *Ascaphus* tadpoles by a "hitching" action of the mouth. The lower labium is planted on the substrate, and the upper extended to find a grip. Then the lower labium moves into position near the upper. A seal is maintained by extensible folds at the corners of the disc. Altig and Brodie report that *Ascaphus* tadpoles move about 10 cm/min. by use of the mouth and disc against "moderate" current. Gradwell (1971a) rigorously analyzed and documented the mechanism of locomotion by mouth and disc in *Ascaphus*. His elegant experimental study largely evaluated the interaction of the gill irrigation cycle and aspects of adhesion with the sucker, but he also examined sucker locomotion by careful observation, by manipulation of anesthetized tadpoles, and by measuring sucker pressures during crawling over a pressure transducer embedded in plastic. He described sucker locomotion as a two-phase cycle—abduction, characterized by the forward thrust of the snout, and adduction, or pulling the snout backward (see fig. 5.2).

Abduction begins with the backward movement of the lower jaw and the lower lip, while the peripheral seal of the sucker is maintained. This opens the mouth by pulling the oral valve away from contact with the upper jaw. Buccal water enters the sucker cavity and reduces its negative pressure. The inspiration phase of the irrigation cycle immediately occurs,

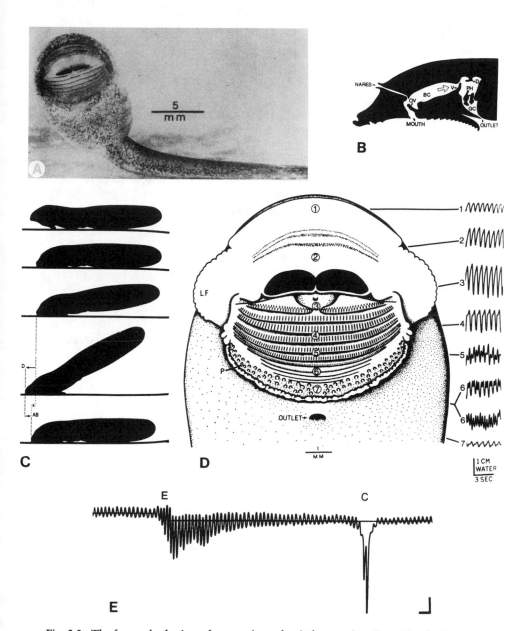

Fig. 5.2. The frog tadpole *Ascaphus* uses its sucker in locomotion (From Gradwell 1971a). A. Tadpole adhering to glass. B. Suction system of tadpole (see text). C. Stages in sucker crawling. D. Sucker morphology (see text). E. Sucker pressure during engagement (E) and crawling (C).

so there is an overall rise in sucker pressure. The orbitohyoid muscles relax as the interhyoideus contracts, raising the buccal floor and increasing buccal pressure. As the mouth opens, transfer of buccal pressure to the sucker cavity reduces suction. The lower lip contact provides friction for thrusting the snout forward, though some suction is maintained. The trunk and tail are raised from the substrate so that the branchial flow during the exhalation phase of irrigation, enhanced by the increased buccal pressure, is unobstructed.

Adduction involves a return movement of the lower jaw, powered by its musculature. Suction is increased by buccal depression and the backflow of water from the sucker to the buccal cavity. The backward-pointing denticles of the upper beak help position the snout in the substratum as the forward-directed denticles of the lower beak may also scrape as sucking pressure diminishes. Crawling and irrigation are coordinated; much irrigation occurs in the resting phase between crawling cycles. Gradwell observed that tadpoles crawl most effectively in still water, but can crawl slowly against a current. Tadpoles usually move in a straight line, since the paired lower jaw muscles exert equal forces. Gradwell observed some locomotion sequences in which forces were unequal, so that one side of the lower jaw was displaced more than the other. This caused a slight change of direction of each hitch of the sucker; tadpoles turn 90 degrees in 7-13 hitches. Periodically tadpoles disengage the sucker by decreasing the buccal pressure and raising the snout. The anterior rim of the sucker buckles from contraction of the levatores mandibulae, as the cartilages of the suprarostral system are lifted to raise the snout. The tadpole swims away to a new site of attachment.

USE OF THE HEAD FOR LOCOMOTION
BY TERRESTRIAL ANIMALS

Amphibian Burrowing

With the exception of caecilians (order Gymnophiona), burrowing in amphibians is limited. Many of the salamanders and some of the frogs thought to burrow in fact follow root channels or burrows formed by other organisms, rather than initiating and forming burrows themselves. This form of locomotion is simply body undulation, often using limbs as well, in contact with the substrate. Further, in many cases, indications that animals burrow are only inferential. For example, three species of Hispaniolan *Eleutherodactylus* are considered head-first burrowers because (1) they call and have been collected in "shallow underground chambers," and (2) they have a patch of cornified skin on the snout and large subarticular (and other) tubercles (Hedges and Thomas 1987). No observation of the animals actually burrowing has been recorded.

Desmognathine salamanders are thought to use their heads to wedge themselves under rocks and into burrows. Wake (1966) noted several modifications of the skull that he considered "streamlining" for swimming and burrowing: skull flattening, including smoothing and flattening of dorsal skull elements and smooth superficial profiles; increased density and articulation of anterior skull elements; and shifts in muscle origins from dorsal to latero-ventral. He intimated that the modification of cranial bones and muscles for skull elevation in desmognathines, in contrast to the norm of simple mandibular depression, might function in burrowing as well as feeding. Martof (1962), Valentine (1963), and Wake (1966) all suggested, based on morphology and observations of *Leurognathus* and *Desmognathus* wedging their heads under rocks (but driven by body undulation and perhaps some limb propulsion) and *Phaeognathus* living in burrows, that desmognathines are active burrowers when necessary, though they often use already-formed burrows and root channels. However, Brandon (1965) tested burrowing in *Phaeognathus*, finding it virtually unable to penetrate even very loosely packed soil. The salamanders "repeatedly lifted the posterior part of the head and pushed against the soil with the snout, but were unable to penetrate the surface." He noted that once in a cavity, salamanders accomplish burrow enlargement and compaction by means of body wall undulation. I therefore infer that salamanders do not actively burrow with their heads, but use preformed burrows that they may enlarge with their bodies. The head may be modified for use as a wedge driven by the body, but it is not likely an active burrowing component. Further, though *Phaeognathus* has almost always been collected from burrows, their elongate bodies, reduced limbs, skull modifications, reduced eyes, and modified eyelids seem to be adaptations for a fossorial existence, but not burrowing per se. Several terrestrial salamanders seem modified for a fossorial existence. Species of *Ambystoma*, too, are reported to be burrowers (Bishop 1943) but this appears to be based on their capture in fossorial situations rather than descriptions of active burrowing. Some *Ambystoma* have head modifications, such as skull flattening, associated with fossoriality.

Emerson (1976) stated that 95% of burrowing anurans (adults) dig into soil hind feet first. However, a few species in several families burrow headfirst. Two use their heads to build nests; two others usually burrow with their hind feet, but occasionally headfirst; the rest burrow headfirst into the substrate and construct underground burrow systems. All use both their heads and their arms in burrowing. Emerson carefully studied the morphology of *Hemisus marmoratum* by dissection, osteological measurement, and film analysis. *Hemisus marmoratum* flexes its head on its vertebral column and pushes its snout into the substrate. The flexion action always initiates burrowing. Once the head is positioned in the soil, the forelimbs move out from the body against the soil, then retract posteriorly. Two actions result: displacement of soil, and forward movement. Emerson hypothesized that there is a causal relationship between pectoral-cranial morphology and head movement. The pectoral girdle is quite anterior in *Hemisus,* shifted over the back part of the head, and is mobile. The cucullaris flexes only the head, rather than also move the pectoral girdle as in *Rana,* and the rhomboideus anterior raises the head as in *Hemisus,* rather than pull the pectoral girdle forward as in *Rana.* There is a large increase in size of the forelimb retractors compared to other frogs, and better developed humeri. The shift in the position of the pectoral girdle and the modifications of cucullaris and rhomboidei facilitate head flexion. Emerson notes that other headfirst burrowing frogs have some similar modifications of these units but not to the extent of *Hemisus.* Emerson does not indicate any modifications of the skull of *Hemisus* that might be associated with burrowing. The evolutionary scenario that Emerson proposed is, first, the shift in muscle insertions, which increases head flexion. Then the anterior shift of the pectoral girdle mechanically couples the girdle and the body. Once the head is flexed, the forelimbs are retracted, the muscles that raise the head contract, and the head functions as a brace. Overlapping vertebrae and the fused first and second presacrals may reduce buckling of the body axis. Emerson noted that *Hemisus* has the modifications of the hind limbs found in backward burrowers but rarely uses them. When *Hemisus* was observed to burrow with its hind feet, it shifted to headfirst burrowing when its body was nearly submerged. Emerson suggests that headfirst burrowing may be a secondary modification (not involving morphological changes of the skull), but it is advantageous in underground movement and provides a much more rapid entry to the soil than does backward burrowing.

Among the gymnophione amphibians (caecilians), burrowing initiated by the head characterizes all taxa. Even the secondarily aquatic typhlonectids do a significant amount of burrowing into the substrate (Moodie 1978; personal observation). The terrestrial caecilians are limbless, elongate, tailless (or nearly so) fossorial members of tropical faunas. Some attention has been paid to their unique mode of undulatory body locomotion (von Schnurbein 1935; Gaymer 1971; Gans 1973a, 1974; Renous and Gasc 1986) and to their musculature (Nishi 1916, 1938; Edgeworth 1935; Kesteven 1944; Lawson 1965; Naylor and Nussbaum 1980; Nussbaum and Naylor 1982), but very little to their method of burrow initiation. Gans (1974) commented briefly on the position of the head relative to the substrate and noted slight side-to-side motion of the head before the pronounced dorso-ventral movements of burrowing. I have studied burrowing in several genera of caecilians through examination of osteology and myology, electromyography, and kinematic analysis of filmed sequences. I will summarize published and some unpublished data in order to present a more complete description of head use in burrowing, so that comparisons can be made to other elongate burrowers.

Many workers have noted the flattened, wedge-shaped morphology of the head (fig. 5.3A), the terminal, usually underslung lower jaw, and the reduced eyes of caecilians, all correlated with a burrowing, fossorial existence. Skulls show variation in shape and extent of stegokrotaphy (dermal roofing) among species, but do not include the vertical keels and lateral canthi found in derived amphisbaenians (see below). The skin characteristically is extensively coossified to the skull from the snout to the parietal ridge, and to the lower jaw. The tip of the snout has a thick epidermal pad, and the nostrils are rimmed with cartilaginous cupulae. It is possible that these components are resilient force cushions or absorbers that reduce stress applied to the skull as the snout initiates the burrow. Many caecilians retain plugs of cartilage at the junctures of the sphenoid and basal elements, which may also absorb stress (Straub 1984). In nearly all species the nasals and premaxillae are fused on either side, and they are heavily bound by connective tissue at midline. The extent of dermal roofing is nearly complete in many taxa by the time a free-living existence begins (see Wake and Hanken 1982).

The head musculature is modified for burrowing, as is the body musculature. Bemis et al. (1983) and Nussbaum (1983) considered the adaptation of the interhyoideus muscle as a significant jaw adductor in all caecilians. Bemis et al. suggest it to be a means of keeping the diameter of the head nearly that of the body, despite a strong bite-feeding mechanism, so that energetic cost of burrowing is minimized. The dorsal head-trunk musculature—the paired m. cutaneous dorsalis (von Schnurbein 1935; Lawson 1965; Bemis et al. 1983 [m. dorsalis of Wiedersheim 1879; m. rectus lateralis of Naylor and Nussbaum 1980; Nussbaum and Naylor 1982]) and m. dorsalis trunci (Naylor and Nussbaum 1980; Nussbaum and Naylor 1982; Nishi 1916; Bemis et al. 1983 [m. intercostalis of Wiedersheim 1879; m. vertebralis of von Schnurbein 1935; m. rectus capitis superior of Lawson 1965])—inserts broadly on the slope of the occiput from the parietal crest to the base of the skull and forms a powerful head extensor-elevator. The paired m. longus capitis et colli (Bemis et al. 1983; Nishi 1938 [m. flexor colli et capitis, Edgeworth 1935]), originating from the basapophyses of the first 12-16 vertebrae (in *Dermophis*) and inserting on the ventral surface of the basal bone below the otic capsules, is a powerful flexor of the neck and head. The levator arcus branchiales and rectus cervicis (Edgeworth 1935; Bemis et al. 1983) would assist in burrowing

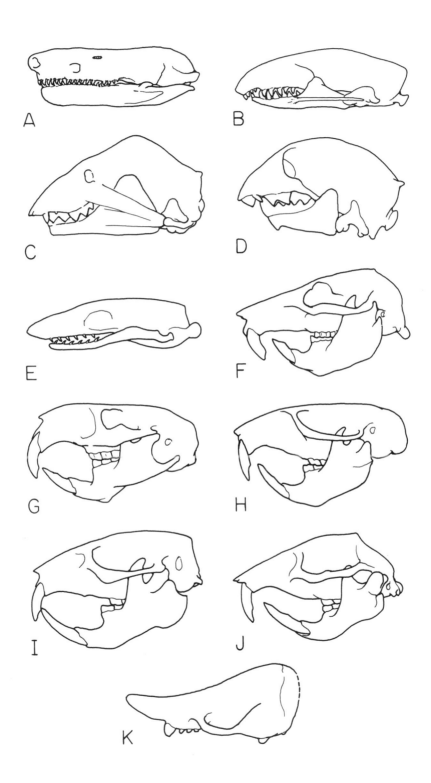

by positioning the hyobranchial and buccal regions tightly so that head-neck diameter is reduced. The m. intertransversarius capitis (Lawson 1965; confirmed by my observations) likely is a postural, perhaps flexion-maintaining, muscle. Head and neck turning, or waving, is facilitated by contraction of the oblique muscles of the body sheath of one side, and, at least in *Dermophis*, a long inferior slip of the m. cutaneous lateralis that inserts on the short, broad, flat first rib (of vertebra two).

Initiation of burrowing usually follows one of two modes, and both have been observed in several species. In the first mode, the head lies on or just above the substrate, and shallow body curves are present, the first beginning at about the twentieth annulus (of a 100-annulus animal). The head usually penetrates the soil at an angle of 45 degrees or less, and virtually all head movement is dorso-ventral, usually elevating the soil above the first several centimeters of the burrow. The animal smoothly descends into the substrate. In the second mode, the head is elevated above the substrate and the neck (see Wake 1980) is strongly arched. The first body curve begins at approximately the twenty-fifth annulus and is a broad semicircle on the substrate. The arched neck and elevated head are waved slightly from side to side, and the snout may touch the soil once or twice before burrowing. The head plunges forcefully into the soil at an angle between 45 and 90 degrees, and the burrow is penetrated deeper into the substrate. The body continues to form lateral curves on the substrate surface, probably to provide more purchase for forceful penetration. The animal disappears much more rapidly and less sinuously in this mode. The first mode seems to obtain when the animal is relaxed, and the soil consistency is known, or at least does not apparently warrant testing. The second mode occurs when an animal is stressed, or when it does more sampling of the substrate.

Burrow formation is by elevation and compaction of the substrate by the head. There is some shaping, but little initial widening, by the body, since its diameter is usually no greater than that of the head at the jaw articulation. Force of penetration is effected by powerful flexion and elevation of the head, coupled with the locomotor mode of coordinated con-

---

Fig. 5.3. *Opposite* Lateral views of skulls of terrestrial burrowers. Note flattened profile of snout-burrowers, extensive ossification, large occipitals, and reduced orbits of all forms, and large jaws and teeth of tooth-diggers. A. *Dermophis mexicanus* (gymnophione amphibian redrawn from Wake and Hanken 1982). B. *Amphisbaenia* (amphisbaenian redrawn from Gans 1974). C. *Diplometopon* (amphisbaenian redrawn from Gans 1974). D. *Agumodon* (amphisbaenian redrawn from Gans 1969). E. *Rhinophis* (uropeltid redrawn from Gans 1973b). F. *Mylospalax* (claw-digging rodent redrawn from Dubost 1968). G. *Ctenomys* (G–J, tooth-digging rodents redrawn from Dubost 1968). H. *Thomomys*. I. *Tachyoryctes*. J. *Spalax*. K. *Xenocranium* (fossil palaeanodont redrawn from Rose and Emry 1983).

traction of the muscles of the body wall sheath and those of the axial skeleton. Once several centimeters of the body are in the burrow, a mechanism similar to that of the hemichordates, uropeltids, and amphisbaenians (see below) obtains. The axial mass contracts into curves within the body wall sheath, and accelerates within the sheath, then the body wall musculature also contracts, effecting some sequential progression as these alternating series of coordinated contractions pass down the length of the body (see Gaymer 1971; Gans 1973a). The integument is annulated, which might aid in position maintenance. The contracted neck or "collar" skin and body wall musculature may act as an anchor following the penetrating stroke.

I have observed several species of caecilians construct their burrows, and have observed their behavior in the burrows, by placing soil between two glass plates separated by a space the diameter of the animal's body, placing the animal on the surface, and observing it in a dark room using red light. Under these conditions, mode 1 is usually used, and the burrow extends from side to side, in the container, deepening until the bottom of the container is explored. Almost always, the burrow is extended to an exit on the surface, so that two apertures are available for use. Within the burrow, the animal characteristically forms one or more enlarged chambers by more extensive head flexion and elevation. These cavities are usually about twice the length and three times the depth of the head. When not moving about in the burrow, the animals usually rest with their heads extended into these chambers, elevated slightly from the substrate—another use of the powerful dorsal head-trunk musculature. I have had animals representing five genera and two families in such apparati for as long as a month each, in order to do burrowing and feeding experiments, and behavior among all taxa observed is quite similar (Wake, in preparation).

The skin of caecilians is smooth and lacks the shield scales and fur present in other burrowing taxa. The epidermis is thicker than that of many other amphibians (personal observation) and has many mucous glands. Other authors (e.g., Gans 1962) suggest that mucous secretions might lubricate the burrows, but I have chemically tested burrow surface soil for mucus and found no more reaction than in soil in which caecilians had never been placed.

A major change in head structure in caecilians, apparently correlated with reduction of vision in the fossorial environment, is the development of a chemosensory tentacle. This structure, in all but the primitive rhinatrematids, has a lumen to the vomeronasal organ and then to the olfactory lobe of the brain. Certain eye structures are adapted for tentacle function—the retractor bulbi, normally of the eye, retracts the protrusible tentacle, and the Harderian gland lubricates its channel (see Billo and Wake 1987, for details). Eyes are variably reduced, but even without lenses, extrinsic and intrinsic musculature, and other components, the eyes are probably functional as photoreceptors (Wake 1985). The olfactory lobes are large and elongate and comprise a major part of the anterior half of the brain; the skull is elongated anteriorly to accommodate them. Skull shape is determined, then, at least in part, by accommodation of increased size of the olfactory components of the brain, as well as by the apparent adaptations (flattening, wedge shape) for burrowing.

There are numerous parallels in structure and function for burrowing in the elongate, limbless amphibians and reptiles (and to a lesser degree in burrowing fishes and animals). However, some of the adaptations for burrowing give a similar result in very different ways—modifications *within* the order Gymnophiona are similar. However, when gymnophiones are compared to limbless fossorial amniotes, it is apparent that different sensory modalities are accented, though vision is usually reduced. Also, bones and muscles are diversely modified to effect flattening and activity, and the integument responds in a diversity of ways that seem to be adaptations for fossoriality, especially burrowing. Phylogenetic constraints determine some of the range of variability, and much use is made in new ways of features present initially for other uses (exaptations).

Reptilian Burrowing

A diversity of reptiles burrow, at least to some degree. Turtles and crocodiles variously use snouts and limbs to dig nests for egg deposition. Several lineages of lizards are elongate, have reduced limbs, and burrow or follow root channels or other preconstructed burrows (pygopodids, cordylids, skinks, *Feylinia*). Snakes are thought to be derivatives of a burrowing lepidosaurian lineage (Underwood 1970). A number of lizards and snakes burrow or otherwise seek cover under the substrate. Mosauer (1932) perspicaciously identified the need "to clearly differentiate between the adaptations of animals to desert conditions and their adaptations to the sand." He separated behavioral and morphological/mechanical features in these contexts, using as an example *Heterodon,* the hognosed snake, which has a highly specialized digging snout but does not live in deserts. He also indicated two major modes of structural change: those that facilitate locomotion in or on sand, and those that protect sense organs and body openings (similar to my rejection of correlates of fossoriality versus those of locomotion per se).

Mosauer (1932) considered species that are modified for locomotion on sand and those that burrow in it. I shall not consider the former, for they do not have specific skull use. There is, however, a grey area of transition. Some of the sand swimmers bury themselves by swimming at an angle into the substrate, with the snout pointed downward and moved from side to side as the limbs and body propel the animal into the sand (e.g., *Phrynosoma*). In several species in which head movement has a limited, but important, burrowing component, since it is primarily a wedge driven into the sand by body locomotion, there are significant modifications of head/skull structure. The snout usually bears a sharp canthus rostralis formed of edges on the rostral and supralabial scales. The lower jaw is countersunk, reducing resistance in burrowing and preventing jaw opening. Scales are usually smooth, and the center is often concave. These generalizations obtain for several lizards and snakes of different families that inhabit loose sand. Mosauer (1932) analogized loose sand to a fluid medium, and considered adaptations for sand burrowing markedly different from those for habitation of moist sand or firmer soil. He considered both of the latter substrate types to be much firmer and resistant, and indicated that blunt, rounded heads with solidified skulls, such as found in *Anniella,* a limbless lizard, are necessary to withstand the resistance of a firm medium. Norris and Kavanau (1966) looked carefully at ecological, morphological, and physiological parameters of burrowing in the shovel-nosed snake, *Chionactis occipitalis.* Its skull is wedge-shaped anteriorly, it has a large medial scale on the lower jaw (which is underslung), and a large postrostral cavity. Of particular interest for this essay are Norris and Kavanau's comments that "the wedge-shaped, dorsoventral flattened snout . . . is pressed into the sand by a loop of the body . . . and the . . . body passed through sand without causing any abrupt changes in pressure." A key feature is that the neck is arched in burrowing so that the rostral scale is below the abdomen. A cavity under the throat is thereby produced, facilitating gular respiration, the mode when burrowing rather than abdominal respiration. They note that several burrowing snakes and lizards have similar adaptations.

Without doubt, the seminal work on the functional morphology of burrowing in reptiles, including head/skull use, is that of Gans. His empirical and theoretical work, based on case studies of amphisbaenians and uropeltid snakes, provides a broad comparative framework for delineating questions of adaptation, functional constraints, general fossoriality versus locomotor mode, and phylogenetic constraints.

Gans summarized much of his work on amphisbaenians in 1974. The group is an assemblage of 130 species, all modified for burrowing. They occur in southern Europe, Morocco, central-to-southern Africa, South America from Panama to Patagonia, the Antilles, northern Mexico, and Florida in both humid and xeric habitats. Amphisbaenians are elongate; most lack limbs and girdles, and have the right lung reduced. They have a number of modifications of the skull: it is heavily ossified and solid, premaxillae are heavy with large facial processes and a large medial maxillary tooth; there are few, large teeth on the dentigerous elements; the stapes is enlarged; and the braincase is completely enclosed by the frontal bones, normally only dorsal elements. Skulls may be rounded or pointed, flattened, vertically keeled, or wedge-shaped with lateral canthi (see fig. 5.3B-D and below). Gans uses biomechanical analyses of amphisbaenian structure and function to examine factors responsible for selection for fossoriality, alternate evolutionary pathways and their conflicts in being fossorial, why some forms recur in different groups, and the limits of geographic ranges of species.

I shall focus on Gans's analysis of the mechanisms of tunneling and the concomitant modifications of the skull. The diameter of a tunnel and the penetrability and compressibility of the resistant soil determine the energetic cost of construction and maintenance. Tunnels are formed by excavating or compacting the soil, or both. Excavation requires removal of soil from the anterior end of the tunnel; compaction does not. Gans notes that skull shape and movements facilitate penetration and tunnel widening, therefore compaction. The ramming penetration of amphisbaenians effects tunneling, and the shape of the head determines the amount of compaction. Given that the head is pushed by a given amount of energy, it penetrates to maximum distance if its shape is a pointed cone. If soil consistency is not uniform (e.g., contains a rock), there will be a local concentration of force at the point of greatest resistance on the cone, tending to turn the head. Modifications of the basic cone shape to resist failure include changing the cylinder to a wedge, which increases rate of increase of area of penetration; making the apex of the cone round; and covering the cone with either a very hard or a resilient substance. Different amphisbaenians make use of each of these mechanisms. As in caecilians and uropeltids, the integument is annulated and loosely attached to the axial mass. Therefore friction of the penetrating stroke is reduced as amphisbaenians bunch the neck skin and fix it against the tunnel well. Using this as a base, the head is accelerated by contraction of the costocutaneous muscles.

Further consideration of head shape by Gans (1974) has to do with distribution among species and their geographic distribution. By far the majority of species (87) have rounded or pointed shapes; 26 have flattened spade-shaped heads; 11 have vertically keeled heads; six have wedge-shaped heads with strong lateral canthi. Spade-snouted and "keeled-headed" species are usually allopatric to each other, but often sympatric to round-headed ones; the group with wedge-shaped heads is allopatric to other amphisbaenians. Those forms which meet the greatest friction in addition have more extensively fused or enlarged head shields in order to reduce shear. Gans (1968, 1969, 1974, 1978) summarizes burrowing patterns as follows: the primitive sequence, characteristic of round-headed forms, is that of the head forced into the soil and the burrow widened by body penetration. One modification of this pattern is the utilization of a two-phase cycle of the head penetrating the soil, then widening the tunnel by elevating the head, ramming soil toward the top of the tunnel, then

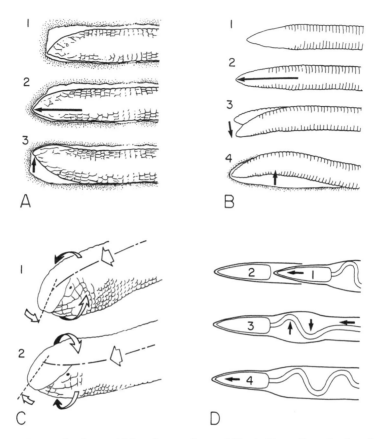

Fig. 5.4. Burrowing in amphisbaenians and uropeltids. A. Tunneling of a shovel-snouted amphisbaenian (from Gans 1974). B. Tunneling of a keel-snouted form (from Gans 1974). C. Oscillatory tunneling in a trogonophid amphisbaenian (from Gans 1974). D. Burrowing progression in a uropeltid (from Gans 1973b).

smoothing the wall with the pectoral region (fig. 5.4A). Spade-snouted forms use that mechanism, and it has apparently evolved independently in three lineages. Two lineages of "keeled-headed" forms widen the tunnel by driving the head alternately to the left and right, and smooth the wall with the sides of the head and trunk, again a two-phase cycle (fig. 5.4B). The wedge-shaped lineage (trogonophids) uses an oscillating stroke to remove soil from the end of the tunnel and to compact it to the wall (fig. 5.4C).

Gans analyzes two-phase digging cycles as a problem in force generation. The force needed to drive a cone into a substrate is a function of the maximum diameter of the cone in contact, friction of the cone, and the soil type. The momentum to sink the cone to depth is the sum of the forces needed to sink the cone at any point. The greatest diameter of the cone is that of its base. If each cycle of cone penetrance also widens the burrow to the diameter of the base, less momentum is necessary for the next ramming stroke. Since any slippage between body wall and burrow limits the potential for building up energy for the penetrating stroke, Gans suggests that there is an advantage to separating the penetrating and widening actions. The spade-snouted and keel-headed amphisbaenians do this by maximizing the shape of the penetrating wedge, and using separate motions to widen the burrow. Since force required to deepen a burrow is a function of burrow diameter, which is correlated to body diameter, the body diameters of amphisbaenians conserve cross-sectional area.

In amphisbaenians, head-raising muscles involved in burrowing occur in a pinnate pattern. The dorsal musculature which pulls the head up inserts on the skull via the nuchal tendon; muscle slips insert on both sides of the neural arches of vertebrae throughout the anterior trunk. This is in contrast to the situation of paired longitudinal muscles in caecilians. Pinnate muscles are more efficient (see Gans 1974). I suspect that the presence of a single occipital condyle in reptiles, rather than the paired condyles of amphibians, provides a less restricted pivot point so that the single insertion of the nuchal tendon is more efficient as well. The spade-snouted amphisbaenians rotate their heads about the occipital condyle, compacting soil into the burrow roof. The keel-headed forms penetrate with the head in a medial position, and widen the burrow by moving the anterior part of the body side to side, bending the head around its rostral tip as a fulcrum. Trogonophids, with their sharp lateral canthi and v-shaped rather than cylindrical bodies, use an oscillating burrowing motion. The head is rotated in either direction around the long axis of the animal (fig. 5.4C). The canthi scrape the burrow end, and the side of the head compacts the soil that is dislodged. The body is u-shaped, rather than round, and the rib tips, or ends of the "u," anchor the body against the torsion of oscillation so that the animal does not simply spin.

Gans discusses a number of modifications of the amphisbaenian skull for burrowing (1960, 1968, 1969, 1974, 1978). In general, they include having the facial portion of the skull anterior to the nasal capsule and the brain sheathed by interlocking bones, and the vibration detector of the ear shifted to the facial portion of the skull via the long extracolumellar process. Eyes are reduced, as in many fossorial taxa. It is significant that amphisbaenians have implemented vibration detection as a major sensory mode, in contradistinction to caecilians, which have utilized olfaction via the nose and the unique tentacle. The penetrating surface is reinforced internally for rigidity, but by different dermal bones in different lineages—indicating convergence, as described by Gans.

A problem in burrowing is the transmission of forces from the occipital condyle to the snout. The posterior part of the skull is reinforced by ossification, sheathing, and interlocking mortise joints, rather than simple butt joints. The braincase is therefore a narrow tubular strut, and the jaw muscles outside the braincase do not increase head diameter significantly (see my analogous comments on caecilians, above).

Gans's work on uropeltid snakes provides an analogous test system for hypotheses about adaptations for burrowing, and the constraints that phylogeny imposes on them. Uropeltids are small tropical rain forest snakes occurring in India and Sri Lanka. They all have pointed heads, a keeled rostrum, and modifications of the axial musculature and the tail (Gans 1973b, 1974, 1976; Gans et al. 1978). The small, conical, wedge-shaped head bears a keratinized ridge, extending in some species half the length of the head. The ridge allows a narrower head in animals of relatively larger size (Gans 1974), serves as a device for stress distribution, and hardens the surface of the head to facilitate penetration. The skull is heavily fused (more than any other snake) and has strongly strengthened premaxillae, choanae roofed by bone, few dentigerous elements, a stout lower jaw, and a projecting occipital condyle (Gans 1973b and fig. 5.3E). The anterior axial musculature is larger and thicker than that posteriorly, includes large quantities of myoglobin and mitochondria, and has other enzymatic and ultrastructural modifications. These muscles apparently are modified for sustained work loads during soil penetration (Gans et al. 1978). The burrowing mechanism is one in which the head simply is driven into the substrate, then the axial musculature (therefore the vertebral column) contracts to form several curves within the widened but straight skin. The axial mass propels the head forward through the external loops of the mass, applying force to the body (effectively the burrow) walls (fig. 5.4D). The burrow formed thus is wider than the widest part of the body, which Gans considers to provide two advantages: it protects against constraining force for an animal carrying embryos or after a large meal, and it allows penetration in nonhomogeneous substrates with roots, rocks, and adherent soils. The burrow can meander in response to differences in compression of various components of the burrow wall.

Uropeltids are constrained biogeographically and phylogenetically (35 species), and most taxa have the adaptations listed above. Some modifications are similar to those of amphisbaenians and caecilians, but many are unique to the lineage, an illustration that convergence, presumed to be dictated by habitats and/or life histories, has different paths, and extensions well beyond the basic pattern of convergence.

Skull Locomotion in Birds

Birds use their skulls, particularly their beaks and associated bones and muscles, in a great diversity of functions. They make nests in a variety of substrates, and they explore the substrate (ranging from water to sand to mud to soil to tree trunks) for food. However, these activities are rarely, if ever, directed locomotor events. There are many anecdotes in the avian literature of use of diverse morphological structures as functional units for breeding (especially nesting), feeding, and locomotion, but the latter rarely specifically involve the beak and skull. Perhaps the best known of these unanalyzed phenomena is the use of the beak by parrots to climb. They use their strong, recurved beaks to hook over wires of a cage (and, apparently, branches of trees in the field) and flex the head on the chest so that the legs gain forward purchase when extended (Welty 1975). This example of skull (beak plus musculature) use in locomotion may well obtain in other groups, and the attention of avian biologists to flight (primarily) and walking and swimming (secondarily) should be extended to more ancillary modes of locomotion.

Mammalian Burrowing and the Skull

Many mammals in several orders dig burrows. Most burrow by means of limb or limb and body action; some use the head as an organ to penetrate the substrate before limb movements dig in; some use the head to compact or transport the soil dislodged by limbs and body; and a few taxa in different groups use their teeth to penetrate the soil and even to extend the burrow. Compared to that available for other classes of vertebrates, there is a veritable wealth of literature on use of the limbs in burrowing, and of skeletal, myological, sensory, and integumental modifications for burrowing in mammals (much summarized by Hildebrand 1985). The literature does not really deal with major questions posed in this context, however: what modifications appear to be for burrowing per se; which are for the fossorial life style in general though they may (or may not) be involved in burrowing; which came first, burrowing (given that it can occur without morphological modification) or fossoriality (which does not require that the animal necessarily construct its own burrow)?

There are several summaries of mammalian modification for fossoriality, particularly those of Dubost (1968a, b), and Nevo (1979), which also summarize much literature. Dubost discussed a diversity of morphological adaptations for subterranean living, including the external aspect, the head, pectoral, and pelvic components, and the special sensory units. He emphasized the morphological similarities among burrowing marsupials (Notoryctes), insectivores (13 genera in three families), and rodents (14 genera in four families), but, like most authors, did not consider digging mammals that do not spend substantial parts of their lives in burrows, such as armadillos and aardvarks. He illustrated several features of the head associated with fossoriality: the flattened snouts with thick digging pads and the pointed snouts with long vibrissae, the reduced and often hidden eyes, short fur, underslung lower jaws, and reduced covered external ears. Several insectivores and rodents dig with their incisors. These teeth, like those of other rodents, are ever-growing; the skulls, especially the premaxillae and the dentaries, are strongly reinforced.

Dubost also summarized trends in eye reduction in fossorial mammals. Covering by skin, lens reduction, and loss of components of accommodation are strikingly similar to the trends in regressive evolution of the eye in caecilians described by Wake (1985) and in hagfish by Feinholm and Holmberg (1975). The ear is not exceptionally developed, but olfaction is "well" developed, as is the tactile sense. Dubost suggested that more research on these sensory modes is needed.

Nevo (1979) evaluated convergence and divergence in the evolution of completely fossorial mammals. Nevo considered that fossorial mammals have converged on several specializations; the morphological ones include a cylindrical body, reductions of appendages, eyes, and ears, hypertrophy of acoustic and tactile senses, and food generalism (herbivory in rodents, insectivory in marsupials and insectivores). Nevo stated that there is considerable adaptive convergence morphologically and ecologically. There is also adaptive divergence in a number of features, and major phylogenetic differences relate to tooth structure and specialization for diets.

Several workers have considered skull and tooth modifications in burrowing rodents. Curiously, many of them fall into difficulty: they restrict their discussions to taxa that use their heads, especially their teeth, in burrowing, but then discuss skull and tooth morphology only in terms of diet and feeding. Agrawal (1967) considered skull modifications in rodents in this manner. He stated that the Oriental rodent genera that he examined seek food outside the burrow, so though "the skull plays a role in the process of digging and . . . has affected its structure," he attributed modification of incisors and protrusion of premaxillae to feeding strategy. He noted that the flattening of the skull, the pointed rostrum, and the anteriorly sloping occiput give increased effectiveness to the shoveling action of the head, and that the increased height of the occiput gives increased surface area for attachment of the highly developed dorsal neck musculature used in digging. Howard and Smith (1952) introduced their discussion of the rate of growth of incisors in *Thomomys* (pocket gophers, family Geomyidae) in terms of use in digging in hard soil and removing rocks, etc., which they suggest should lead to a high rate of incisor growth. (There are many comments in the literature about pocket gophers using their incisors to dig.) They found a greater rate of growth than in other rodents reported in the literature (upper incisors in *Thomomys*, 0.62 mm/day, 8.91 inches/year; lowers 0.99 mm/day, 14.19 inches/year; versus $\bar{x} = 0.276$ mm/day for seven reports for uppers in other taxa, $\bar{x} = 0.41$ mm/day for ten reports of lower incisors). Howard and Smith observed that gophers in cages used their incisors to dig in their cages on soil that was too hard to dig with the claws. They did not do the obvious experiment of measuring tooth growth in gophers presented with different substrates and food types, or those prevented from digging.

There have been few attempts to compare features of the skulls of burrowing taxa within and among lineages. Agrawal (1967) and Dubost (1968a, b) included several species in their analyses, which were done as broad comparisons. Examination of the skulls in figure 5.3F, G, H, I, and J shows several convergent features. Flattened skulls, elongate nasals, reduced orbits, and massive maxillae and dentaries (and articulations) characterize burrowing rodents. Elongate incisors are features of tooth diggers (compare the relative incisor lengths in 3G, a hand-digger, with the other skulls, all tooth-diggers).

However, a recent study by Lessa and Thaeler (1989) is a masterful analysis of morphological and ecological variation in one lineage of mammals, the pocket gophers of the family Geomyidae. They perform a morphometric analysis of components of the osteology and musculature of jaws and forelimbs, and identify two directions of morphological specialization, one toward claw digging and the other toward tooth digging, even among species that use both methods. This idea accounts for the major patterns of variation in both forelimb and skull shape, in the context of allometric variation. They find an inverse correlation between the development of characters associated with tooth digging and claw digging, the former associated with narrower, more procumbent incisors, anteriorly extended glenoid fossae, and enlarged jaw musculature. The Thomomyini are more specialized for tooth digging, and the Geomyini for claw digging, though one geomyine, *Cratogeomys*, also uses its incisors for digging. It has developed the modifications for tooth digging, but not as extremely as in the thomomyines. Lessa and Thaeler note that the two modes of digging have very different ecological consequences. Claw digging is associated with a narrow niche (sandy soils); tooth digging with a much broader spectrum of niches. An important conclusion is that only in some cases does morphological specialization lead to narrowing of the niche. For example, tooth digging appears to provide the potential for an expansion of ecological niche width.

Two studies worth contrasting because of their similarity of questions and approaches, though published more than 40 years apart, are those of Orcutt (1940), who compared the anatomy of a geomyid pocket gopher (*Geomys bursarius*) to the white rat (*Rattus norwegiensis*, family Moridae), and Bekele (1983a, b), who compared the mole-rat (*Tachyoryctes splendens*, family Rhizomyidae) to the black rat (*Rattus rattus*). The goal of both studies was to assess the nature of modification for fossoriality by comparing a tooth-and-limb digging rodent with a nonburrowing rodent.

Orcutt noted that most muscles of the pocket gopher are increased markedly in thickness, but less so in width, especially in the neck. There is little increase in length, except for the adductors and the depressor of the jaw, which Orcutt correlates with "loosening and cutting soil." He also described irregular bony outlines that provided greater muscle attachment surface in the fossorial form.

Bekele also described cranial morphology and added a quantitative analysis of the jaw and cervical muscles and a functional interpretation of their use in the fossorial species. The mole-rat (*Tachyoryctes*) skull (fig. 5.3I) is heavier, broader, and deeper. The nasal bones end in line with the premaxillae rostrally, and the rostrum is more compact, shorter, and broader. The mole-rat has a constricted interparietal and a strong triangular sagittal crest. The mole-rat's zygomatic arch is wider and stouter, giving increased areas for muscle attachment at either end. The palate is constricted rostrally; the internal pterygoid fossa and a number of aspects of the occipital are modified for muscle attachment. The lower jaw of the mole-rat is much more robust and deeper, with a high coronoid process and a strong attachment of the two halves at the median symphysis. The upper and lower incisors are very large and pro-odont (outwardly projecting) in the mole-rat. Bekele (1983a) noted that muscle origins, and often insertions, especially the jaw adductors and depressor, are more extensive in the mole-rat. The temporal muscle is significantly larger in the mole-rat, the masseter in the black rat. Bekele's extrapolated analysis of function indicates that all jaw muscles except the posterior deep masseter produce more force in the mole-rat.

Bekele (1983b) noted that mole-rats have short, compact cervical vertebrae, black rats long, wide ones. Cervical muscle weights show larger extensors in the mole-rat and larger lateral muscles in the black rat. The deeper skull of the mole-rat is deemed to increase the efficiency of the occipital muscles and the amount of work they perform. Transverse bending moments are similar in the two species, but the moment of the cervical extensors of the mole-rat is nearly twice that of the black rat (0.39 versus 0.21). Bekele discussed alternative modes of muscle action for lifting and pushing soil with the head and found none of the models logical, based on muscle efficiencies and field observations of the animals. Bekele constructed a static mechanical model to evaluate the differences in osteology and musculature. He noted that several aspects of muscle morphology were not considered, and that the actual physiological situation is not known. An analysis of muscle forces, based on their lines of action in lever systems, shows marked differences in forces produced by the same muscles in the two forms. The mole-rat compensates for reduced efficiency of force use (due to the long pro-odont incisors increasing the resistance arm) by increasing leverage of the temporal muscle. Bekele concluded that the increased width and depth of the skull and dentary for larger muscle attachment areas minimize the mechanical disadvantage of the resistance arm at the incisors. The total force applied at the incisors by the mole-rat is about twice that exerted by the black rat. The cross-sectional area of the incisors in the mole-rat is twice that of the black rat. But Bekele noted that the mole-rat exerts less pressure with the incisors than the black rat. Curiously, he concluded that the mole-rat has less specialization of the incisors for use on hard materials than the black rat, and the black rat is specialized in efficiently applying more incisor pressure than the mole-rat. Bekele suggested that this is associated with the seed-eating habits of the black rat. To me, this is another retreat to conclusion based only on feeding mechanics, for which so much more is known, and it provides no real attempt to consider utilization of the system in digging.

Much of the conjecture by Bekele on functional aspects of burrowing in *Tachyoryctes* is dependent on the excellent observations and comparative analysis of burrowing in three genera of mole-rats (*Tachyoryctes*, family Rhizomyidae; and *Heliophobius* and *Heterocephalus*, family Bathyergidae) by Jarvis and Sale (1971; see fig. 5.5B, C, D). They found considerable similarity in the method of digging and the burrow patterns among the three genera. All of the mole-rats dig with their well-developed pro-odont incisors. Their lips are enlarged to prevent soil entering the mouth. Lateral folds of the upper lips are nearly in contact when the mouth is opened; they lie in the space behind the upper incisors as the mouth closes, so that in any position, soil is precluded. The snout is large and flattened, and is used in packing soil. Valvular external nares keep soil from entering the nasal cavities. The jaw musculature is heavy; the bite is strong, including in digging. *Tachyoryctes* digs with forward and upward sweeps of the lower incisors to cut away the soil surface. The animal braces with its laterally rotated hind feet during biting. It pushes dislodged soil under its body with its forefeet and then turns around and compacts the soil with one side of its face (see above discussion of cervical musculature) and its forelimb. It pushes the dirt out of the burrow, then turns around to resume digging.

Burrowing in *Heliophobius* is similar, except that soil transport is via the hind legs. The animal digs its nose and upper incisors into the top of the burrow for balance, and kicks the dirt out of the burrow backward with its feet. *Heliophobius* is solitary, so each animal digs its own burrow. *Heterocephalus*, which is colonial, has a similar pattern, except that it transports soil backward with both front and hind feet. Also, in *Heterocephalus*, animals take turns doing the digging to extend the burrow system. All of these animals stop digging periodically to groom their fur and clear their incisors of soil. Tucker (1981) also described the burrowing behavior of *Heterocephalus* in some detail. He discussed other morpho-

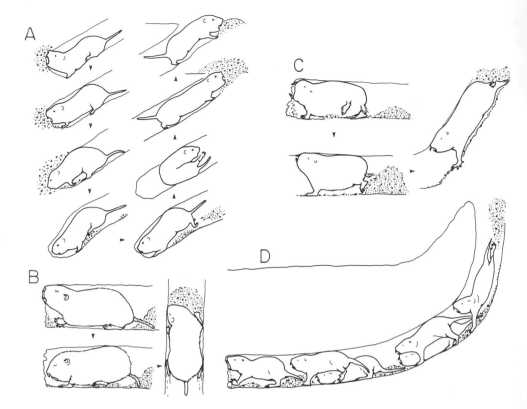

Fig. 5.5. Burrowing in rodents. A. *Arvicola,* showing tooth use, head compaction, and soil transport by the head (redrawn from Airoldi et al. 1976). B. *Tachyoryctes,* showing tooth use and soil transport by the head (redrawn from Jarvis and Sales 1971). C. *Heliophobius,* showing tooth use and soil transport by the rear feet (redrawn from Jarvis and Sales 1971). D. *Heterocephalus,* showing communal digging and tooth use (redrawn from Jarvis and Sales 1971).

logical and behavioral attributes of burrowing, especially the very loose and generally thin skin, and the large cutaneous sensory areas. Many of the latter lie on the head and face in the areas most exposed to mechanical stimuli. Some of these, however, have different degrees of exposure in burrowing than in feeding. For example, the naso-labial patch is relatively shielded during burrowing with the mouth open, but exposed, because the oral cavity is closed, during investigative and social behavior. Tucker also proposed a functional analogy of the loose skin of *Heterocephalus* to the situation in amphisbaenians (and therefore caecilians and uropeltids) in which the body wall musculature and integument are effectively separated from the trunk. However, Tucker's own statements that emphasize differences in their respective burrowing modes demonstrate the limitations of the analogy.

Several other workers have reported on various aspects of burrowing in rodents, particularly the use of the incisors in digging and the head in compacting soil and shoving it to the surface. Airoldi et al. (1976; see fig. 5.5A) and Casinos et al. (1983) reported this for the arvicolids *Pitymys* and *Arvicola*. Nevo (1979) reported that *Spalax* uses incisors and front feet to dig, kicks back the soil with hind feet, and compacts both soil to be excavated and the tunnel walls with its head. It then shoves the soil to the surface with its head. Gasc et al. (1985) noted that both *Spalax* and *Arvicola* have wedged-shaped heads, ankylosed cervical vertebrae, and very reduced eyes associated with fossoriality. In discussing the description of Airoldi et al. (1976) of the digging-clearing cycle in *Arvicola,* which emphasizes the protraction of the head and the extension of the neck, followed by tearing of the soil by jaw closure and retraction of the head, Gasc et al. noted that the upper and lower incisors act as a tool (a post-hole digger?), for the head can rotate as much as 180 degrees on the axis of the body. They contrasted this mode to that of *Spalax:* the specific actions of teeth and head differ, as do the time sequences. Use of the lower incisors in scraping predominates, and soil is elevated and compacted by the shovel-like aspect of the dorsum of the head.

Gasc et al. (1985) plea that careful analysis of patterns of burrowing be made before generalizations about convergence are assumed. Substantive investigation, which has only begun, reveals significant differences in bone structure, incisor use, myology, including muscle activity, and other aspects of digging among taxa superficially presumed to be very similar. Gasc et al. (1986) support these contentions with morphological and x-ray cine data applied to vector analysis of digging in the golden mole, *Eremitalpa granti,* family Chrysochloridae (fig. 5.6). It burrows in very loose sand, using its front feet to dig and its flattened and rostrally narrow head and its shoulders to compact sand. They note that the lower jaw is underslung and the eyes and external ears are covered. Most head and forelimb movements are in the parasagittal plane. Gasc et al. describe burrowing in terms of (1) initial penetration, in which the head is plunged into the sand and the front feet begin to dig, and (2) progression or forward movement coupled with buttressing. They consider head morphology only in passing, focusing on that of the limbs. Even buttressing, which appears to be largely a function of the dorsum of the head and the neck and ventrally the chest, is dealt with in terms of forelimb movement rather than the coupling of the osteology and myology of the head. Gasc et al. noted that buttressing is the main adaptive feature for digging in loose, collapsible soil. They even state that "from a biomechanical point of view,

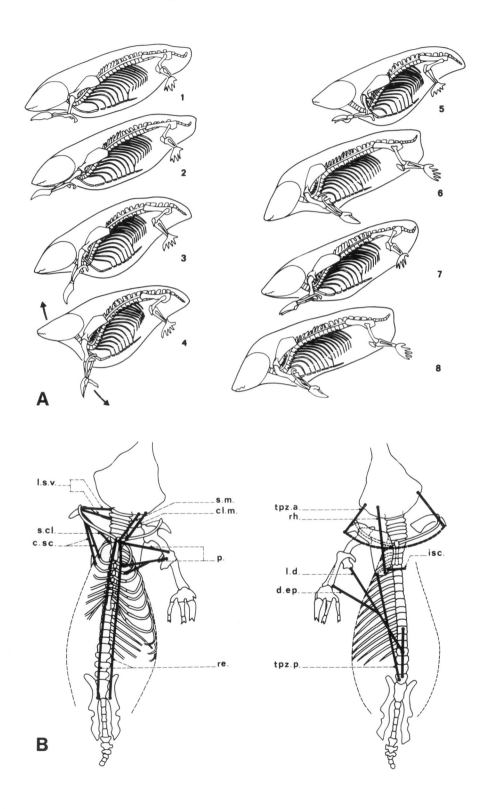

the head and cervical column represent the intersection of two sets: the forelimb system and the trunk–hind limb one." They comment that body displacements dictate the penetration and path of the snout through the sand.

Curiously, Gasc et al. mention the useful study of another chryso-chlorid, *Chrysochloris asiatica*, the Cape Golden Mole, by Puttick and Jarvis (1977) only in the context of use of forelimbs in digging. In fact, that rather careful study described the adaptive morphology of the species, which includes numerous modifications of the forelimb and shoulder, and their musculature, but also the powerful and enlarged dorsal neck muscu-lature, the enlarged occiput for its insertion, vertebral modifications to ac-commodate the musculature, reduced eyes and ears, and the hard leathery pad on the muzzle. More significant, Puttick and Jarvis analyze burrow-ing in terms of a power stroke, which involves coordinated up-and-down thrusts of the forelimbs and strong upward thrusts of the head. They state that the head is used to clear a space in front of the burrowing animal by displacing soil. The recovery stroke is simply repositioning of the forelimbs and the head. This is not dissimilar to the description of burrowing in *Eremitalpa* (Gasc et al. 1986), though cast in different terms. Still, the Gasc et al. study is a pioneering effort to apply modern techniques and analysis to a controlled laboratory study of burrowing.

A useful study of the morphology of fossoriality is that of Rose and Emry (1983). Examining the Oligocene palaeanodonts *Epoicotherium* and *Xenocranium,* they were struck by their skeletal specializations for fos-soriality which equal or exceed those of extant fossorial mammals, and by their convergence with a number of chrysochlorid characteristics (see above). Their skulls have expanded, domed occiputs with broad lambdoid crests, hypertrophy of the malleus-incus and other ear units, reduced eyes, and a flattened, shovel-shaped rostrum, upturned in *Xenocranium* (fig. 5.3K). The skull is heavily fused and buttressed. There appears to be a single small incisor on each ramus of the lower jaw. The second through fifth cervical vertebrae are fused. There are numerous modifications of the forelimbs. Rose and Emry conclude that the skull modifications suggest that the snout was used for digging to bore through the soil, and that the

Fig. 5.6. *Opposite* Kinematics of digging in the rodent *Eremitalpa* (from Gasc et al. 1986). A. Schematics of buttressing and digging phases drawn from x-ray cinematography. B. Muscle lines of head and pectoral systems (left, ventral; right, dorsal). Abbreviations: cl.m., cleido-mastoideus; c.sc., costo-scapularis; isc., interscapularis; l.s.v., levator scapulae ventralis; re., rectus abdominis; rh., rhomboideus; l.d., latissimus dorsi; d.ep., dorso-epitrochlearis; p., p. occipitalis and p. cervicalis; s.cl., subclavius; s.m., sterno-mastoideus; tpz.a., trapezius, pars anterior; tpz.p., trapezius, pars posterior.

occipital crest and fused cervical vertebrae indicate that the head was used to compact the walls and roof of the burrow. They note the strong similarity of the shape of the snout of *Xenocranium* to the shovel-snouted amphisbaenians, and suggest that a similar mode of burrow compaction was used. They also conclude that vision was reduced and hearing of low-frequency sound was amplified, both characteristic of fossorial animals. Finally, they indicate that these palaeanodonts were probably the most specialized "rapid-scratch" burrowers that ever lived.

We therefore see a suite of modifications for burrowing among several lineages of mammals from at least the Oligocene. This pattern of convergence includes small size, diverse amplifications of forelimb and pectoral girdle and their myology, reduced eyes, covered ear openings, and short fur. Cervical vertebrae are often short and stout, and occasionally fused. Dorsal neck musculature is stout, and the skull is modified for massive insertion of those muscles. The skull is usually massive, often widened, and is well structured and buttressed, particularly in the rostral region. The skull is often flattened and shovel-shaped. Many mammals that use their snouts and heads for digging and compacting have thick, hairless pads of the integument, a feature not emphasized in this discussion. Both taxa that use their incisors to dig and those that use their snouts fall into two shape classes, regardless of taxonomic affiliation: snouts may be pointed, or they are wedge-shaped with underslung lower jaws. The species that use their incisors for breaking soil all have large, ever-growing incisors, massive dentaries, and hypertrophied jaw adductors and depressors with extensive origins and often broad insertions. As Lessa and Thaeler (1989) point out, tooth digging appears to facilitate greater niche breadth than does claw digging. Many taxa have a number of similar morphological adaptations for burrowing and for fossoriality. I hasten, however, to reiterate the warning of Gasc et al. (1986) that similarity of structure may mask great diversity of function.

ADAPTATIONS OF THE SKULL FOR LOCOMOTION: SUCKERS VERSUS SHOVELS

Suckers

Common (redundant) adaptations of the skull for locomotion occur in several groups. The development of suckers, or adhesive structures, occurs in several aquatic taxa, notably a diversity of catfish and their relatives, and certain frog tadpoles. All of these forms share an ecological correlate: life in rapidly moving mountain streams. It is reasonable that the development of suckers follows a common scenario in these remotely related lineages. First, components of the mouth, or less commonly, the trunk adjacent to the pectoral fins, develop a mechanism for pressure reduction in the mouth and buccal, or parapectoral, cavities in order to effect near-vacuum adhesion to the substrate. Enlarged "lips" and dilated oral musculature are morphological correlates of this behavior. Adaptation of suckers for locomotion is rarer, but seems correlated with life in fast-moving streams at high altitudes or latitudes. In both fishes and amphibian tadpoles, the mode of locomotion is a convergence on a hitching mode, involving releases of suction, lower-jaw projection and propulsion, and sometimes coordination of activity of head suckers and pectoral or pelvic structures to effect anterior progression. Cartilages and bones of the anterior part of the skull, and their associated musculature and integument and their derivatives, are rather similarly modified to effect dual cycle respiratory and concomitant locomotor pumps.

Shovels

There are suites of modifications of the skull and its associated structures for burrowing that appear across vertebrate taxa, whether in aquatic or terrestrial environments. Skulls are often flattened anteriorly; they may have keels. The nose may be reinforced by keratinized cones (amphisbaenians, uropeltids) or by a suite of cartilaginous nasal capsules, with deep, resilient, coossified integument, and fused bony elements (gymnophiones, amphisbaenians, mammals), or by heavily ossified, well-buttressed rostra with well-developed flattened integumentary pads (several mammals). Heads are usually narrower than bodies, even in the most elongate forms (gymnophiones, amphisbaenians). A number of skull modifications for burrowing per se and fossoriality in general are common among various amphibians, reptiles, mammals, and even among a few fish. The flattened, shovel-like snout has been mentioned for each taxon. Many taxa have an underslung lower jaw so that the mouth is not opened by friction during burrowing. Fish, amphibians, reptiles, and mammals that burrow all characteristically have pronounced occiputs for insertion of dorsal cervical musculature for extension and retraction of the head during burrowing. There exist diverse modes among vertebrate lineages for reinforcement of skull components to effect (1) more extensive areas for origin and insertion of musculature; (2) coossification of integument to skull, apparently to reduce shear during burrowing; and (3) conical penetration of the snout or, conversely, flattened, wedge-shaped penetration by the rostrum of the substrate. Among and within lineages, different skeletal elements (nasals, premaxillae, incisors, for example) may be modified for similar use. Use of the incisors as digging tools is a uniquely mammalian characteristic. Yet, there are differences among tooth diggers in jaw and muscle morphology and actions that indicate how superficial the general convergence is, and that tooth use indeed evolved several times within rodent groups, as well as among the orders of mammals.

Several features of the skull and head seem to be characteristics of fossoriality rather than adaptations for burrowing. Integuments are modified so that edges that would provide resistance to tunnel walls are reduced or absent. Amphibian skins are smooth, and mucus-moistened to a greater or lesser degree (more in frogs and salamanders, less in gymnophiones). Scalation in squamates and amphisbaenians is smooth, and scales of the head may be enlarged, presumably for protection and friction reduction (and reinforcement for burrowing when it is actively used). The pelage of fossorial mammals is short, thick, and soft, or much reduced—again, presumed to reduce friction. However, the bodies of gymnophiones, amphisbaenians, and uropeltids are annulate, presumably to increase grip on burrow walls. Penetration therefore may be very different functionally from locomotion in burrows.

Sensory modalities are variously emphasized among burrowing animals. Eyes in most fossorial taxa are reduced, their sockets small and sometimes lost completely. In some gymnophiones, the eyes are completely roofed by dermal bone, though there is morphological evidence that they might be functional photoreceptors (Wake 1985). Usually another sensory modality is emphasized and often it is hypertrophied. Olfaction is the dominant mode in gymnophiones. The nostrils are large, sometimes valvular, and the olfactory lobes compose a large part of the mass of the brain. The unique chemosensory tentacle is an evolutionary experiment in cooption of structures involved in vision and olfaction (Wake 1985; Billo and Wake 1987) in other amphibians (and vertebrates in general). The skull is modified in providing an aperture for its tip and a bony canal in the maxilla, and sometimes the premaxilla, for its course, and in provision of expanded sites of origin for its musculature. Both fossorial reptiles and mammals make more use of olfaction than vision, but both groups predominantly emphasize modifications of the ear. Amphisbaenians, in particular, have restructured the ear and it is highly vibration-sensitive, perhaps with some loss of hearing acuity. Some mammals have expanded the ear components, variously the malleus-incus or the otic capsule and its contents, so that vibratory and/or acoustic acuity is implemented. At the same time, the head and skull are modified to protect ear function. Gymnophiones and amphisbaenians lack a tympanum, which obviously prevents damage to such a structure and which further smooths the outline of the head. Fossorial mammals characteristically lack external ears or pinnae, and the external auditory meatus is small and covered by fur, also reducing resistance to the head. Many mammals also increase tactile sensitivity by increasing number and length of vibrissae. In *Heterocephalus*, the naked mole-rat, hair is virtually absent, but patches of vibrissae are distributed over the body. This implementation violates the generalization of streamlining the surface of the body. I know of no study of wear on vibrissae during burrowing, but they are clearly well maintained in many fossorial mammals. It would be interesting to know whether the vibrissae of fossorial mammals (1) grow faster, (2) are shed and replaced more often, or (3) are more flexible than those of other mammals.

GENERAL CONCERNS

Which came first—fossoriality, that is, living underground for much of the life of the animal, or burrowing, in order to get underground? Some inferences can be made, if one accepts certain assumptions about the polarity of both morphological features and behaviors as noted below. I have already noted that there are forms that live underground, and even burrow, without apparent modification of the body for these activities (e.g., some salamanders, some lizards and snakes, some mammals). Many taxa in both aquatic and terrestrial habitats go underground without burrowing by following root channels, for instance, or crevices in rock piles. I therefore infer that the primitive morphology is the generalized, unmodified one, and that following already constructed channels is the primitive behavior. The derived behavior, then, is active burrowing, and the derived morphology includes modifications for subterranean life without burrowing (e.g., eye reduction, body elongation) and also the modifications for burrowing per se. Character state transitions must be carefully analyzed within lineages because of the diversity of morphologies and behaviors represented by various taxa.

Whether burrowing preceded fossoriality, or vice versa probably differs in different lineages. I hypothesize that in many lineages, burrowing preceded fossoriality. It is possible that animals that were feeding generalists nosed about in the substrate in search of prey, or followed plants to their roots. Exploitation of litter and subsurface prey might have allowed selection for features that effected prey capture and manipulation, and only incidentally burrowing at first. Conversely, in other animals fossoriality may have preceded burrowing. The subterranean existence provides an equilibrated environment with reduced predation (Nevo 1979). As animals utilized such environments, selection may have favored extension of burrows, compaction of the walls of burrows to make them more permanent, and soil transportation from the burrow. The team-digging of extended burrows by the colonial naked mole-rats may well be a highly derived behavioral expression of morphological and social structure, and feeding ecology, as Jarvis and Sales (1971) noted. At the same time, it is clear that the resistance of the medium is very important to locomotor activity. Specific characteristics of the substrate (grain size, moisture or its absence, etc.) are major determinants of burrowing effectiveness, as seen in examples ranging from amphioxus to moles. The use of suckers in fast-moving water by diverse fish and frog tadpoles is another example of a convergent response to similar ecological conditions that impose constraints but provide behavioral "opportunities."

These various evolutionary trends suggest that some of the morphological (and probably behavioral) features associated with locomotor phenomena are "exaptations" (Gould and Vrba 1982), or features present as modifications (adaptations) for a particular role, or even due to another role but not involved in it, that are therefore available for use in new ways. Such evolutionary/phylogenetic "baggage" is maintained, but not as a consequence of selection for a particular role. The presence of ever-growing incisors in rodents, generally assumed to be a modification for feeding on hard cellulose materials, and their utilization for breaking the soil to burrow, is an example of such an exaptation. The development of sucking discs in some fishes and tadpoles is another exaptation. The suckers presumably developed as holdfasts for position maintenance in fast-moving streams, but in the rare instances discussed above, are utilized for locomotion.

Analysis of such modifications of morphology and behavior for specific functions also calls for another warning about the nature of adaptations. Optimization models abound in the literature, and it is often assumed (though, fortunately, less frequently recently) that highly specialized organisms are optimally "fit" to their environments. However, specialization does not often yield full optimization. There are often trade-offs, and specialization for certain kinds of functions can result in reduced efficiency of other functions. Gans (1974) noted, for example, that the cranial deformation for burrowing in amphisbaenians through flattening of the anterior part of the skull reduces the space available for the olfactory apparatus and shifts the tooth rows to a position less efficient for crushing and biting. He noted that the ear is concomitantly restructured, with probable loss of auditory function, and the extracolumella is elongated as a compensation for the cranial modifications for burrowing. This example is useful in two other contexts. First, the elongated extracolumella is therefore an exaptation, and increased vibratory sensitivy is effected; and second, I infer that Gans believes that modifications for burrowing clearly preceded implementation of the vibration-sensory mode. These several examples are, I believe, indicators of the way evolutionary morphologists are likely to approach questions of adaptation in the future.

It is clear from this discussion that many questions about the structure and function of the skull as a locomotor organ remain unanswered. Aquatic animals that require fast-moving water, and terrestrial animals that live underground, are not easy to examine experimentally. Yet, the handful of recent studies that approach questions of function of the skull in locomotion indicates that the technology is available. It is a matter now of the availability of the animals and the investigator's patience, innovativeness, and ability to ask good questions. Obviously, some generalizations about skull use in locomotion are indicated. But, as Gasc et al. (1985) note, assumptions about convergence are many and superficial. Detailed idiographic studies are necessary to make available data other than the anecdotal, to provide the empirical base for generalization, and to allow a clearer delineation of pattern and process in evolution.

ACKNOWLEDGMENTS

I thank my colleagues Bill Fink, George Lauder, Axel Meyer, Ned Johnson, Jim Patton, Don Straney, David Wake, and Richard Wassersug for discussion and commiseration about the state of investigation of the skull as a locomotor organ. I especially thank Karen Klitz for preparing the illustrations. I am grateful to the National Science Foundation for supporting my work on the biology of the fossorial gymnophiones, and that of many of us who investigate adaptation and convergence in phylogenesis and evolution.

REFERENCES

Agrawal, V. C. 1967. Skull adaptations in fossorial rodents. Mammalia 31 (2): 300–312.

Airoldi, J.-P., R. Altrocchi, and A. Meylan. 1976. Le comportement fouisseur au campagnol terrestre, *Arvicola terrestris scherman* Shaw (Mammalia, Rodentia). Revue suisse de zoologie 83 (2): 282–286.

Alexander, R. McN. 1965. Structure and function in the catfish. Journal of Zoology, London 148: 88–152.

Altig, R., and E. D. Brodie, Jr. 1972. Laboratory behavior of *Ascaphus truei* tadpoles. Journal of Herpetology 6 (1): 21–24.

Annandale, N., and S. L. Hora. 1922. Parallel evolution in the fish and tadpoles of mountain torrents. Records of the Indian Museum, Calcutta 24: 505–509.

Bainbridge, R. 1983. Problems in fish locomotion. In *Fish Locomotion,* R. W. Blake, ed. New York: Cambridge University Press, pp. 13–32.

Bekele, A. 1983a. The comparative functional morphology of some head muscles of the rodents *Tachyoryctes splendens* and *Rattus rattus.* I. Jaw muscles. Mammalia 47 (3): 395–419.

————. 1983b. The comparative functional morphology of some head muscles of the rodents *Tachyoryctes splendens* and *Rattus rattus*. II. Cervical muscles. Mammalia 47 (4): 549–572.

Bemis, W. E., K. Schwenk, and M. H. Wake. 1983. Morphology and function of the feeding apparatus in *Dermophis mexicanus* (Amphibia: Gymnophiona). Zoological Journal of the Linnean Society 77: 75–96.

Benjamin, M. 1986. The oral sucker of *Gyrinocheicus aymonieri* (Teleostei: Cypriniformes). Journal of Zoology, London B 1: 211–254.

Billo, R., and M. H. Wake. 1987. Tentacle development in *Dermophis mexicanus* (Amphibia, Gymnophiona) with an hypothesis of tentacle origin. Journal of Morphology 192 (2): 101–111.

Bishop, S. C. 1943. *Handbook of Salamanders*. Ithaca, N.Y.: Comstock.

Brandon, R. A. 1965. Morphological variation and ecology of the salamander *Phaeognathus hubrichti*. Copeia: 67–71.

Breder, C. 1926. Locomotion of fishes. Zoologica 4 (5): 159–312.

Brien, P., M. Poll, and J. Bouillon. 1959. Éthologie de la reproduction de *Protopterus dolli* Blgr. Annali Royal Belgique, ser. 8, vol. 71: 3–21.

Casinos, A., J.-P. Gasc, S. Renous, J. Bou. 1983. Les modalités de fouissage de *Pitymys duodecimcostatus* (Mammalia, Arvicolidae). Mammalia 47 (1): 27–36.

Dubost, G. 1968. Les mammifères souterrains. Revue d'écologie et de biologie du sol 5 (1): 99–197.

Edgeworth, R. H. 1935. *The Cranial Muscles of Vertebrates*. Cambridge: Cambridge University Press.

Emerson, S. B. 1976. Burrowing in frogs. Journal of Morphology 149 (4): 437–458.

Feinholm, B., and K. Holmberg. 1975. The eyes in three genera of hagfish (*Eptatretus, Paramyxine,* and *Myxine*)—A case of degenerative evolution. Vision Research 15: 253–259.

Foss, G. 1963. *Myxine* in its natural surrounds. In *Biology of* Myxine, A. Brodal and R. Fange, eds. Oslo: Scandinavian University Books, pp. 42–45.

————. 1968. Behavior of *Myxine glutinosa* L. in natural habitat: Investigation of the mud biotope by a suction technique. Sarsia 31: 22–13.

Gaige, H. T. 1920. Observations upon the habits of *Ascaphus truei* Steineger. Occasional Papers of the Museum of Zoology, University of Michigan 84: 1–9.

Gans, C. 1960. Studies on amphisbaenids (Amphisbaenia, Reptilia). I. A taxonomic revision of the Trogonophinae and a functional interpretation of the amphisbaenid adaptive pattern. Bulletin of the American Museum of Natural History 119: 129–204.

————. 1962. The legless tetrapod caecilian poses questions for research. Natural History 71: 26–27.

————. 1968. Relative success of divergent pathways in amphisbaenian specialization. American Naturalist 102: 345–362.

————. 1969. Amphisbaenians—Reptiles specialized for a burrowing existence. Endeavour 28: 146–151.

————. 1973a. Locomotion and burrowing in limbless vertebrates. Nature 242 (5397): 414–415.

———. 1973b. Uropeltid snakes—Survivors in a changing world. Endeavour 32: 60–65.

———. 1974. *Biomechanics: An Approach to Vertebrate Biology*. Philadelphia: J. B. Lippincott Co.

———. 1976. Aspects of the biology of uropeltid snakes. In *Morphology and Biology of Reptiles*, A. d'A. Bellairs and C. B. Cox, eds. Linnean Society Symposium Series 3. Dorchester: Dorset Press, pp. 191–204.

———. 1978. The characteristics and affinities of the Amphisbaenia. Transactions of the Zoological Society of London 34: 347–416.

Gans, C., H. C. Dessauer, and D. Baic. 1978. Axial differences in the musculature of uropeltid snakes: The freight-train approach to burrowing. Science 199: 189–192.

Gasc, J.-P., S. Renous, A. Casinos, E. Laville, and J. Bou. 1985. Comparison of diverse digging patterns in some small mammals. In *Vertebrate Morphology*. H.-R. Duncker and G. Fleischer, eds. Fortschritte der Zoologie 30. Stuttgart: Gustav Fischer, pp. 35–38.

Gasc, J.-P., F. K. Jouffroy, and S. Renous. 1986. Morphofunctional study of the digging system of the Namib Desert golden mole (*Eremitalpa granti namibensis*): Cinefluorographical and anatomical analysis. Journal of Zoology, London A 208: 9–35.

Gaymer, R. 1971. New method of locomotion in limbless terrestrial vertebrates. Nature 234: 150–151.

Gould, S. J., and E. S. Vrba. 1982. Exaptation—A missing term in the science of form. Paleobiology 8: 4–15.

Gradwell, N. 1971a. *Ascaphus* tadpole: Experiments on the suction and gill irrigation mechanisms. Canadian Journal of Zoology 49: 307–332.

———. 1971b. Observations on jet propulsion in banjo catfishes. Canadian Journal of Zoology 49: 1611–1612.

Greenwood, P. H. 1986. The natural history of African lungfishes. In *The Biology of Lungfishes*, W. E. Bemis, W. W. Burggren, and N. E. Kemp, eds. Journal of Morphology 1 (suppl.): 163–180.

Hardisty, M. W., and I. C. Potter. 1971a. The behavioral ecology and growth of larval lampreys. In *The Biology of Lampreys*, vol. 1, M. W. Hardisty and I. C. Potter, eds. New York: Academic Press, pp. 85–126.

———. 1971b. General biology of adult lampreys. In *The Biology of Lampreys*, vol. 1, M. W. Hardisty and I. C. Potter, eds. New York: Academic Press, pp. 127–206.

Hedges, S. B., and R. Thomas. 1987. A new burrowing frog from Hispaniola, with comments on the *inoptallus* group of the genus *Eleutherodactylus* (Anura: Leptodactylidae). Herpetologica 43 (3): 269–279.

Hildebrand, M. 1984. Digging and crawling without appendages. In *Analysis of Vertebrate Structure*, 2d ed., M. Hildebrand, ed. New York: John Wiley and Sons, pp. 463–484.

———. 1985. Digging of quadrupeds. In *Functional Vertebrate Morphology*, M. Hildebrand, D. M. Bramble, K. R. Liem, and D. B. Wake, eds. Cambridge, Mass.: Belknap Press, pp. 89–109.

Howard, W. E., and M. E. Smith. 1952. Rate of extrusive growth of incisors of pocket gophers. Journal of Mammalogy 33 (4): 485–487.

Hubbs, C. L., and I. C. Potter. 1971. Distribution, phylogeny, and taxonomy. In *The Biology of Lampreys,* vol. 1, W. M. Hardisty and I. C. Potter, eds. New York: Academic Press, pp. 1–65.

Jarvis, J. V. M., and J. B. Sale. 1971. Burrowing and burrow patterns of East African mole-rats *Tachyoryctes, Heliophobius,* and *Heterocephalus.* Journal of Zoology, London 163: 451–479.

Johnels, A. G., and G. S. O. Svensson. 1954. On the biology of *Protopterus annectens* (Owen). Arkiv für Zoologie 7: 131–164.

Johnson, R. D. O. 1912. Notes on the habits of a climbing catfish (*Arges marmoratus*) from the Republic of Colombia. Annals of the New York Academy of Science 22: 327–333.

Kemp, A. 1986. The biology of the Australian lungfish, *Neoceratodus forsteri* (Krefft 1870). In *The Biology of Lungfishes,* W. E. Bemis, W. W. Burggren, and N. E. Kemp, eds. Journal of Morphology, 1 (suppl.): 181–198.

Kerr, J. G. 1900. The external features in the development of *Lepidosiren paradoxa.* Transactions of the Royal Society of London 192: 299–330.

Kestevin, H. L. 1944. The evolution of the skull and the cephalic muscles. Part II. The Amphibians. Memoirs of the Australian Museum, Sydney 8 (3): 133–236.

Knight-Jones, E. W. 1952. On the nervous system of *Saccoglossus cambrensis* (Enteropneusta). Philosophical Transactions of the Royal Society of London B 236: 315–354.

Lawson, R. 1965. The anatomy of *Hypogeophis rostratus* Cuvier. Part II. The Musculature. Proceedings of the University of Newcastle upon Tyne. Philosophical Society 1 (5): 52–63.

Lessa, E. P., and C. S. Thaeler, Jr. 1989. A reassessment of morphological specializations for digging in pocket gophers. Journal of Mammalogy 70 (4): 689–700.

Lindsey, C. C. 1978. Form, function, and locomotory habits in fish. In *Fish Physiology,* vol. 7, W. S. Hoar and O. J. Randall, eds. New York: Academic Press, pp. 1–100.

Martof, B. S. 1962. Some aspects of the life history and ecology of the salamander *Leurognathus.* American Midland Naturalist 67 (1): 1–35.

Minckley, C. O., and H. E. Klaassen. 1969. Burying behavior of the plains killifish, *Fundulus kansae.* Copeia (1): 200–201.

Moodie, G. E. E. 1978. Observations on the life history of the caecilian *Typhlonectes compressicaudus* (Dumeril and Bibron) in the Amazon basin. Canadian Journal of Zoology 56 (4): 1005–1008.

Mosauer, W. 1932. Adaptive convergence in the sand reptiles of the Sahara and of California. Copeia (2): 72–78.

Naylor, B. G., and R. A. Nussbaum. 1980. The trunk musculature of caecilians (Amphibia: Gymnophiona). Journal of Morphology 166: 259–273.

Nevo, E. 1979. Adaptive convergence and divergence of subterranean mammals. Annual Reviews of Ecology and Systematics 10: 269–308.

Nikolsky, G. V. 1963. *The Ecology of Fishes*. New York: Academic Press.

Nishi, S. 1916. Zur vergleichenden Anatomie der eigentlichen Ruckenmuskeln. Morphologisches Jahrbuch 50: 167–318.

———. 1938. Muskeln des Rumpfes. In *Handbuch der vergleichenden Anatomie der Wirbeltiere*, vol. 5, L. Bolk, E. Goppert, E. Kallius, and W. Lubosch, eds. Berlin: Urban and Schwarzenberg, pp. 351–446.

Noble, G. K. 1929. The adaptive modifications of the arboreal tadpoles of *Holophryne* and the torrent tadpoles of *Staurois*. Bulletin of the American Museum of Natural History 58 (7): 291–334.

Norman, J. R. 1931. *A History of Fishes*. London: Ernest Benn.

Norris, K. S., and J. L. Kavanau. 1966. The burrowing of the Western shovel-nosed snake, *Chionactis occipitalis* Hallowell, and the underground environment. Copeia (4): 650–664.

Nussbaum, R. A. 1983. The evolution of a unique dual jaw-closing mechanism in caecilians (Amphibia: Gymnophiona) and its bearing on caecilian ancestry. Journal of Zoology, London 199: 545–554.

Nussbaum, R. A., and B. G. Naylor. 1982. Variation in the trunk musculature of caecilians (Amphibia: Gymnophiona). Journal of Zoology, London 198: 383–398.

Orcutt, E. E. 1940. Studies on the muscles of the head, neck, and pectoral assemblages of *Geomys bursarius*. Journal of Mammalogy 21 (1): 37–52.

Piavis, G. W. 1971. Embryology. In *The Biology of Lampreys*, vol. 1, M. W. Hardisty and I. C. Potter, eds. New York: Academic Press, pp. 361–400.

Puttick, G. M., and J. V. M. Jarvis. 1977. The function of anatomy of the neck and forelimbs of the Cape Golden Mole, *Chrysochloris asiatica* (Lipotyphla, Chrysochloridae). Zoologica africana 12 (2): 445–458.

Renous, S., and J.-P. Gasc. 1986. The burrowing of gymnophiones (Amphibia) a morpho-functionally founded hypothesis of the comparison with other vertebrates. Zoologische Jahrbuch Anatomie 114: 95–130.

Ritter, W. 1902. The movements of the Enteropneusta and the mechanism by which they are accomplished. Biological Bulletin 3: 24–30.

Rose, K. D., and P. J. Emry. 1983. Extraordinary fossorial adaptations in the Oligocene palaeanodonts *Epoicotherium* and *Xenocranium* (Mammalia). Journal of Morphology 175 (1): 33–56.

Sawyer, H. W. 1959. Burrowing activities of the larval lampreys. Copeia: 256–257.

Schnurbein, A. F. von. 1935. Der Bewegungsapparat von *Hypogeophis*. Beitrag zur Kenntnis der Gymnophionen XXIII. Morphologisches Jahrbuch 75: 315–330.

Strahan, R. 1963. The behavior of *Myxine* and other myxinoids. In *Biology of Myxine*, A. Brodal and R. Fange, eds. Oslo: Scandinavian University Books, pp. 22–32.

Straub, J. O. 1984. Aspects of the cranial anatomy of *Grandisonia diminutiva* Taylor. Mémoir de la Société zoologique de France 43: 55–63.

Trueman, E. R., and H. D. Ansell. 1969. The mechanisms of burrowing into soft substrata by marine animals. Oceanography and Marine Biology Annual Reviews 7: 315–366.

Tucker, R. 1981. The digging behavior and skin differentiations in *Heterocephalus glaber*. Journal of Morphology 168: 51–71.

Underwood, G. 1970. The eye. In *Biology of the Reptilia*, vol. 2, C. Gans and T. S. Parsons, eds. New York: Academic Press, pp. 1–97.

Valentine, B. D. 1963. The plethodontid salamander *Phaeognathus:* Collecting techniques and habits. Journal of the Ohio Herpetological Society 4 (1–2): 49–54.

Wake, D. B. 1966. Comparative osteology and evolution of the lungless salamanders, family Plethodontidae. Memoirs of the Southern California Academy of Science 4: 1–111.

Wake, M. H. 1980. Morphometrics of the skeleton of *Dermophis mexicanus* (Amphibia: Gymnophiona). Part I. The vertebrae, with comparisons to other species. Journal of Morphology 165 (2): 117–130.

———. 1985. The comparative morphology and evolution of the eyes of caecilians (Amphibia: Gymnophiona). Zoomorphology 105 (5): 277–295.

Wake, M. H., and J. Hanken. 1982. The development of the skull of *Dermophis mexicanus* (Amphibia: Gymnophiona), with comments on skull kinesis and amphibian relationships. Journal of Morphology 173 (2): 203–223.

Wassersug, R. J., and W. F. Pyburn. 1987. The biology of the peret toad, *Otophryne robusta* (Microhylidae), with special consideration of its fossorial larva and systematic relationships. Zoological Journal of the Linnean Society 91: 137–169.

Webb, J. E. 1973. The role of the notochord in forward and reverse swimming and burrowing in the Amphioxus *Branchiostoma lanceolatum*. Journal of Zoology, London 170: 325–338.

Webb, J. E., and M. B. Hill. 1958. The ecology of Lagos Lagoon. IV. On the reactions of *Branchiostoma nigeriense* Webb to its environment. Proceedings of the Royal Society of London 241: 355–391.

Welty, J. C. 1975. *The Life of Birds,* 2d ed. Philadelphia: W. B. Saunders.

Wiedersheim, R. 1879. *Die Anatomie der Gymnophionen*. Jena: Gustav Fischer Verlag.

6

Structural Basis of Hearing and Sound Transmission

R. Eric Lombard and Thomas E. Hetherington

INTRODUCTION

ALL ACTIVE, FREE-LIVING METAZOANS have complex sense organs located in the head, the part of the animal encountering the environment first during normal locomotion. Vertebrates are among the most active of animals and cephalization in them is as much a consequence of the evolution of sense organs as it is of feeding and respiration. This is particularly true of the neurocranium, that part of the skull housing the olfactory, visual, and stato-acoustic organs as well as that part of the central nervous system evolved to process input from them—the three primary vesicles of the brain.

In this chapter we consider in schematic format the structural components of the vertebrate skull related to hearing and sound transmission from the interrelated perspectives of function and evolution. These perspectives provide a logical if not always provable explanation for the location and configuration of skull features related to hearing which otherwise are inscrutable.

The fundamental building block of hearing in vertebrates is the hair cell (fig. 6.1). Hair cells are autapomorphous for vertebrates, occurring in no other animals. All hair cells develop from ectodermal placodes and remain epithelial in adults where they occur interspersed with supporting cells in neuroepithelial patches that contain anywhere from tens to hundreds of thousands of hair cells.

Over the past twenty years we have begun to learn about the general response properties of hair cells, but though a basic picture has emerged, cells from only a very limited number of taxa and end organs have been examined. Present knowledge has been most recently reviewed by Ashmore (1988). Hair cells are transducers: They change displacement at their apical end into an electrical potential that results in a chemical discharge at synapses at their basal end. The chemical discharge in turn initiates an electrical potential in a nerve fiber to the brain. The specific displacement

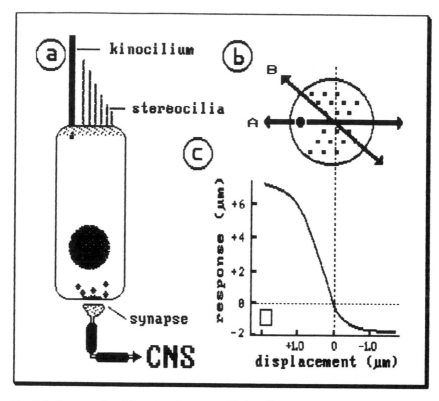

Fig. 6.1. Structural and functional aspects of hair cells. a. General structure of a hair cell. In life, the kino- and stereocilia would project partly into an acellular matrix contained within a fluid space. b. Apical schematic view of a hair cell showing the relationship of the apical projections to the axis of maximum response (arrow a). Displacements away from this axis (arrow b) result in reduced response as a function of the cosine of the angle from the axis. c. Graph illustrating the relation between displacement and response for a generalized hair cell. The response to displacements of the stereocilia toward the kinocilium are much greater in magnitude and opposite in sign from displacements away from the kinocilium. Redrawn from Hudspeth and Corey (1977).

to which the cells are sensitive is shear of their sterocilia relative to the apical surface of the cell; either the cell can be moved relative to the stereocilia or vice versa (fig. 6.1).

Individual cells are limited in the range of displacement variables to which they are sensitive. They have a limited dynamic range, responding to displacements over about three orders of magnitude from 3×10^{-10} to 2×10^{-7} m. The highest best frequency of response so far measured— about 350 Hz—occurs in some of the electrically tuned cells in a turtle basilar papilla, but this is unusual; most respond best only to frequencies below 100 Hz (Art and Fettiplace 1987). Finally, individual hair cells, though having an axis of stimulation to which they are most sensitive, cannot detect the direction of a signal source.

Morphological studies over the past 20 years have demonstrated obvious as well as subtle variation in the structure of hair cells from different acousticolateralis structures. Three major hair cell morphs are known (types I, II, and lenticulate) and several subtle variations in cell constituents have been described (Lewis et al. 1985). For example, the length of the stereociliary bundle varies, being generally longer in vestibular than in auditory epithelia, but bundle length also may vary in a regular way within auditory epithelia. This latter variation appears to be functionally correlated with best frequency of sensitivity (Turner et al. 1981). This variation in structure and in response properties indicates that evolution has taken place in hair cells; hair cells are not a singular type and have diversified in evolutionary time. Nevertheless, the presently known response properties of hair cells are not broad enough to account for the known range of hearing abilities of vertebrates. In fact, hair cells, talented though they may be, are best thought of as being rather limited with respect to the requirements of hearing. In ourselves, for example, the ear is sensitive to sound frequencies of from 15 to 15,000 Hz, detects sound amplitude over six orders of magnitude in part of that range, and detects the direction of the sound source. Clearly, the hair cells of our inner ear are receiving help in overcoming their limitations. Much of this help comes from the attributes of auxiliary nonneural structures, most of which are either made of the skull and nearby structures or influence the form of the skull and nearby structures. These auxiliary structures can be thought of as signal conditioners. Their function is to transform the incoming acoustic signal into a form to which the hair cells can respond (fig. 6.2).

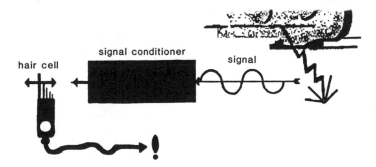

Fig. 6.2. In vertebrate hearing a signal conditioner is necessary to alter incoming sound into a form to which hair cells can respond.

In this chapter we consider the evolution and function of representative auxiliary nonneural signal conditioners in vertebrates. The evolution of the diversity of vertebrate hearing abilities has come about primarily through the evolution and diversification of these auxiliary structures rather than through the evolution of the hair cells. Some evolution of the cells has occurred to be sure, but apparently as a later refinement rather than as an early, fundamental change within the evolution of any particular hearing system. The representatives we review have been chosen to demonstrate that auxiliary hearing structures are at once similar in function but diverse in origin and history so as to display the range of solutions vertebrates have found to detect sound in the environment.

EARLY EVOLUTION

Surface neuromast organs, where groups of hair cells are embedded in the surface ectoderm and directly confront the aquatic environment at their apical end, are generally considered the most primitive hair cell placement presently occurring in vertebrates, though Northcutt (1989) clearly demonstrates that the surface neuromasts of many Recent taxa are likely secondarily derived through reduction by paedomorphosis. In surface neuromasts, the stereocilia are coupled to the fluid of the environment by a gelatinous cupula. A more derived condition is to have neuromasts within canals beneath the skin: the lateral line system. These canals are open to the aqueous environment only at selected points and thus the contained hair cells (again covered with a cupula) confront the environment indirectly. The lateral line system of canals and openings is a signal conditioner functioning to configure its hair cells to detect certain types of environmental fluid displacements, but its exact role in the adaptive biology of fishes is somewhat enigmatic. The lateral line has been shown to be used in detecting local water displacements for close-range obstacle detection in some fishes (Dijkgraaf 1963) and small surface waves in others (Schwartz 1974). Physiologically, lateral line receptors respond best to displacements (or the derivatives of displacement: acceleration or velocity) of 20 to 100 Hz with thresholds in the range of 1×10^{-7} to 1×10^{-9} m (Sand 1981; Coombs and Janssen 1990).

Surface neuromasts and lateral lines occur in most gnathostome fish and in amphibians that have an aquatic phase to their life history. The lateral line canal system on the head is often embedded totally or partially within the bones of the skull, forming a prominent and often specific pattern found even in the earliest vertebrate fossils (fig. 6.3). Thorough reviews of the pattern of surface neuromasts and lateral lines in Recent taxa,

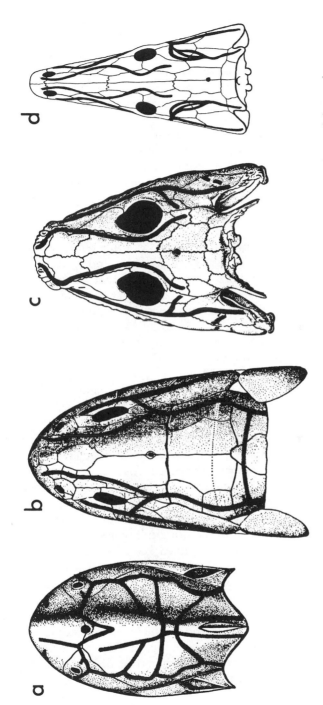

Fig. 6.3. Lateral line canals in the skulls of some fossil vertebrates. The various skull bones are shown in outline and the canals are indicated by heavy lines. a. *Anglaspis*, a Paleozoic jawless fish and member of the earliest group of vertebrates with a fossil record. Skull is about 3 cm long. b. *Eusthenopteron*, a Paleozoic sarcopterygian fish related to the lineage from which tetrapods evolved. Skull is about 10 cm long. c. *Palaeogyrinus*, a Paleozoic amphibian related to the lineage leading to amniotes. Skull is about 20 cm long. d. *Trematosaurus*, a Mesozoic amphibian related to the lineage leading to modern amphibians. Skull is about 50 cm long. Redrawn from Romer (1974).

their ontogeny, diversity, and possible phylogeny maybe found in Coombs et al. (1988) and Northcutt (1989).

In vertebrate embryos, the paired otic labyrinths of the inner ear begin as fluid-filled, epithelial vesicles formed by involution of the otic placodes of the surface ectoderm. The vesicles form lateral to the hind brain just dorsal to the hyoid arch and pouch. Subsequently, each vesicle is transformed into the adult configuration of otic fluid–filled chambers and semicircular ducts. This general developmental sequence is believed to reflect the evolution of the internalized membranous labyrinth from surface neuromasts and lateral line (fig. 6.4, nos. 1, 2). In sharks and rays, the labyrinth maintains a tenuous connection to the environment via a duct piercing the roof of the chondrocranium marking its mode of development (fig. 6.11, ED).

Within gnathostomes, three semicircular ducts and two major chambers, the utricle and saccule, invariably result from differentiation of the otic vesicle. In agnathans fewer semicircular ducts and chambers are formed. The otic semicircular ducts occur in orthogonal planes of space and are confluent with the chamber of the utricle. The utricle is in turn connected to the more ventral saccule by a duct. Five neuroepithelia containing hair cells are associated with these structures: one with each otic semicircular duct (cristae) and one each with the utricle and saccule (maculae). In each, the kinocilium and stereocilia of each hair cell are generally embedded in a covering material that is in contact with the fluid of the labyrinth. The otic labyrinth in this basic form is a signal conditioner constructed to enable its contained hair cells to detect the attitude and movements of the animal with reference to its environment (fig. 6.5). This is the reverse of surface neuromasts and the lateral line, where the function is the detection of movements of the environment with reference to the animal. Isolation from environmental displacements is thus necessary for the labyrinth, since the same transducers are utilized, and it is achieved by internalization (fig. 6.4). Whereas in surface neuromasts and lateral lines shear results from the movement of the stereocilia relative to the cell, in these labyrinthine end organs it results from displacement of the cell relative to its stereocilia. The hair cells are coupled to the general tissues of the head and thus are moved or are positioned with the head. The otic fluid in the labyrinth, on the other hand, is free to flow, and owing to its inertia lags in its displacement relative to that of the animal. Shear at the apex of the hair cell results. This shear is configured by the shape of the ducts and cupula for the otic semicircular ducts and by the inclusion of otoconia to enhance differential inertia in the utricle and saccule. This particular functional mode, where shear depends on coupling of the hair cells to the head, demands that this coupling be as rigid as possible. This requirement is likely the explanation for periotic connective tissue which binds the laby-

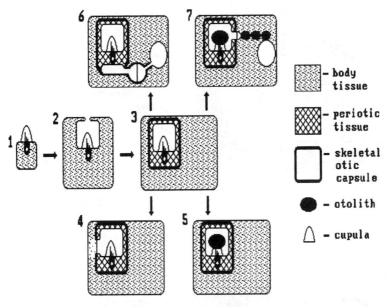

Fig. 6.4. The major configurations of hearing structures in fishes. *Center row:* a plausible sequence in the early evolution of the otic region prior to the origins of hearing mechanisms. 1. The surface neuromast in which the apical projections of the hair cells are embedded in a gelatinous cupula which is in direct contact with the fluid environment. 2. Internalization of the neuromast such as in the lateral line or the early stages in the evolution of the membranous labyrinth (and also seen in embryogenesis). Contact with the environment is less direct. 3. Isolation of the otic neuroepithelia as in the membranous labyrinths of vertebrates. Here the fluid space (otic fluid) lies within a skeletal otic capsule and is bound to it by periotic tissue. This is a vestibular structure. *Lower row:* two types of displacement detectors used in hearing by fishes. Both are evolved from vestibular structures. 4. The direct cupular mechanism of the macula neglecta of carcharhinid sharks where a membrane-lined opening of the skull occurs. 5. The direct otolithic mechanism of the saccular macula of sharks. *Upper row:* two types of pressure detectors found in fish in which the swim bladder is used as a pressure transducer. In both, the parts inside the otic capsule are derived from vestibular structures 6. The bulla mechanism of clupeids. Gas in the bulla pulsates against a membrane which moves fluid which displaces the cells. 7. The Weberian ossicle mechanism of ostariophysine fish. Gas in the swim bladder pulsates against the Weberian ossicles, which move fluid which displaces an otolith.

rinth to a skeletal otic capsule which in turn is bound to the braincase of the skull (figs. 6.5 and 6.6). It also may be that as a dense and hence acoustically reflective tissue, the otic capsule also evolved to further isolate the labyrinthine receptors from environmental displacements.

With the primitive gnathostome labyrinth just outlined as a starting point, the stage is set for the evolution of hearing; yet it would seem that all the wrong props are in place. The transducer, the labyrinthine hair cell,

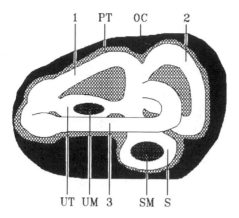

Fig. 6.5. Schematic illustration of the left membranous labyrinth showing a lateral view of the basic parts found in all gnathostomes (1, 2, 3: the otic semicircular ducts. UT: utricle. S: saccule). The otic capsule (OC) may closely follow the shape of the membranous labyrinth (especially on its internal surface). The periotic tissue (PT) binds the labyrinth to the otic capsule. The two primitively vestibular maculae, UM and SM, repeatedly give rise to auditory epithelia in the evolution of hearing.

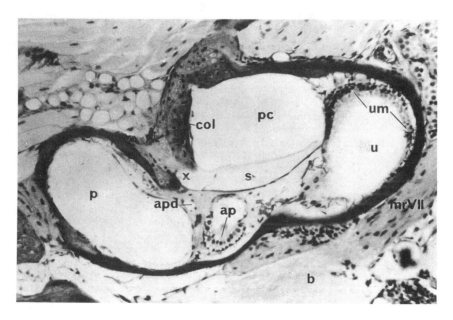

Fig. 6.6. Photomicrograph of a frontal section through the otic capsule and labyrinth of the salamander, *Batrachoseps attenuatus.* Anterior is to the right and lateral is toward the top of the page. Note the bone of the capsule following the shape of the labyrinth in some regions and the periotic connective tissue between the labyrinth and the capsule. Portions of the membranous labyrinth: p, posterior semicircular duct; u, utricle; s, saccule. Sensory neuroepithelia: ap, amphibian papilla; um, utricular macula. Periotic fluid spaces: apd, amphibian periotic duct; pc, periotic cistern; x, junction of the duct and cistern. Col: the movable plate of skeletal tissue in the fenestra ovalis; b, brain.

is configured to detect very low frequency displacements produced by the movements of the animal over a limited range of amplitudes. In the labyrinth these hair cells are integral functional parts of vestibular end organs, and as a consequence of their functional role are isolated from the environment, the source of sound. Thus, from the very beginning it would appear that the theme for auditory evolution is to make do from what is available rather than to aim for what would be "best." For example, there is no functional logic that would dictate that hearing organs be placed at the caudal end of the skull. That they are there very likely has everything to do with the early evolution of a receptor suitable for the dynamics of primitive aquatic locomotion and nothing to do with the functional necessities of hearing. As the examples discussed in later sections will show, this is a theme maintained throughout the evolution of hearing structures in vertebrates.

It would also appear that, given the starting conditions, auditory receptors have evolved "inside out," from the presumptive acoustic labyrinthine hair cells out to the environment. Isolation of labyrinthine hair cells was not (and still is not) perfect. For some, a weak coupling to the environment through an isolation flaw could be exploited by natural selection to initiate the formation of a hearing organ. Subsequent evolution would involve the improvement of the sensitivity and fidelity of this coupling in a way so as not to introduce environmental "noise" to the remaining preponderance of cells dedicated to the vestibular function of the labyrinth. In some vertebrates, parts of the saccular or utricular maculae have been coupled to the environment for audition. In others, novel maculae or papillae derived from the primitive saccular or utricular maculae then have evolved for hearing (fig. 6.7). In many, more than one macula may be

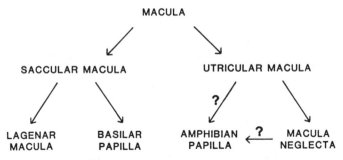

Fig. 6.7. Plausible evolutionary relationships among the sensory neuroepithelia, which in at least some taxa are related to hearing. The evolutionary derivation of the amphibian papilla is less certain than the others. Also, the basilar papillae of amphibians and amniotes may not be homologous. The amphibian and basilar papillae are always related to sound perception when they occur. The others are involved in sound perception in some taxa and solely in vestibular function in others.

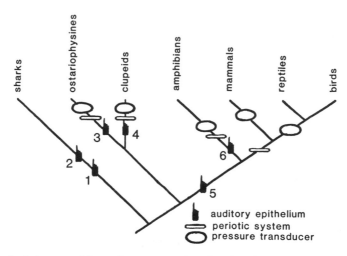

Fig. 6.8. A phylogeny of the major taxa mentioned in this chapter and the origins of some auditory structures in vertebrates. The ostariophysines and clupeids are both major groups of actinopterygian boney fish. The most reasonable estimates for the evolutionary origins of major components of the hearing systems in these groups are indicated by icons placed on the phylogeny. All three major components—auditory neuroepithelia, periotic fluid systems, and pressure transducers—have evolved more than once. 1. Saccular macula. 2. Macula neglecta. 3. Saccular macula. 4. Utricular macula. 5. Basilar papilla. 6. Amphibian papilla. The lagenar macula is involved in hearing in some actinopterygian taxa as well.

involved. Figure 6.8 illustrates the phylogenetic relationships of the taxa considered in the remainder of this chapter and, in schematic form, the most parsimonious phyletic origins of auditory function for hair cells and some auxiliary structures. Groups of hair cells dedicated to audition can be seen to have evolved several times. Diverse means of improving the coupling between the auditory hair cells and the environment have evolved in vertebrates, as well as similar solutions achieved multiple times in parallel, also schematically illustrated in figure 6.8. In the following sections we shall examine the evolution and function of some of the better-known auxiliary structures in each of these taxa.

AUDITORY STRUCTURES IN FISHES

In open water, sound radiates from a simple, monopolar pulsating source in spherically spreading, longitudinal waves consisting of an oscillating displacement of water particles and a concomitant oscillation of pressure. Figure 6.9 graphs particle displacement as a function of distance from a simple pulsating source for a variety of sound frequencies all at the same source strength. Quite evident is the expected decrease in displacement

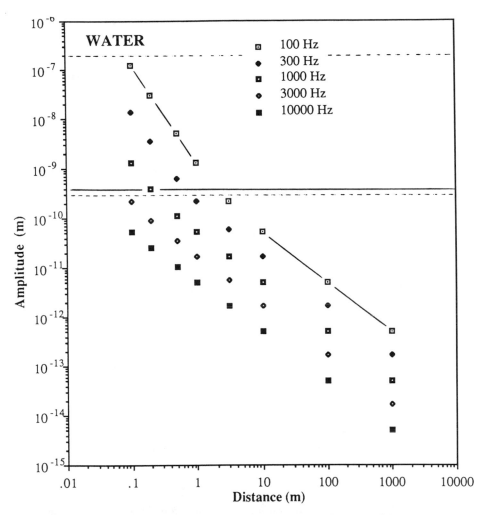

Fig. 6.9. Graph of water particle displacement amplitude as a function of distance from the source for several frequencies of sound. The sound source for each is a pulsating sphere of small size with a strength of 1×10^{-6} Watts. Such a source in air would measure 72 dB re .00002 N/m² at 10 cm, approximately a normal speaking voice. The dashed lines delimit the general sensitivity range of a hair cell. The solid line is the rough boundary between the near and far fields equal to wavelength/$2p$. In the near field, displacement amplitude is greater than would be expected. The relationship between displacement and distance in the near field would be different for other kinds of sources (Van Bergeijk 1966). This is an idealized case. In the real world, sound would suffer excess attenuation as a result of temperature gradients, physical obstacles, etc., and the magnitude of some of these effects would vary with frequency. Equations used to generate points are listed in the appendix.

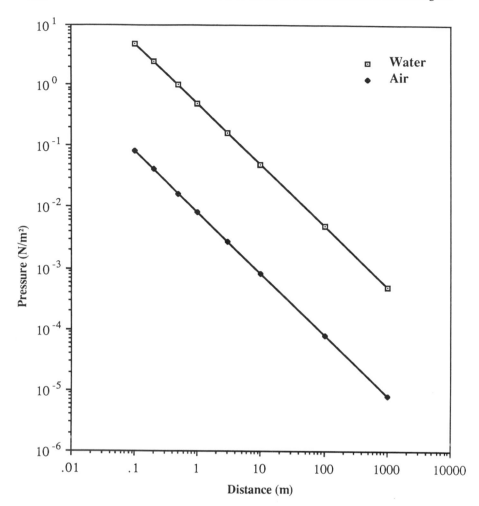

Fig. 6.10. Graph of pressure as a function of distance from the source for the same sound source as shown in figure 6.9. The relation of pressure with distance is shown for both air and water. As in figure 6.9, this is an idealized example. Equations used to generate points are listed in the appendix.

amplitude with increase in frequency. Also evident is that the decrease in displacement amplitude with distance from the source is not uniform. Far from the source, displacement is decreasing proportional to 1/distance: the far field. Very near to a simple pulsating spherical source the decrease is proportional to 1/distance^2: the near field. The transition zone occurs at about wavelength/2ρ and so is farther from the source at lower frequencies (Van Bergeijk 1966). Pressure decreases uniformly at 1/distance from the source for all frequencies (fig. 6.10).

As a whole, the body of a neutrally buoyant aquatic vertebrate is the same density as its environment. If the organism were structurally homogeneous it would be translucent to sound waves; all parts would oscillate in phase and with the same amplitude as the surrounding water. In order to detect the displacement component of a sound wave, hair cells must be placed such that apical shear is created as a consequence of local differential densities. In order to detect the pressure component of a sound wave, a pressure-to-displacement transducer is needed between the environment and the hair cells, since they are not in themselves pressure-sensitive. Below we describe examples of these two mechanisms as they occur in fishes.

Displacement Detection

Carcharhinid sharks respond to sounds between 40 and 800 Hz and are most sensitive between 40 and 200–300 Hz (Nelson 1967). They have auditory organs that detect the displacement component of sound and are capable of detecting displacements of about 5×10^{-10} m at threshold (Banner 1967; Corwin 1981). This figure is probably not meaningfully different from the experimentally determined threshold value known for isolated hair cells of 3×10^{-10} m (Ashmore 1988) and is perhaps slightly more sensitive than intact lateral-line hair cells (1×10^{-9} m, Coombs and Janssen 1989). This indicates a remarkably good coupling between the hair cells in the labyrinth used in sound detection and the surrounding water medium.

Two maculae are known to be involved in hearing in *Carcharhinus*, the macula neglecta and the cranial portion of the saccular macula, and though both directly detect the displacement component, the two function differently (Corwin 1981). Sharks have a unique tube in the labyrinth, the posterior canal duct, connecting the posterior vertical semicircular duct with the saccular chamber (fig. 6.11). The kinocilia and stereocilia of the macula neglecta hair cells project into the lumen of the connecting duct where they are covered by a gelatinous cupula. All the hair cells have the functional axis aligned with the duct and the duct itself is aligned with a membranous opening in the roof of the otic capsule, the "fenestra ovalis" (fig. 6.11). The "fenestra ovalis" lies at the base of a depression in the cartilaginous skull roof which is filled with a mucoid connective tissue. The arrangement of these structures provides a low-impedance, confined, and directed path for the displacements of sound waves to reach the stereocilia of the hair cells in the macula neglecta (fig. 6.11; and in schematic form in fig. 6.4, no. 4). In this system the cupula is well coupled to the displacements of the environmental fluid and the hair cells are not, being instead better coupled to the denser skull. Thus, in a sound field the cupula oscillates at a greater amplitude than the hair cells (and perhaps out of phase as well), creating shear of the stereocilia relative to the cell. This functional

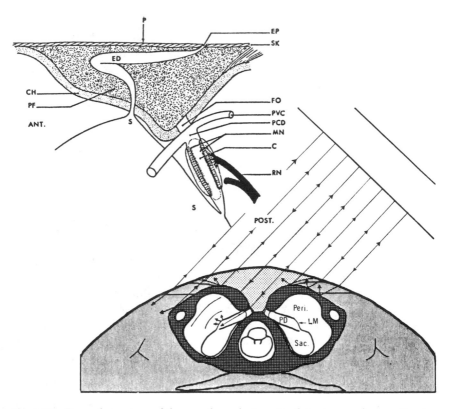

Fig. 6.11. General structure of the macula neglecta as it relates to sound perception in some sharks. *Upper:* Schematic illustration of the macula neglecta showing its orientation with respect to the roof of the otic capsule and the "fenestra ovalis" (FO). The macula neglecta (MN) lies on two sides of the posterior canal duct (PCD), which contains a cupula (C) and connects the posterior vertical canal (PVC) with the saccule (S). The nerve branch from the macula is shown (RN). The "fenestra ovalis" lies in the roof of the otic capsule of the chondrocranium (CH) in a region where it is depressed and filled with mucoid tissue (PF). This tissue is covered only by skin (SK). Also shown is the endolymphatic duct (ED), a remnant of development retained only in sharks and rays which opens to the environment at the endolymphatic pore (EP). Reprinted with permission from Fay et al. (1974). *Lower:* Schematic cross section through the otic capsules and braincase of a shark illustrating how the macula neglecta sense organ might be directionally sensitive. Only sound impinging on the "fenestra ovalis" along the axis of the posterior canal duct (PD) is transmitted to the macula neglecta (LM). The saccule and periotic space are illustrated as well. Reprinted with permission from Corwin (1977).

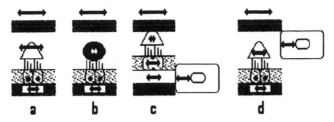

a   b   c   d

Fig. 6.12. Ways in which hair cells are able to detect sound in vertebrates. In all, the length of the arrow indicates relative amplitude of displacement. (a) and (b) are direct displacement mechanisms in which displacements of the environment are coupled to the neuroepithelium. (c) and (d) are indirect: pressure changes are transduced to displacements. (a) and (b) are modified from Corwin (1981). a. The direct cupular mechanism. Here the cupula (middle arrow) is well coupled to the otic fluid in which it lies. The otic fluid is well coupled to the environment in which the displacements of the sound occur (topmost arrow). The hair cells are coupled to the skull (bottom arrow), a dense tissue which is less well coupled to the environment. Essentially, the cupula is moving relative to the cells, and shear results. This mechanism occurs in the macula neglecta of sharks. b. The direct otolith mechanism. Here the very dense otolith or otoconial mass (middle arrow) is less well coupled to the displacements of sound in the environment (upper arrow) than the skull to which the hair cells are coupled (bottom arrow). Essentially, the cells are moving relative to the otolith or otoconia. This mechanism is believed to occur in the saccular macula of sharks and the lagenar and saccular maculae of many actinopterygian fishes. c. The indirect cellular mechanism. Here the hair cells (lower left arrow) are coupled to the displacements created by the transducer (right arrow) from the pressure component of sound. Other tissues (skull and cupula) are less well coupled (upper arrow). Essentially, the cells are moving relative to the cupula. This mechanism occurs in the utricular macula of clupeid fishes and the basilar papilla and its derivatives in amniotes (where the cupula is called a tectorium). d. The indirect cupular mechanism. Here the cupula (upper left arrow) is coupled to the displacements created by the transducer (right arrow) from the pressure component of sound. Other tissues (skull and hair cells) are less well coupled (bottom arrow). Essentially, the cupula is moving relative to the cells. This mechanism occurs in the saccular macula of ostariophysine fish (where the cupula is in fact an otolith) and the amphibian and basilar papillae of frogs (where the cupula is called a tectorium).

mode is schematically illustrated in figure 6.12. Experimental evidence (Corwin 1981) indicates that this receptor detects the higher frequencies sharks are capable of hearing well (125–300 Hz).

Saccular, utricular, and lagenar maculae are overlain by a solid otolith or a mass of separate otoconia. The calcium salts which form the bulk of these otoliths or otoconia in various taxa have densities ranging from 2.6 to 3.3 g/cm³, values more than two to three times greater than for any other vertebrate tissue save bone (Carlström 1963). In sharks the saccular macula is overlain by polycrystalline, aragonite otoconia mixed with exogenous sand (Maisey 1987). This receptor form is schematically shown in figure 6.4, no. 5. The more cranial portion of the saccular macula has been found to detect the lower frequencies of sound to which sharks are most sensitive, < 125 Hz, and is thought to do so in the manner depicted schematically in figure 6.12 (Corwin 1981). In this mechanism, the otoconial mass is poorly coupled to the environmental fluid, owing to its high density, and thus oscillates at very reduced amplitude compared to the surrounding tissues of the head, including the hair cells. As in the cupular mechanism above, phase differences can occur as well. The result: shear of the stereocilia relative to the apical hair cell surface is created as the hair cells are oscillated at a higher amplitude and/or out of phase with the otoconial mass.

A wide taxonomic diversity of fishes is known to be capable of detecting the displacement component of sound (Hawkins 1981), but only a small fraction of fish species have been studied so far (about 30 out of $>30,000$). In skates and rays, the otoconial mechanism of sound displacement detection appears to occur in the utricular macula (Budelli and Macadar 1979) and the same mechanism but with a solid otolith may be widespread in the lagena of actinopterygians. Among fish, the cupular mechanism has been described only for *Carcharhinus*. However, in many cases the exact mechanism and sensory macula used in each are not necessarily known. Modifications of the skull related to the detection of displacements associated with sound such as that described for the shark macula neglecta have not been described in any other taxon. In no case examined so far are fishes sensitive to the displacement component of sound much above 250 Hz, and the frequency of best sensitivity is always below this figure. Given the displacement threshold of the hair cell and the physical facts of displacement amplitude as a function of frequency and distance from the source, this is not surprising. For a sound source of moderate intensity such as is shown in figure 6.9 only frequencies below 300 Hz would have displacements above threshold at any significant distance from the source.

Pressure Detection

A gas bubble in a liquid will pulsate in response to the fluctuating pressure component of a sound wave in the liquid. Several lineages of actinopterygian fishes have evolved hearing mechanisms that take advantage of this fact. In each, the swim bladder, a gas-filled vesicle originally functioning in buoyancy and/or respiration, is used to fill the role of the pulsating gas bubble. When the bladder or a special part of it pulsates, the wall is displaced as a function of the frequency and amplitude of the sound and the physical characteristics of the bladder itself. The displacements created by this transduction mechanism are then coupled to the hair cells of the labyrinth.

The various coupling mechanisms and maculae involved in different taxa indicate that hearing mechanisms involving the transduction of pressure to displacement via the swim bladder have evolved more than once in fishes. Two of the more elaborate transducing mechanisms known for fishes are the bulla mechanism of clupeids and the Weberian ossicles of ostariophysines (figs. 6.4, 6.6, 6.7). Not only are the connections between the bladder and the labyrinth made differently, the macula involved in each is different and the mechanism whereby shear at the hair cells is created is different as well.

Of the hearing mechanisms evolved to take advantage of the swim bladder, one of the best studied is that of the clupeid fishes. Most of our knowledge of this system comes from the work of Gray (summarized in Blaxter et al. 1981). In these animals, thin, paired anterior extensions of the swim bladder project to the otic region of the skull (figs. 6.4, 6.13). Each ends as a gas bubble enclosed in a boney bulla formed from the prootic of the otic capsule. Inside each bulla the gas bubble is separated from a periotic fluid space by a membrane. From the bulla, the periotic fluid space enters the otic capsule, where it forms close relationships with the utricular and saccular maculae. The utricular macula is subdivided and in part connected to the membrane of the gas bulla by an elastic thread.

Oscillations in pressure cause the gas in the bulla to expand and contract. In rarefaction, the gas expands and the membrane of the bulla bulges against the periotic fluid. Expansion takes place mainly at the membrane because elsewhere the gas is constrained by the bone of the bulla. The periotic fluid in turn flows through the opening into the otic capsule, where its movement causes displacement of the middle and posterior parts of the utricular macula away from the periotic space. On compression the process is reversed. As a result, the hair cells of the middle and posterior parts of the macula are displaced and shear is created at their apices (fig. 6.12c). Experimentally, herring detect sounds up to around 1,000 Hz with thresholds at 5 to 6 $\times$ 10^{-3} N/m^2 at their most sensitive frequencies (Enger 1967).

In ostariophysine fishes, the gas in the swim bladder as a whole responds to the pressure component of the sound wave (fig. 6.4, no. 7). At the cranial end of the bladder a portion of the dorsal wall is specialized to displace as the contained gas expands and contracts. A bilateral set of three bones, the Weberian ossicles, connects the bladder wall to an unpaired periotic fluid sinus at the back of the skull. The ossicles are modified portions of the cervical axial skeleton and are arranged such that they amplify the movements of the bladder wall as delivered to the periotic sinus. The periotic sinus in turn is adjacent to a transverse canal filled with otic fluid, which is confluent with the saccular chambers of both labyrinths. Oscilla-

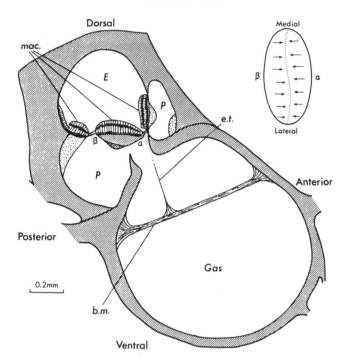

Fig. 6.13. Schematic section through the bulla and utricular macula of a clupeid fish. The gas in the bulla expands and contracts in the pressure changes of the sound field. This causes the bulla membrane (b.m.) to displace, which moves periotic fluid (P) through the opening into the otic capsule. This movement displaces parts of the utricular macula (mac.). The apices of the macular hair cells project into the otic fluid of the membranous labyrinth (E). A thin thread (e.t.) connects the bulla membrane to part of the macula. Inset upper right shows the orientation of the axis of stimulation for the hair cells of the central macula. Reprinted with permission from Best and Gray (1980).

tion of the bladder wall thus causes displacement of the otic fluid in the saccule. The saccular otolith, which in ostariophysines is flattened and fluted, is coupled to the otic fluid and is thus displaced as well, causing shear at the apices of the hair cells in the saccular macula (fig. 6.12d). Note that the final mechanism of producing shear at the hair cells is different from that in clupeids (cf. fig. 6.12c and d). In one the cells move relative to the tips of the stereocilia, in the other the tips of the stereocilia move relative to the cells.

In ostariophysines, low thresholds of from 1×10^{-2} to 1×10^{-3} N/m² can extend to 2,000–3,000 Hz, considerably higher frequencies than in fishes without special auditory adaptations of the swim bladder or fishes with displacement sensitivity only (Hawkins 1981; Coombs 1981). The mechanism by which this wider frequency sensitivity is achieved is unknown, but a good bet is that, just as in terrestrial systems (see below), it stems from the mechanical properties of the transduction and displacement delivery systems and not from the hair cells. The biological significance of broad-range frequency sensitivity in fishes is not known, but it is likely not the most important correlate of a pressure-to-displacement transduction mechanism. The pressure thresholds known for these fishes indicate that they can detect the pressure component of moderately intense sounds well into the far field. For example, for a 300 Hz tone at a source strength of 1×10^{-6} Watts, a displacement detector such as the shark papilla neglecta would detect the sound at a distance of about 1 m (figs. 6.9, 6.10). A pressure-transduced detector such as the saccular macula of ostariophysines would detect the same sound at a distance of 500 m or more.

Given this advantage, it is not surprising that mechanisms to detect the pressure component of sound have arisen more than once within actinopterygians. On the other hand, pressure-transduced systems have the disadvantage that they are not directionally sensitive: a gas bubble pulsates equally no matter what the direction of incoming sound. Perhaps for this reason all fishes with pressure transducers tested so far also have at least one macula disposed to detect the displacement component of sound (Fay 1981, 1984). Theoretically, displacement-sensitive maculae can be directionally sensitive if the hair cells are differentially oriented and their responses integrated by the nervous system (Schuijf 1981; Fay 1984).

In summary, two different mechanisms for detecting sound have evolved in fishes. The first, displacement detection, appears to be widespread and has resulted in the least modification of the otic and surrounding region of the skull. Structural modifications of the skull correlating with the otolithic form of this mechanism are unknown at present, though a low-density channel from the hair cells to the environment might be expected. Structural modifications of the skull related to the cupular form of this mechanism would be similar, though the channel would lead from the cupula to the environment as in the shark papilla neglecta rather than from the cells. Modifications of the otic region related to the second mechanism, pressure detection and transduction to displacement, are less subtle. Here the otic region is sometimes highly modified, as in the formation of the bulla by the prootic in clupeids. At the very least the skull contains openings for the passage of periotic and/or otic fluid systems as channels to provide access for the auditory hair cells to the displacement transducer.

TERRESTRIAL HEARING

For an identical source strength, the displacement amplitude for any given frequency is greater in air than in water at the same distance from the source (figs. 6.9, 6.14). In other words, if an organism had a displacement detector equally competent in air and water, an identical signal would be detectable further from the source in air than in water. If detection threshold is taken as the threshold of hair cells, 2×10^{-10} m, then the 100 Hz sound source in these examples would be detectable at about 3 m in water (fig. 6.9) and 100 m in air (fig. 6.14). Pressure amplitude is greater in water than in air at any given distance from the source (fig. 6.10). In other words, if an organism had a pressure-transducing mechanism equally competent in air and water, an identical signal would be detectable further from the source in water than in air. For the example in figure 6.10, a detector with a threshold of 1×10^{-3} N/m^2 at 100 Hz would detect the signal at about 400 m in water and about 10 m in air.

An expectation from these simple observations might be that terrestrial animals would evolve hearing mechanisms designed to detect the airborne displacement component of sound. They have not. The average body density of any vertebrate is comparable to that of water, close to 1 g/cm^3; that of air is about 0.001 g/cm^3, a thousandfold difference. This means that a terrestrial animal faces the problem of being somewhat opaque to airborne sound, the reverse general problem faced by aquatic animals. About 99.99% of the acoustic energy impinging on a terrestrial organism is reflected from its surface back to the environment; the coupling between the organism and the fluid environment is poor. Displacements transmitted into the body flesh are reduced by nearly two orders of magnitude (about 35dB). For the 100 Hz example used above, the threshold distance would not be near 100 m as expected, but about 1–2 m.

Given these complications it is not surprising that the most acute aerial hearing in terrestrial vertebrates occurs in animals with pressure transducers. Some tetrapods do have hearing mechanisms that are displacement-sensitive. These occur in organisms of several taxa, generally fossorial, which have evolved mechanisms to couple the ear to the terrestrial substrate as well as retain a reduced aerial displacement sensitivity. Because the earliest as well as most recent terrestrial pressure-transduction mechanisms involve components of the neuro-, splanchno-, and dermatocranium, the evolution of hearing has had a much more pronounced impact on the structure of the skull than in aquatic vertebrates. In the following sections we briefly outline the evolution of structure and func-

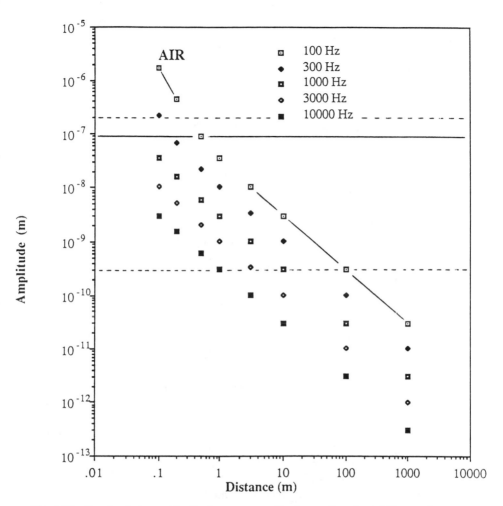

Fig. 6.14. Graph of air particle displacement amplitude as a function of distance from the source for several frequencies of sound. The sound source for each is a pulsating sphere of small size with a strength of 1×10^{-6} Watts. Such a source would measure 72 dB re .00002 N/m² at 10 cm, approximately a normal speaking voice. The dashed lines indicate the general sensitivity range of a hair cell. The solid line is the rough boundary between the near and far fields equal to wavelength/2ρ. In the near field, displacement amplitude is greater than would be expected. This is an idealized case. In the real world sound would suffer excess attenuation from temperature gradients, physical obstacles, etc., and the magnitude of some of these effects would vary with frequency. Equations used to generate points are listed in the appendix.

tion in the early tetrapods and then consider the otic features of various Recent taxa as exemplars of both pressure and displacement-sensitive mechanisms.

EARLY TETRAPODS

Figure 6.8 illustrates present conceptions of the evolution of auditory hair cell populations, and the periotic channels and pressure transducers which couple the cells to the environment in some major taxa of vertebrates. Two populations of hair cells are uniquely associated with aerial hearing in tetrapods: the basilar papilla and the amphibian papilla. In both, the hair cell stereocilia are embedded in a gelatinous tectorial structure. Present notions of their evolutionary derivations are illustrated in figure 6.7. The basilar papilla, present primitively in all classes of tetrapods and the sarcopterygian fish *Latimeria,* is generally believed to be homologous in all (Fritzsch 1987; Fritzsch and Wake 1988) but may have evolved independently in amphibians and amniotes (Wever 1974). The amphibian papilla, on the other hand, unambiguously occurs only in Recent Amphibia.

Two basic gross patterns of periotic fluid systems are found in tetrapods: that of amphibians and that of amniotes (reviewed in Lombard and Bolt 1979; Fritzsch and Wake 1988). In amphibians, the periotic system is configured such that the cupulae of the two auditory papillae are set into motion relative to more stable hair cells when the periotic fluid is oscillating (fig. 6.12d; and fig. 6.15, nos. 5. and 6). In amniotes, it is configured such that the hair cells of the basilar papilla are set in motion relative to a more stable tectorium by oscillations of the periotic fluid (fig. 6.12c; and fig. 6.15, nos. 2, 3, and 4). Structurally and functionally, the two are sufficiently different that separate evolutionary origins are almost certain, as pointed out by Wever (1976).

Three configurations of pressure-transduction structures are found in living tetrapods (Lombard and Bolt 1979): those of amphibians; reptiles plus birds; and mammals (fig. 6.15). All are similar structurally in that each involves a superficial air space on the side of the skull that is bounded by head tissues but open to the pharynx medially by a tube and is separated from the environment laterally by a thin tympanic membrane. This is the middle ear cavity. In all three the tympanic membrane is structurally coupled to an opening in the wall of the otic capsule, the fenestra ovalis or oval window, by a bone or chain of bones, the middle ear ossicle(s). At the oval window, the periotic system abuts the middle ear ossicle fitted in the opening. In general, pressure fluctuations of the incoming acoustic signal cause the tympanic membrane to vibrate. The displacements of these vibrations are transmitted to the oval window by the middle ear ossicle(s),

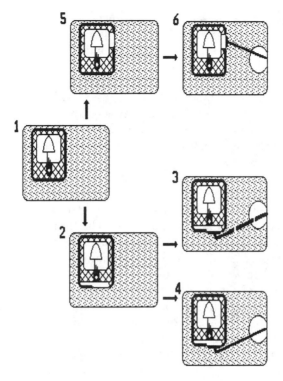

Fig. 6.15. Some hearing mechanisms in terrestrial vertebrates. All involve the basilar papilla only and assume homology of that papilla throughout tetrapods. Structural conventions as in figure 6.4. 1. At the starting point, the hair cell icon represents the evolution of the basilar papilla from a vestibular neuropithelium. *Lower sequence:* the evolution of amniote hearing mechanisms. 2. The amniote form of a periotic fluid system which places the auditory neuroepithelium between two fluid spaces. 3. The mammalian pressure transducer (middle ear cavity and tympanic membrane) is connected to the periotic system by a chain of three ossicles. 4. The pressure transducer of reptiles and birds (middle ear cavity and tympanic membrane) is connected to the periotic system by a single ossicle. *Upper sequence:* the evolution of the amphibian hearing mechanism. 5. The amphibian form of the periotic system in which the hair cells remain coupled to the skull. 6. The amphibian pressure transducer (middle ear cavity and tympanic membrane) is connected to the periotic system by a single ossicle.

where they are passed to the periotic system and thence to the hair cells/ tectoria. Structural evidence from both recent and fossil tetrapods indicates that the three pressure-transducing systems had separate origins (figs. 6.8, 6.15). That of the amphibians is the oldest, dating to the Late Paleozoic (Bolt and Lombard 1985); that of mammals the youngest, arising in the Late Mesozoic (Allin 1986). It is also conceivable that in both amphibians and reptiles pressure-transducing middle ears have arisen more than once (Lombard and Bolt 1979; Lombard and Bolt 1988).

Considering these attributes together indicates an evolutionary scenario in which the first step in aerial hearing was the evolution of hair cell epithelia only weakly coupled to the displacement component of sound because of the density difference of tissue and air. This coupling was improved by the evolution of periotic channels coupling the neuroepithelia to the wall of the otic capsule at an oval window. Periotic systems evolved twice, once in the amphibians ancestral to modern amphibians, and once in the amphibians or earliest amniotes prior to the divergence of the lineage leading to mammals. A middle ear pressure transducer coupled to the oval window then evolved once within the Amphibia and twice within amniotes: early in the reptiles ancestral to modern reptiles and birds and later in the reptiles ancestral to mammals. The formation of these middle ear structures in each of the three cases involved the same head tissues, accounting in part for their similarity, but at different times in the structural history of tetrapods, accounting in part for the differences. At the same time some of the similarity in the three results from the restricted structural options available for a pressure transducer that must match the impedances of air and otic fluids. Likewise, some structural difference results from alternative options in other aspects of acoustical function such as sound localization, time resolution, or frequency tuning.

GENERAL DESIGN AND FUNCTION
OF THE TETRAPOD TYMPANIC EAR

The tetrapod tympanic ear can be considered both an acoustic pressure transducer, transducing sound pressure into displacements within the inner ear, and an impedance-matching device, minimizing the loss of acoustic energy as it passes from a low-impedance medium (air) into a high-impedance medium (inner ear fluids). Features of the tympanic ear related to its pressure-transducing function will be considered first.

Transducing aerial sound pressure into fluid displacements deep within the head requires a structural system with a movable, exposed collector (tympanum) overlying an air-filled chamber (middle ear cavity) (figs. 6.16, 6.17). The compressibility of air within the ear cavity allows movement of the tympanum in response to fluctuations of sound pressure on its external surface. The tympanum is typically a thin, low-mass membrane held in tension within a supportive framework. It is usually derived from both the epidermal and dermal layers and is largely fibrous. In amphibians, reptiles, and birds it is externally convex, and in mammals externally concave. The tympanum is supported along its margin by a variety of elements in the

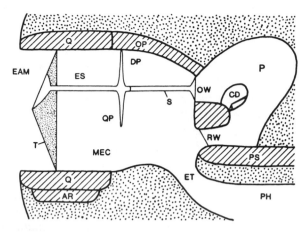

Fig. 6.16. Diagrammatic representation of the tetrapod tympanic ear, based on a generalized lizard, in transverse section. The tympanum (T), is externally convex and attached to an extrastapes (ES). Processes of the extrastapes also often contact the opisthotic (OP) via a dorsal process (DP) and the quadrate (Q) via a quadratic process (QP; this process does not contact the quadrate in the transverse plane depicted in the diagram). The extrastapes connects to the stapes (S) that has an expanded footplate in the oval window (OW). All parts of the stapes lie within the middle ear cavity (MEC). Motion of the stapedial footplate produces displacement waves within the periotic fluids in the periotic channel (P) that exit at the round window (RW), impinging back on the air-filled middle ear cavity. The auditory end organ within the cochlear duct (CD) is stimulated by fluid motion effects. The middle ear cavity communicates with the pharynx (PH) via a eustachian tube (ET). AR, articular bone; EAM, external auditory meatus; PS, parasphenoid. After Henson (1970).

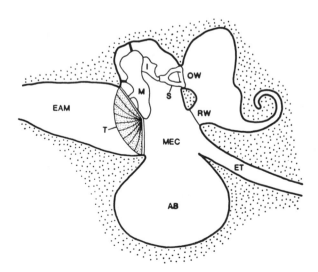

Fig. 6.17. The middle ear of a generalized mammal in transverse section. The tympanum (T) is externally concave and connected to a three-part ossicular chain consisting of a malleus (M), an incus (I), and a stapes (S). An auditory bulla (AB), an extension of the middle ear cavity (MEC), is often observed. EAM, external auditory meatus; ET, eustachian tube; OW, oval window; RW, round window.

different tetrapod groups. In anuran amphibians support is provided by a circular tympanic annulus evolved from part of the palatoquadrate, the primitive upper jaw of gnathostomes (Bolt and Lombard 1985). In many reptiles and birds the quadrate (fig. 6.16), also evolved from part of the palatoquadrate, forms much or part of the supporting frame (Henson 1974). Various adjacent skull elements, especially the squamosal, and interconnecting ligaments also support the tympanic margin of many reptiles and birds. In contrast, the mammalian tympanum is supported by the tympanic (or ectotympanic) bone derived from the dermal angular bone of the primitive tetrapod lower jaw (Allin 1986) that completely encircles the tympanum except at its most dorsal point (Moore 1981).

The middle ear cavity connects to the pharynx via eustachian tubes (figs. 6.16, 6.17), thereby allowing communication between the middle ear cavities on either side. In many species this communication allows the middle ear to act as a directionally sensitive pressure-gradient receiver (Michelsen 1971). Motion of a tympanum will be affected by pressure fluctuations on both its external surface (produced by aerial sound) and internal surface (produced by pressure waves resulting from motion of the contralateral tympanum and traveling through the pharynx and eustachian tubes). Sound waves coming from different directions will have different effects on the external surfaces of the two tympana, and the interaction between external and internal pressures (that may increase or decrease tympanic motion) will be dependent upon the wavelength (or frequency) of the sound signal. Therefore, the precise movement of a tympanum in a pressure-gradient system will be dependent on the direction and frequency of the sound. Pressure-gradient function of the tympanic ear has been demonstrated in anuran amphibians (Capranica and Michelsen 1988) and some birds (Hill et al. 1980), and is probably widespread among smaller species where small head size minimizes acoustic shadow effects and differences in timing that can provide directional cues for larger animals. Although larger tetrapods may employ shadow effects or differences in timing for sound localization, eustachian tubes are still commonly observed. In some forms, however, such as many mammals, the eustachian tubes are narrow and typically collapsed, thereby allowing little communication between the two middle ear cavities.

The volume of the middle ear cavity has important implications for the frequency response of the middle ear (see below), and therefore varies among tetrapods. The most dramatic variation is observed in mammals, where in some, such as certain gerbilline and heteromyid rodents (Lay 1972; Webster and Webster 1975), the floor of the middle ear cavity may be greatly expanded to form a large auditory bulla (fig. 6.17). The walls of the tetrapod middle ear cavity are formed, depending on the species, by muscle, connective tissue, cartilage, or bone. Mammals provide a good example of the latter condition. Most have middle ear cavities largely surrounded by a variety of skeletal elements that differ among groups. The diverse patterns of bones supporting the middle ear cavity probably result from the independent evolution of auditory bullae (that form a large portion of the ear cavity volume) within the different mammalian lineages (Novacek 1977). In many mammals, the tympanic bone extends medially from the tympanum to form part or much of the floor of the middle ear cavity and also a significant portion of the bullar walls. Numerous other bones, however, including the entotympanic, squamosal, basisphenoid, basioccipital, exoccipital, alisphenoid, and smaller elements that appear temporarily during development, may contribute to the bullar walls (Novacek 1977). These elements, as well as others in the otic region, may fuse in various combinations. For example, in many mammals the tympanic, squamosal, and petrosal bones fuse to form the temporal bone (Moore 1981). Fusion of skull elements surrounding the middle ear cavity and tympanum may protect against artifactual fluctuations in air pressure produced by motion of surrounding tissue during swallowing or breathing (Henson 1961).

The otic capsule also may display specializations that are functionally important in hearing. In mammals, for example, the inner ear is encased primarily within the anterodorsal (petrous) portion of the periotic bone, which typically consists of very dense bone (Moore 1981). This portion of the periotic bone may be acoustically isolated from surrounding tissues to limit bone conduction of sound to the inner ear along routes other than the middle ear. In bats, which are well known for their echolocating abilities, there is a wide gap between the periotic and basioccipital bones, as well as smaller gaps between the periotic and other skull bones (Henson 1970). Such gaps are filled with loose connective tissue, adipose tissue, or blood sinuses and presumably dampen high-frequency signals passing toward the otic region from the larynx during sound emission. This arrangement therefore would limit interference between emitted sounds and returning echoes. In cetaceans, the periotic-tympanic bone complex often is isolated from the rest of the skull by sinuses extending from the middle ear cavity and filled with a foam of small air bubbles trapped in oil and mucus (Fraser and Purves 1960). These sinuses may reflect underwater sound passing toward the inner ear along routes other than the middle ear ossicles (see below), and, by allowing independent sampling of sound intensity at two different points (left and right head surfaces), may aid in directional analysis of sound signals.

Tympanic motion produced by fluctuations in external sound pressure is relayed to a single auditory ossicle or a chain of ossicles attached to the

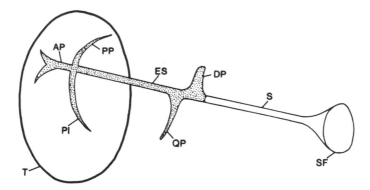

Fig. 6.18. The stapes (S) and extrastapes (ES) of a lizard. The view is medial, posterior, and dorsal. Note the dorsal process (DP) and quadrate process (QP) of the extrastapes that typically attach to the paroccipital crest of the opisthotic and quadrate respectively, and the several processes (AP, anterior process; PI, pars inferior; PP, posterior process) that extend beneath and attach to the inner surface of the tympanum (T). SF, stapedial footplate.

internal surface of the tympanum and passing through the middle ear cavity toward the inner ear (figs. 6.16, 6.17, 6.18). In all tetrapods except mammals there is a single element, the stapes. This element is often called the columella, but because we consider it very likely that in all tetrapods it is homologous to the primitive hyomandibula, we use the term stapes. The stapes typically connects laterally to a cartilaginous extrastapes (fig. 6.18). The junction between the two elements generally is a tight connection allowing little mobility. The extrastapes usually is broadly connected to the tympanum and has several processes (fig. 6.18). Typically there is a dorsal, ascending process that attaches to the otic capsule; for example, in anuran amphibians such a process connects to the parotic crest of the prootic (Jaslow et al. 1988), and in many reptiles a similar process attaches to the paroccipital process of the opisthotic (Wever 1979). Other processes may attach to the quadrate and elements of the hyoid arch. In reptiles and birds there are often numerous processes that extend from the distal portion of the extrastapes and radiate within the tympanum (fig. 6.18). These processes probably act to stiffen the tympanic membrane as well as transmit motion from a wide area of it to the stapes (Wever 1979).

Medially the extrastapes is continuous with the typically bony shaft of the stapes. The latter extends through the middle ear cavity to an expanded stapedial footplate lying in the oval window of the otic capsule (fig. 6.16). In some species with small middle ear cavities the stapedial shaft passes through connective tissue and muscle. For example, in anuran amphibians only the lateral half or at most two-thirds of the stapes lies within the middle ear cavity (Jaslow et al. 1988). In most nonmammalian tetrapods the stapedial footplate is roughly circular and has a ventral hinge on the otic capsule. This hinge may be cartilaginous, as in many amphibians (Jaslow et al. 1988), or ligamentous, as in birds (Gaudin 1968). Considerable variation in the precise shape of the stapedial footplate is observed in tetrapods, but there is little information on the functional significance of such variation.

In mammals there are three auditory ossicles, and the evolution of this more complicated ossicular chain provides an interesting challenge for the functional and evolutionary morphologist (see Allin [1986] for a current perspective). The malleus is the most distal of the three ossicles, and it possesses an elongated manubrium embedded in the tympanum (fig. 6.17). In many adult mammals (and immature individuals of other species) an anterior process of the malleus makes a fibrous connection with the tympanic bone. Ligaments may also bind the malleus to the tympanic. Such connections between the malleus and tympanic bone may minimize relative motion between these elements and lower the risk of damage to the tympanum (Henson 1974). Proximally the malleus articulates with the incus, and the latter has a long process that extends medially to articulate with the stapes (fig. 6.17). The incudomalleolar and incudostapedial joints are typically of the synovial variety and freely mobile. The stapes has an expanded footplate that fits into the oval window. Ligamentous tissues between the incus and walls of the middle ear cavity and between the stapes and the rim of the oval window probably stabilize both of these elements.

Having described the general features of the tetrapod tympanic ear that make its pressure-transducing function possible, we now discuss features related to its impedance-matching function. To compensate for the high degree of reflection of acoustic energy at the air/tissue interface (see above), two basic strategies have evolved. One strategy is to collect sound energy over a relatively large area of the head surface, represented by tympanic area, and converge this energy onto a relatively small opening into the inner ear, the oval window (fig. 6.16). In many tetrapods the ratio of tympanic area to oval window area is close to 20, but the value varies considerably among and within taxa. For example, the lizard *Crotaphytus collaris* has a ratio of 13.3 (Wever and Werner 1970), and ratios among birds and mammals range from 11–47 and 14–60, respectively (Schwartzkopff 1957; Henson 1974). Because this value is not the only determinant of energy transfer (see below), such variation does not necessarily imply different efficiencies in sound reception.

The second strategy employed to minimize problems of impedance matching involves the arrangement of the auditory ossicle or ossicles into a lever system that amplifies the force of tympanic motion caused by fluctuations in sound pressure. The various processes of the extrastapes appear

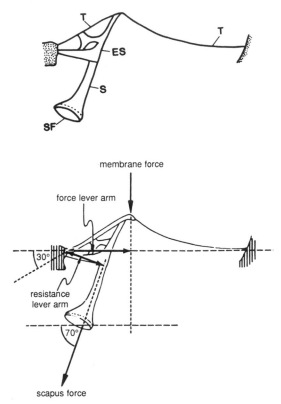

Fig. 6.19. *Top:* Diagrammatic representation of the middle ear of the boreal owl (*Aegolius funereus*) in transverse section. Processes of the extrastapes (ES) are attached to the tympanum (T), and the footplate (SF) of the stapes (S) would fit into the oval window. *Bottom:* The avian middle ear represented as a lever system. The diagram is based on the configuration depicted above. Tympanic motion produces rotation of the extrastapes and a basically linear, pistonlike motion of the stapes and stapedial footplate. Parts of the extrastapes act as lever arms, and because the force lever arm is longer than the resistance lever arm, the force of footplate motion is amplified. From Norberg (1978).

to contribute to the lever function in nonmammalian tetrapods. For example, Norberg (1978) proposes that in birds the extrastapes undergoes a rotational motion when the tympanum moves inward, and this extrastapedial motion causes a simple linear motion of the stapedial shaft (fig. 6.19). Because the extrastapedial-stapedial complex has an oblique orientation with respect to the tympanum, the complex acts as a lever system with a lever arm ratio of about 1.6. Similarly, experiments by Wever and Werner (1970) on the lizard *Crotaphytus collaris* suggest that the arrangement of the extrastapedial processes associated with the tympanum forms a rotating lever system that produces an amplification of about 2.14. Again, the stapes is assumed to move as a simple piston. However, it appears unlikely that the stapes moves only in a linear, pistonlike fashion. Gaudin (1968) observed transverse movements of the stapes in several avian species, and speculated that the stapedial footplate rotated about its ventral, ligamentous hinge with the otic capsule (fig. 6.20). The stapedial footplate of anuran amphibians also rocks about a ventral hinge with the margin of the oval window (Jaslow et al. 1988). The location of a fulcrum

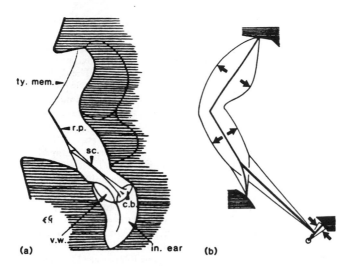

Fig. 6.20. Function of the avian middle ear as envisioned by Gaudin (1968).
a. Diagrammatic representation of the avian middle ear in transverse section. b.
Motion of the middle ear elements in response to sound. The arrows show the
direction of motion, and the thin lines the extremes of excursion. Rather than move as
a piston, the footplate of the stapes (c.b.) swings back and forth about a ventral hinge
with the otic capsule. Because the force lever arm (consisting of the extrastapes and
much of the stapes) is much longer than the resistance lever arm (consisting of the
stapedial footplate) greater amplification is produced than depicted in figure 6.19. in.
ear, inner ear; r.p., rostral process of the extrastapes; sc., scapus; ty. mem.,
tympanum; v.w., vestibular window. From Gaudin (1968).

close to the oval window would produce greater force amplification because the stapedial footplate is such a short lever arm compared to the
stapedial shaft and extrastapes.

The precise lever arrangement and movements of the ossicular chain
of nonmammalian tetrapods is therefore not totally understood, although
it is clear that some amplification of tympanic force occurs. Multiplying
the areal (tympanic to oval window) ratios and lever arm ratios provides a
value that generally describes the effectiveness of a given middle ear in
impedance matching. For example, Norberg (1978) calculated a value of
56 for the owl *Aegolius funereus,* and Wever and Werner (1970) calculated
a value of 26.6 for the lizard *Crotaphytus collaris.* In both cases the majority of the amplification occurred from areal convergence (35 for the owl
and 13.3 for the lizard), but it needs to be emphasized that the lever function of the ossicular chain (especially the possible lever movements of the
stapes itself) is still poorly understood and perhaps underestimated. Also,
such analyses disregard a possible lever action within the tympanum itself,
in which its curvature and buckling tendency may amplify force acting on

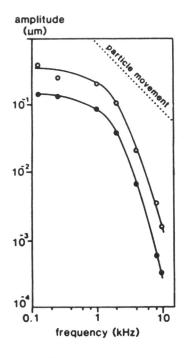

Fig. 6.21. Motion of the tympanum (open circles) and stapedial footplate (solid circles) of the ringed turtledove *Streptopelia risoria* in response to sound of different frequencies applied at 100 dB SPL. The dashed line shows the theoretical amplitude of particle displacements at the sound intensity. Both tympanic and stapedial motion are less than particle motion at all frequencies. Tympanic motion is greater than stapedial motion at all frequencies, suggesting that stapedial force is amplified as much as five times during middle ear function. This amplification may be produced by leverage action of the extrastapedial-stapedial complex combined with a tympanic lever system based on tympanic buckling. It also could be produced by the lever system envisioned by Gaudin (fig. 6.20). After Saunders and Johnstone (1972).

its center (Khanna and Tonndorf 1972). Saunders and Johnstone (1972) found that the amplitude of stapedial motion was 10–12 dB less than that of the tympanum in the ringed turtledove, *Streptopelia risoria* (fig. 6.21). This suggests that force of stapedial movement may be amplified as much as five times by a tympanic lever system (Kuhne and Lewis 1985).

Lever action in the mammalian ossicular chain is better understood. Motion of the tympanum produces motion of all of the ossicles along the same axis (Khanna and Tonndorf 1972). The manubrium acts as an in-lever arm, and the long process of the incus and the stapes together act as an out-lever arm. The manubrium is typically longer than the latter two elements by a factor of 1.2–3.5 (Henson 1974), so the force of motion of the tympanum is amplified accordingly. As with nonmammalian tetrapods, convergence of tympanic area onto oval window area provides a greater amount of amplification, with areal ratios of mammals ranging from 14 to 60 (Henson 1974). Combining lever and areal ratios for some representative mammals—humans, domestic cats, and a heteromyid rodent (*Dipodomys merriami*)—provides a total amplification of about 18, 65, and 97 respectively (Khanna and Tonndorf 972; Webster and Webster 1975). Additional amplification of the force of ossicular motion may result from the buckling properties of the curved mammalian tympanum (Khanna and Tonndorf 1972).

Responsiveness of middle ear ossicles may be modulated by one or more middle ear muscles in tetrapods. In many cases the major function of such muscles remains speculative, but they generally appear to provide protection against high-intensity sound damage to the inner ear (especially during vocalization) and also may enhance detection of sound signals within naturally important frequency ranges by sharpening the bandpass properties of the middle ear (Wever and Vernon 1960; Oeckinghaus and Schwartzkopff 1983).

STRUCTURAL SPECIALIZATIONS FOR FREQUENCY TUNING

Any mechanical system will have a resonant frequency at which loss of energy during transmission is minimal. Mass and stiffness of structures cause energy losses, but the effects are opposite with respect to frequency. Loss due to mass increases with frequency, whereas loss due to stiffness decreases with frequency. At a certain frequency, the resonant frequency, these loses cancel out and the only energy loss is related to friction, which is far less than that associated with mass and stiffness. The resonant frequency, at which energy transmission to the inner ear is maximally efficient, can be set by modification of the mass and/or stiffness of the middle ear.

Figure 6.22 displays the frequency responses of the middle ears of some representative tetrapods obtained by measuring motion of the sta-

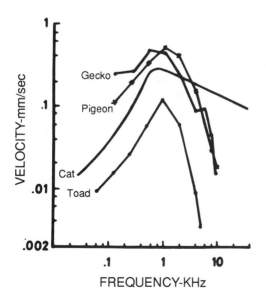

Fig. 6.22. Frequency responses of the middle ears of several tetrapods obtained by measuring motion of the stapedial footplate. All of the middle ears are acting as bandpass filters with both high- and low-frequency roll-offs. The severity of the roll-off, however, varies among species. After Saunders and Johnstone (1972).

pedial footplate (Saunders and Johnstone 1972). The response patterns are similar, showing a resonant frequency near 1 kHz, and roll-offs at the high- and low-frequency ends, produced, respectively, by mass and stiffness effects. The resonant frequency of the middle ear is often linked to frequencies of importance to the animal, such as frequency of mating call (Capranica 1976), and, because of mass effects, may vary with body size (Moffat and Capranica 1978; Pinder and Palmer 1983).

Studies on mammals provide some of the best examples of modifications of the middle ear for high- and low-frequency sensitivity. Many mammals are very sensitive to both high- and low-frequency sound. Sensitivity to low-frequency sound has been produced not by increasing the mass of the auditory ossicles but rather by reducing the stiffness of the ossicular chain (Moore 1981). Retention of low-mass ossicles has allowed reasonable sensitivity to high-frequency sound, while the reduced stiffness has enhanced low-frequency sound reception. Webster and Webster (1975) found that heteromyid rodents have reduced ossicular ligaments and middle ear muscles, and increased middle ear volumes, the latter achieved by enlargement of the bullae (fig. 6.23); all of these features reduce the stiffness of the middle ear. Enlarged auditory bullae are found in many mammals, including carnivores (Hunt 1974) and some primates (Cartmill 1975), and presumably are specializations for maximizing low-frequency sound sensitivity in these animals as well. Some mammals have bullar cavities divided into two chambers with a narrow connection between them (Moore 1981). At low frequencies, the effective volume of the middle ear probably includes both chambers. At frequencies above the resonant frequency of the secondary chamber farthest removed from the tympanum, only the volume of the first chamber effectively contributes to the impedance of the middle ear, and this acts to stiffen the middle ear. This partitioning of the middle ear cavity therefore minimizes impedance problems, and enhances hearing, at both low and high frequencies.

Bats use high-frequency sound emissions for purposes of sonar, and these mammals provide the best-studied example of a middle ear specialized for high-frequency sound reception (Hinchliffe and Pye 1969; Henson 1970). The ossicles are small and light, and the tympanum is also small and very thin. The incudostapedial joint is frequently fibrous, and the malleus, incus, and stapes are tightly bound to the walls of the middle ear cavity, the former by its anterior process, the latter two by numerous ligaments. The middle ear volume is small, with little expansion of the bullae. All of these modifications act to stiffen the middle ear and increase responsiveness to high-frequency signals. The small tympanic area compromises impedance matching related to convergence of tympanic area onto the smaller area of the stapedial footplate, but this is compensated for by a

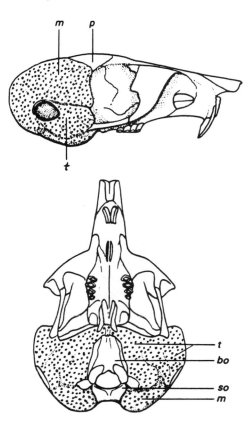

Fig. 6.23. Lateral (top) and ventral (bottom) views of the skull of the heteromyid rodent *Dipodomys merriami* showing the extraordinary size of the auditory bullae (stippled portion) found in some rodents. Such enlarged bullae increase the volume of the middle ear cavity, thereby decreasing stiffness of the middle ear and increasing its responsiveness to low-frequency sounds. bo, basioccipital; m, mastoid part of the bulla; p, parietal; so, supraoccipital; t, tympanic part of the bulla (petrosal and tympanic bones). After Vaughan (1986)

relative lengthening of the manubrium compared to the lever arm formed by the incus and stapes. The middle ear muscles of bats are also relatively large. They may provide an important protective function during sound emission, but may also enhance high-frequency sensitivity by further stiffening the ossicular chain (Henson 1970).

NONTYMPANIC ACOUSTIC RECEPTION IN TETRAPODS: GENERAL ASPECTS

Although the standard pressure-transducing tympanic ear is widespread among tetrapod vertebrates, there are many species that utilize nontympanic mechanisms for acoustic reception. Many of these species live where acoustic signals can readily penetrate the head tissues with little energy loss due to problems of impedance mismatching. In fossorial or aquatic situations, for example, substrate or waterborne sound is much more readily coupled to body tissues than aerial sound. There have been, therefore, various evolutionary modifications of the middle ear associated with fossorial and aquatic habits. However, several surface-living species also lack tympanic middle ears and appear to utilize nontympanic pathways for aerial sound reception. Nontympanic reception of aerial sound can be practical because energy loss during transmission from air to tissue is frequency-dependent. As discussed above in relation to the frequency response of tympanic middle ears, transmission of low-frequency energy is less impeded by mass than transmission of high-frequency energy. Low-frequency sound signals, therefore, may be effectively absorbed by various body tissues lacking the low mass and stiffness often associated with tympanic middle ears. Accordingly, many of the tetrapods that utilize nontympanic mechanisms for aerial sound reception appear to be most responsive to low-frequency sound.

When considering the structural and mechanical basis of nontympanic acoustic reception, it is reasonable to group together all of the acoustic signals that may effectively penetrate head and body tissues, including low-frequency aerial sound, ground vibrations, and waterborne sound. In humans, nontympanic reception of vibrations and sound has been termed bone conduction hearing. Tonndorf (1972) demonstrated two major types of bone conduction hearing in humans, and these are relevant to understanding nontympanic reception in all tetrapods.

One type is an inertial mode, in which displacements of acoustic signals entering the head shake the entire otic region, producing relative motion between the loosely suspended auditory ossicles and otic capsule, thereby producing displacements at the oval window that then stimulate acoustic end organs of the inner ear (fig. 6.24a). Since differential displacement occurs at the oval window, this inertial mode results in the production of fluid movement within the perilymphatic channels of the inner ear comparable to that produced by tympanic hearing. The inertial mode also can operate at the level of the acoustic end organ, in a manner conceptually similar to that described in displacement hearing in fishes (see above). In this variant, as the otic capsule is displaced by absorbed wave energy, overlying tectorial structures will move relative to the hair cells. Whether the displacement amplitude of the tectorial structure is greater than that of the hair cells or vice versa depends on whether an amniote or amphibian inner ear is being stimulated in this fashion. In amniotes, the tectorium is more tightly coupled to the capsule; in amphibians, it is more tightly coupled to the hair cells. In either case, the relative amplitudes are the reverse of those produced by normal tympanic stimulation.

A second type of bone conduction is a deformational mode, in which absorbed acoustic waves deform or move the walls of the otic capsule or middle ear ossicles to produce fluid displacements in the inner ear

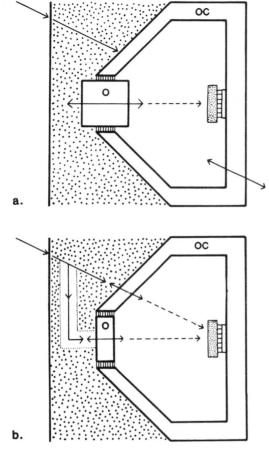

Fig. 6.24. Different possible modes of nontympanic acoustic reception in tetrapods. An otic capsule (OC) surrounds an inner ear containing an acoustic end organ (right inner surface of the capsule). A middle ear ossicle (O) lies within an oval window on the left side of the capsule, and acoustic energy from the environment (represented by the arrow passing from the left) is penetrating the head tissues. a. The inertial mode. Acoustic energy entering the head tissues produces motion of the otic capsule. A loosely attached, massive ossicle moves relative to the otic capsule, generating fluid motion within the inner ear (dashed line) that stimulates the end organ. b. The deformational mode. Acoustic energy penetrating the head produces motion of the walls of the otic capsule or middle ear ossicle, thereby generating fluid motion within the inner ear (dashed line) that stimulates the end organ. Ossicular motion in such cases is often linked to passage of acoustic energy along a low-attenuation route to the ossicle (clear channel around arrows leading to ossicle). Vertebrates may employ any combination of these modes for nontympanic acoustic reception, which may operate over different frequency ranges.

(fig. 6.24b). These displacements of the periotic fluid in turn cause displacement of the hair cells relative to the tectorium. It is likely that a number of tetrapods use specific variations of this general deformational mode as a component of their hearing mechanism. In some cases acoustic energy is channeled along specific, low-attenuation routes from the surface of the body to a movable ossicle positioned in an oval window (fig. 6.24b). For example, the intramandibular fat body of the mandible of toothed whales (Odontoceti) appears effectively to conduct high-frequency signals to the middle ear ossicles (see below). Such a strategy is analogous to tympanic ear function, in which acoustic energy is transmitted along a tympanic-ossicular route and introduced into the inner ear at a specific point (the oval window). It is important to remember that more than one mode may be utilized in the same animal, especially because different modes may be

effective over different frequency ranges. For example, in humans, an inertial mechanism is responsible for reception of bone-conducted sound of
low frequency (below about 1 kHz), whereas otic-deformation is responsible for reception of higher frequencies (Tonndorf 1972).

In previous discussions of the evolution of the tympanic ear (see
above), the advantages of responding to sound pressure versus sound displacement were stressed. When discussing mechanisms of nontympanic
sound reception it is difficult to determine whether one is dealing with
pressure or displacement sensitivity. Studies of underwater hearing in fishes
have linked pressure-transduction capabilities to air-filled or low-density
cavities that will pulsate under the influence of fluctuations of sound pressure. In fishes lacking such morphological systems, displacement effects
have been assumed to underlie auditory responses (Fay and Popper 1980).
In most studies of underwater sound reception in aquatic tetrapods, pressure has been considered the important acoustic parameter, even though
fishlike pressure-transducing configurations may be typically absent. Most
researchers have assumed that underwater sound pressure would produce
motion of middle ear elements or other head tissues in a manner analogous
to tympanic ear function in air. Perspectives of researchers studying fish
hearing have therefore been very different from those of workers examining aquatic hearing in tetrapods. In terrestrial animals sound pressure is
also considered the important parameter for nontympanic sound reception. Wever (1979, 1985), for example, considered any nontympanic
middle ear structures of amphibians and reptiles to be responding to pressure. Yet without an underlying air-filled space, pressure-induced motion
of receptive surfaces may be similar to motion produced by displacement
effects. Therefore, hypotheses employing pressure sensitivity of nontympanic structures may often represent a misapplication of models of tympanic ear function. The question of pressure or displacement sensitivity
should be experimentally determined, perhaps using standing wave apparati that spatially separate these two parameters (Hawkins and MacLennan
1976; Hetherington and Lombard 1982).

NONTYMPANIC RECEPTION OF SUBSTRATE
VIBRATIONS AND AERIAL SOUND

Many tetrapods that utilize nontympanic strategies for acoustic reception
are fossorial, and may use the same mechanisms for detection of both
ground vibrations and aerial sound. It is likely that middle ear morphology
of many of these species is shaped primarily by functional demands for
seismic sensitivity. In many cases, elements of the standard tympanic ear
are modified and incorporated into a system especially effective for vibra-

tion reception and generally less effective for sound reception. However, loss in sound sensitivity is mainly restricted to high frequencies, and such species retain significant sensitivity to low-frequency sounds. Reduction and/or modification of tympanic ear structures is quite widespread among amphibians, reptiles, and certain fossorial mammals. However, nontympanic pathways of acoustic reception unassociated with the tympanic ear have also evolved, especially in amphibians. Because modified tympanic ear elements are more commonly associated with nontympanic reception, such cases will be discussed first.

Modifications of the Tympanic Ear

A common evolutionary modification of the middle ear of fossorial vertebrates includes the loss of a tympanum and middle ear cavity. An auditory ossicle or ossicles are retained, but often increase in mass and show new connections to skeletal elements or other tissues contacting the substrate. The massiveness of such ossicles suggests that they function as part of an inertially sensitive system. Alternatively, the derived connections of such ossicles suggest that they may serve to transmit acoustic energy along a specific pathway from the head surface and associated tissues to the inner ear. Experimental investigations are few, but it is possible that both strategies are used, perhaps operating over different frequency ranges.

Reptiles, especially fossorial forms, provide many examples of modified tympanic ears. Snakes and amphisbaenians (limbless reptiles either placed in their own suborder or considered lizards) have evolved similar strategies of acoustic reception. Both groups often display fossorial habits and both lack tympanic ears. No tympanum is found. No middle ear cavity exists, although in snakes small spaces may be observed along the shaft of the stapes, and Wever (1979) claims that they are air-filled and represent remnants of a middle ear cavity. A stapes is retained, and both snakes and amphisbaenians exhibit clear linkages between the stapes and mandible, either directly or via the quadrate. In snakes the stapes is attached to the quadrate via cartilages or bones (fig. 6.25) that may represent remnants of stapedial processes and the extrastapes (McDowell 1967). In amphisbaenians the stapes is typically a short, heavy element. An extrastapes is connected to the lateral end of the stapes, and often extends anteriorly along the lateral surface of the mandible under the labial scales (fig. 6.26.).

Physiological studies have found that the inner ear of snakes is very sensitive to ground vibrations (Hartline 1971). Because the lower jaw of snakes is often in contact with the substrate, it is possible that ground vibrations produce motion of the mandible that is transmitted to the quadrate and stapes. A similar mandibular pathway may also function in am-

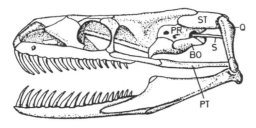

Fig. 6.25. *Top:* Lateral view of the skull of a snake (genus *Python*) showing the stapes (S) connecting laterally to the quadrate (Q). BO, basioccipital; PR, prootic; PT, pterygoid; ST, supratemporal. After Henson (1974). *Bottom:* Schematic diagram of the middle ear of a generalized snake in frontal section. The stapes (S) has an expanded footplate in the oval window (OW) that generates fluid motions that stimulate the acoustic end organ in the cochlear duct (CD). Note the circular flow of fluid motion (arrows) back to an extension of the periotic system (the pericapsular recess, PR) surrounding the lateral portion of the stapes. Snakes, and turtles as well, lack a round window but employ this different strategy for release of pressure waves generated by ossicular motion. Laterally and posteriorly the stapes contacts the quadrate (Q), usually via one or more intervening cartilages (IC). The articulating surfaces of the quadrate and stapes are typically cartilaginous (stippled portions). After Wever (1979).

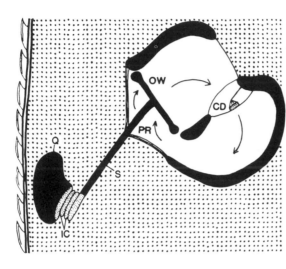

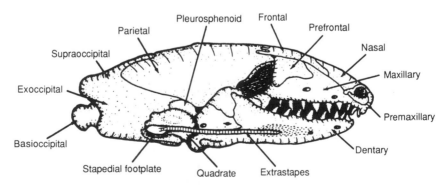

Fig. 6.26. Lateral view of the skull of the amphisbaenian *Amphisbaena manni* showing the extension of the extrastapes along the lower jaw. After Wever (1979).

phisbaenians; Gans and Wever (1972) found that vibrations applied to the labial scales readily produced inner ear responses, presumably via the extrastapedial-stapedial route. The snake and amphisbaenian middle ear is capable of detecting aerial sound as well. Severing the connection between the stapes and quadrate significantly reduced inner ear responses to sound in snakes (Wever and Vernon 1960). These workers also demonstrated, by placing a stimulus sound tube over different parts of the head, that the sound reception was taking place directly over the quadrate and not through the lower jaw. Gans and Wever (1972) established that head and jaw surfaces of amphisbaenians can also absorb aerial sound energy that is transmitted to the inner ear via the extrastapes and stapes. Snakes and amphisbaenians are most sensitive to relatively low frequencies (Wever 1979), and this would be expected because problems of impedance-mismatching associated with the unspecialized head tissues would be most significant at higher frequencies.

Snakes and amphisbaenians may also employ inertial mechanisms for acoustic reception. Ground vibrations penetrating the head may cause motion of the stapes relative to the otic capsule and inner ear fluids. In some specialized burrowing snakes, such as certain species of the family Typhlopidae, the stapedial footplate is exceptionally large, and a short stapedial shaft is loosely attached to the quadrate by a ligament (Wever 1979). This loose anchoring suggests that vibrations are not relayed directly to the stapes, and that the latter acts only as an inertial element. Some amphisbaenians also show exceptionally massive stapes (Wever 1979) that probably act as inertially sensitive elements.

Other reptiles that are largely or partially fossorial show various modifications (including loss) of the standard tympanic ear. Several lizards of the agamid family lack a tympanum and a middle ear cavity, and the extrastapes is embedded in the skin of the lateral head surface or in the depressor mandibulae muscle underneath the skin (Wever 1979). A more common phenomenon found in many lizards (and many anuran amphibians as well), is that of the "hidden" tympanum, in which a fibrous membrane attached to the extrastapes is not external but covered with skin and sometimes muscle tissue. Some horned lizards of the genus *Phrynosoma,* for example, have a thick hidden tympanum, and the extrastapes has a broad contact with the quadrate. *Sphenodon punctatus,* the only living representative of the reptilian order Rhynchocephalia, provides another good example. An external tympanum is absent, but the extrastapes, which has a broad articulation with the quadrate, connects distally to a tough fibrous membrane lying beneath the skin fairly high up on the lateral surface of head, posterior to the squamosal and upper portion of the quadrate (Gans and Wever 1976). The depressor mandibulae muscle overlies part of the fibrous membrane. As in the case of snakes, the broad connection between the extrastapes and quadrate in these species probably aids in detection of vibrations penetrating the lower jaw. And, although Wever (1979) dismisses the possibility that the quadrate may act as a route for sound transmission, the broad connection of the extrastapes to the quadrate suggests that aerial sound energy may be absorbed by tissues in the vicinity of the quadrate. As suggested by its frequent connection to the extrastapes, the depressor mandibulae muscle tissue may also function in sound absorption. Instances of hidden tympana do not necessarily imply nontympanic reception of sound, simply because a type of tympanum is associated with the extrastapes. However, the relationship of the extrastapes to the quadrate and other nearby tissues suggests that alternative pathways of sound absorption and transmission may be involved.

Although most reptiles displaying nontympanic strategies for acoustic reception tend to be fossorial, the largely arboreal chameleons (family Chamaeleonidae) provide an interesting exception. They lack a tympanum, but usually possess a well-defined middle ear cavity, stapes, and extrastapes (Wever 1979). Many species have a well-developed anterior process of the extrastapes that attaches by a ligament to an expanded, platelike extension of the pterygoid bone (fig. 6.27). The pterygoid plate

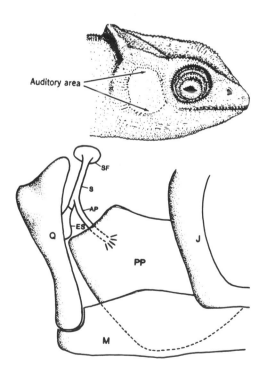

Fig. 6.27. *Top:* Lateral view of the head of the chameleon *Chamaeleo senegalensis* showing the acoustic receptive area (auditory area) of the lateral head surface. After Wever (1979). *Bottom:* The middle ear and associated skeletal elements of *C. senegalensis* in lateral view. The auditory area in the diagram above lies over a platelike extension of the pterygoid (pterygoid plate, PP). An anterior process (AP) of the stapes (S) attaches to the inner surface of the pterygoid plate. The stapes also contacts the quadrate (Q) via an extrastapes (ES). M, mandible; J, jugal; SF, stapedial footplate.

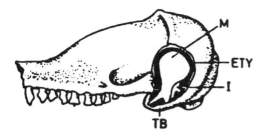

Fig. 6.28. Lateral view of the skull of a golden mole (*Chrysochloris trevelyani*) showing the massive auditory ossicles. Such ossicles probably act as inertial elements for reception of ground vibrations penetrating the head of this fossorial mammal. ETY, epitympanic recess; I, incus; M, malleus; TB, tympanic bulla. From Henson (1974).

lies below the skin of the lateral head surface (fig. 6.27), and appears to act as a site for sound reception. Severing the connection between the extrastapes and pterygoid plate decreases microphonic responses to low-frequency sound (below about 1 kHz) by up to 28 dB (Wever 1968). a posterior process of the extrastapes connects via a ligament to the depressor mandibulae muscle, suggesting that the latter may also serve as an area of sound absorption.

Examples of nontympanic reception are rare in terrestrial mammals. Certain fossorial mammals, such as the golden moles (family Chrysochloridae) appear to use an inertially sensitive configuration for vibration sensitivity. The auditory ossicles are massive (fig. 6.28), and vibration of the head would probably produce significant differences in motion between the stapes and otic capsule.

Terrestrial tetrapods therefore provide several examples of evolutionary modification of tympanic ear elements and their incorporation into a nontympanic system of acoustic reception. Inertial strategies employing massive ossicles are common among fossorial species, but retained ossicles also frequently establish new connections for transmission of acoustic signals to the inner ear. For example, extrastapedial connections to the mandible and quadrate appear important for reception of substrate vibrations entering the lower jaw when the latter contacts the ground. Aerial sound reception also seems to occur through a variety of lateral head tissues, including the lower jaw surface, quadrate region, and depressor mandibulae muscle. Sensitivity, however, is probably restricted to lower sound frequencies.

Alternative Middle Ear Systems: Amphibian Examples

Whereas amniotes have used elements of a tympanic ear to evolve nontympanic systems, a unique middle ear system termed the opercularis system has evolved in the frogs and salamanders. The opercularis system consists of an opercularis muscle and an operculum (Hetherington et al. 1986). The opercularis muscle originates on the pectoral girdle and inserts on the operculum, a typically cartilaginous element lying within the oval window of the inner ear (figs. 6.29, 6.30). The opercularis system is present in metamorphosed frogs and salamanders. Most adult frogs and toads possess both a tympanic middle ear and an opercularis system (fig. 6.30), but reduction and loss of the tympanic ear is often observed (Jaslow et al. 1988). Several species lack a tympanum; the extrastapes merely is embedded in unspecialized epidermis and dermis on the side of the head. In others, all traces of a tympanic ear are gone, including the middle ear cavity and stapes. This condition has arisen independently in several lineages of anurans, and there are no consistent factors (such as fossoriality or voicelessness) that are correlated with loss of the tympanic ear (Jaslow et al. 1988). The other orders of amphibians, the salamanders and the caecilians, completely lack tympanic ears (Jaslow et al. 1988). Terrestrial salamanders possess only an opercularis system. The limbless, fossorial caecilians lack a pectoral girdle and an opercularis system, and possess only a single large otic element, apparently homologous to the stapes, that probably functions in inertial reception of ground vibrations (Wever 1985).

The opercularis system merits close scrutiny as a good prospect for nontympanic reception of sound. The operculum is typically a platelike element that moves about a cartilaginous hinge on the otic capsule (Hetherington et al. 1986). The opercularis muscle is a largely tonic muscle (Becker and Lombard 1977) that in terrestrial situations is maintained in tension (Hetherington and Lombard 1983). Such a tensed muscle would act as a taut structural connection between the operculum and shoulder girdle.

Originally, the opercularis system was proposed to act in reception of ground vibrations (Kingsbury and Reed 1909). Presumably, vibrations entering the forelimb would pass along the opercularis muscle to the operculum and inner ear. Other functional hypotheses have been proposed, including some suggesting that the system acts to modulate responsiveness of the tympanic ear of those anurans that possess both middle ear systems (Lombard and Straughan 1974; Wever 1985). However, morphological evidence suggests that the operculum does not influence motion of the stapes (Hetherington et al. 1986), and functional linkage of the opercularis system to the tympanic ear is not generalizable to all amphibians; many anurans and all salamanders lack tympanic ears. It therefore is unlikely that the opercularis system acts as part of a pressure-transducing middle ear, and recent experimental work has demonstrated that it can indeed function in reception of ground vibrations by transducing substrate displacements into fluid displacements within the inner ear. Removal of the opercularis muscle in bullfrogs (*Rana catesbeiana*) depresses inner ear re-

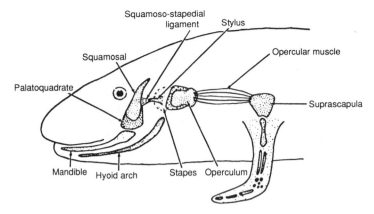

Fig. 6.29. The opercularis system of a salamander, an amphibian lacking a tympanic ear and possessing only this middle ear complex. The area of the otic capsule anterior to the operculum (circumscribed by a dashed line) represents a fused larval stapes (see fig. 6.31). After Kingsbury and Reed (1909).

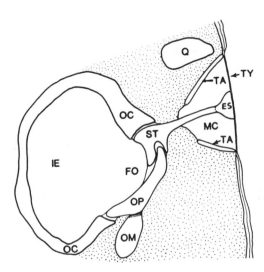

Fig. 6.30. The otic region of an anuran amphibian displaying the relationship between the elements of the two middle ear complexes, the tympanic ear and the opercularis system, of many anurans. This figure represents a frontal view, and compresses features normally observed at different levels into one plane to provide a general view of middle ear structure. Anterior is toward the top. The footplate of the stapes (ST) typically articulates with the operculum (OP), but the morphology of the articulation suggests that the two elements move independently in the oval window (or fenestra ovalis, FO). ES, extrastapes; IE, inner ear; MC, middle ear cavity; OC, otic capsule; OM, opercularis muscle; Q, quadrate; TA, tympanic annulus; TY, tympanum. From Hetherington (1987).

sponses to vibration (Hetherington 1988). Additional measurements have shown that substrate motion affecting the forelimb and shoulder girdle is effectively transferred to the operculum via the tensed opercularis muscle (Hetherington 1988). Movement of the operculum in the oval window appears to produce waves within the inner ear fluids that then stimulate certain end organs of the inner ear. The amphibian opercularis complex essentially acts as an inertially sensitive system; inertial differences between the loosely attached operculum and inner ear are simply magnified by attaching the operculum to a distant body region affected differently by ground vibrations.

Given that the opercularis system is also the only middle ear complex of many amphibians, can it also function as a nontympanic receptor of aerial sound? Lombard and Straughan (1974) observed that removal of the opercularis muscle in certain frogs decreased midbrain responses to sound below about 1 kHz. If we assume that the opercularis system does not modulate function of the tympanic ear, this suggests that the system was directly involved in reception of these lower frequencies. Hetherington (1989) found that disruption of the opercularis system in salamanders, which lack tympanic ears, depresses inner ear responses to sound, especially at frequencies below about 1 kHz. Evidence therefore suggests that indeed the opercularis system can act as an alternative pathway for sound reception, although the precise mode of its function needs to be clarified. Sound absorbed by the shoulder region may, via the opercularis muscle, produce motion of the operculum. Walkowiak (1978) found that brain responses to sound were highest when a sound tube was placed over the shoulder region of *Bombina bombina,* an anuran lacking a tympanic ear. It is also possible that absorbed sound may produce differential motion of the head and body, such that the operculum, anchored to posterior body regions, will move relative to the inner ear and skull (Hetherington 1989). Lastly, it is possible that sound, especially at lower frequencies, may produce substrate motion that can then be detected via the opercularis system in the standard manner—a case of "hearing through your feet." All of these mechanisms could actually be used; the effectiveness of any one may depend on the specific circumstances in which the animal may find itself.

There is evidence that amphibians utilize additional nontympanic pathways for sound reception besides the opercularis system. Vlaming et al. (1984) suggested that sound localization depends on three routes of sound transmission to the middle ear. These separate pathways all would act to modify pressure within the middle ear cavity, and therefore modify tympanic motion, depending on the direction of the sound. The tympanic ear acts as one pathway. Eggermont (1988) suggested that the opercularis system could be another, although it is unclear how this system could affect pressures within the middle ear cavity. Evidence exists that external sound can penetrate into the mouth cavity of frogs, and that the latter serves as another entrance port for sound affecting tympanic motion (Vlaming et al. 1984). Another possible route could be via the lateral body wall and respiratory system. Narins et al. (1988) have found that sound pressure can produce significant motion of the body wall overlying the lungs in the frog *Eleutherodactylus coqui*. In essence, the body wall acts as a tympanum, and pressure changes within the lungs could then pass forward via the respiratory tract to the middle ear cavity and affect tympanic motion. Changes in lung pressure also could produce motion of other body tissues near the lungs that might be relayed (perhaps via the opercularis system) to the inner ear. Also, pressure effects in the lungs could be transferred to the endolymphatic sac system that extends from the inner ear into the vertebral canal (Narins et al. 1988). The anuran tympanic ear therefore may not function as an independent pressure transducer, but may typically interact with other sound-absorbing tissue systems. Furthermore, other systems (such as the respiratory pathway described above) may act as pressure transducers independent of the tympanic ear.

MECHANISMS OF AQUATIC HEARING IN TETRAPODS

Problems of impedance matching are minimal underwater, so a variety of auditory mechanisms that are not practical for aerial hearing, and which are often similar to those of fossorial species, can be employed. Most aquatic tetrapods had terrestrial ancestors that possessed tympanic middle ears, and these tympanic ears have generally been retained but modified for underwater hearing. As a result, major differences are found between hearing mechanisms of fishes and aquatic tetrapods. Amphibians provide a contrast with other aquatic tetrapods, however, because many amphibians have aquatic larvae that completely lack tympanic ears, and some aquatic adults retain this condition (Hetherington 1987). Therefore, hearing in larval and some aquatic adult amphibians involves structures and mechanisms that have not been derived from the tympanic ear; these will be discussed first.

Amphibians: Examples of Strategies Unrelated to a Tympanic Ear

Most amphibians display some aquatic habits during their lives. Many species that have some terrestrial habits as adults have thoroughly aquatic larval stages, so the opportunity exists to analyze acoustic reception in the same species across the water-air transition. If we consider aquatic amphibians an approximate model of primitive, aquatic prototetrapods, such information could contribute to an understanding of the evolution of aerial hearing. Unfortunately, there has been little functional analysis of hearing in aquatic larvae or adults, so the opportunity provided by amphibians has not been adequately exploited. However, available evidence suggests that both pressure- and displacement-transducing mechanisms are used in aquatic hearing (Hetherington and Lombard 1982).

Significant qualitative differences are found between the middle ear structures of aquatic (including larval and adult) and terrestrial amphibians. The tympanic ear and opercularis system develop only at or after metamorphosis (Hetherington 1987), and are clearly associated with terrestrial habits. Two basic middle ear patterns are observed among larval amphibians, one in salamanders and caecilians, and the other in anurans, and these patterns imply significantly different strategies for underwater hearing. In most salamanders, the stapes develops early and is a mobile element during much of the aquatic larval period (Kingsbury and Reed 1909). It is generally a broad, platelike structure lying in the oval window and attached anteriorly to the quadrate by a ligament (fig. 6.31). At metamorphosis, the stapes of most salamanders fuses to the otic capsule (fig. 6.29); it appears to have no acoustic function in this condition. At this time an operculum (see above) develops in the oval window posterior to the fused stapes. In caecilians, there appears to be little difference between the middle ear of larval and metamorphosed forms. In both, an often very large, platelike stapes rests in the oval window, attached by a ligament (or connected via an articulation) with the quadrate. It is therefore very similar to the stapes of most larval salamanders.

The stapes found in larval salamanders, and larval and adult caecilians, probably functions as an inertial element, moving relative to the otic capsule and generating stimulatory waves in the inner ear fluids when

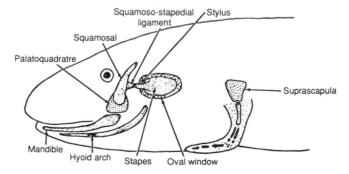

Fig. 6.31. The middle ear of a larval (aquatic) salamander. The large stapes, loosely anchored to the squamosal or palatoquadrate by a ligament, probably acts as an inertially sensitive element for acoustic reception. After Kingsbury and Reed (1909).

acoustic signals penetrate the head. Such an inertial system could be responsive to underwater sound or ground vibrations, so adult caecilians, which are generally either fossorial or aquatic, simply retain the larval configuration of the stapes. Terrestrial salamanders, however, possessing limbs and usually keeping the head off the substrate, lose a functional stapes and develop an opercularis system that is capable of transducing substrate motion (and probably low-frequency aerial sound) into fluid motion within the inner ear (see above).

The middle ear of anuran larvae differs from that of salamander and caecilian larvae. No middle ear elements are observed; rather, the oval window is a large, lateral opening in the otic capsule. In some anurans, a strand of ligamentous tissue, termed the bronchial columella (Witschi 1949), connects the lungs to the round window. It no doubt acts as part of a pressure-transducing system, conducting pulsations of the lungs produced by fluctuations in sound pressure to the inner ear fluids. This pattern is analogous to that of fishes with pressure-sensitive mechanisms and is the opposite of the standard mode of stimulation via the tympanic ear of adult anurans, in which acoustic energy enters at the oval window and exits at the round window.

Anuran larvae may also respond to sound displacements. The large, empty oval window may act as a channel of reduced attenuation, allowing sound waves to enter the otic capsule and affect certain end organs directly (Hetherington 1987). The oval window is closely applied to a branchial chamber that opens posteriorly to surrounding water, and this may facilitate transmission of waterborne sound into the inner ear. It is therefore possible that anuran larvae, like some fishes described above, have both pressure- and displacement-sensitive mechanisms. During metamorphosis and the initiation of terrestrial habits, mobile middle ear elements (operculum and stapes) develop within the oval window, acting to transmit acoustic energy to the inner ear that underwater could enter either through the round window (via a pressure-transducing complex) or directly through the oval window.

Modified Tympanic Ears of Aquatic Tetrapods

Aquatic tetrapods whose ancestors possessed tympanic middle ears adapted for aerial hearing have evolved various mechanisms for hearing underwater sound. Some continue to use the tympanic middle ear as a pathway for absorbed sound energy. Because pressures associated with waterborne sound are higher than those associated with aerial sound, underwater sound waves should readily produce motion of a tympanum overlying an air-filled middle ear cavity. Other aquatic tetrapods have taken advantage of the general impedance match between body tissue and water to evolve enlarged ossicles that act as inertial elements or alternative pathways (usually including tympanic ear elements at some point) to transmit sound energy to the inner ear. Understanding mechanisms of aquatic hearing in tetrapods is difficult because many species are amphibious, spending time both in water and on land, and it is difficult to dissect apart those characteristics linked with aerial hearing from those associated with underwater hearing. The problem is compounded by a general lack of experimental studies and a dependence on inferences drawn from morphological description.

All of the reptilian subclasses have some aquatic species. Most turtles spend considerable time in water and display modified tympanic ear morphologies. Their skulls are heavily ossified and possess a clear otic notch. In many species the margin of the tympanum is almost completely supported by the quadrate bone anteriorly and the squamosal posteriorly (Henson 1974; Wever 1979). The middle ear cavity is also largely encased in bone, with the quadrate forming much of its medial wall. A stapes and extrastapes are found, but there are no other stapedial processes. The extrastapes is typically a broad, disklike plate of cartilage attached to the tympanum. Such a middle ear could act as a pressure transducer underwater. The rigid support of the tympanum and anchoring of the stapes to the quadrate could be specializations to accommodate the increased pressures associated with underwater sound.

Sea turtles are among the most aquatic species of turtles. In *Chelonia mydas,* the middle ear cavity is greatly reduced (fig. 6.32) and apparently filled with mucous material (Hadžiselmovic and Anđelić 1967). The extra-

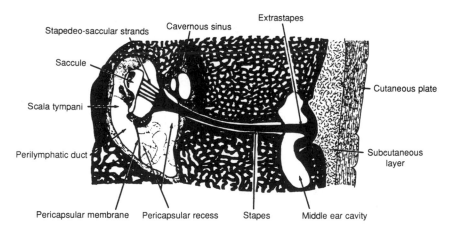

Fig. 6.32. Frontal view of the middle ear of the sea turtle *Chelonia mydas.* The reduced middle ear is typically filled with a gelatinous substance. After Wever (1979).

stapes is attached to connective tissue underneath the heavily ossified scales of the head. The stapes is not an exceptionally massive element, and its shaft extends through a thick layer of bone and is firmly ankylosed to the quadrate (Henson 1974). The sea turtle middle ear cannot be readily categorized as either a pressure- or displacement-transducing system. Because the reduced middle ear cavity is not air-filled, pressure-transducing capabilities would be limited, and because the stapes is not exceptionally large, its effectiveness as an inertial element responding to penetrating kinetic energy would be restricted. Such a middle ear probably acts to relay motion of overlying tissues produced by pressure and/or displacement energy components of underwater sound.

Crocodilians display aquatic habits, but possess well-developed tympanic ears that do not seem specialized for underwater hearing. Crocodilians, like turtles, have heavily ossified skulls, and also possess a bony tympanic margin and bone-enclosed middle ear cavity. The stapes, however, is not exceptionally large or firmly anchored to the quadrate, and both it and the extrastapes display the various processes observed in terrestrial lizards. This contrasts with the middle ear morphologies of the extinct mosasaurs (very large aquatic lizards) and some living aquatic lizards. The middle ears of mosasaurs were similar to those of turtles (McDowell 1967). The extrastapes was a broad, platelike element, the stapes was fixed to the quadrate, and the small middle ear cavity was largely encircled by the quadrate. This same pattern is observed in certain varanid lizards that show aquatic habits, such as *Lanthanotus borneensis* (McDowell 1967). It is likely that the middle ear of mosasaurs functioned like that of sea turtles, the platelike extrastapes acting to transmit motion of head tissues produced by displacement and/or pressure energy associated with underwater sound.

The extinct ichthyosaurs, which were aquatic, fishlike reptiles of the Mesozoic, possessed middle ears completely different from those of other aquatic or amphibious reptiles. The stapes was a massive element (Romer 1974). There was no oval window and the stapes simply abutted the opisthotic and basioccipital elements. Laterally, the stapes broadly contacted the quadrate, and there was no evidence of a middle ear cavity. If the stapes functioned in sound reception at all, its massiveness suggests that it acted as an inertial element transducing the displacement component of sound penetrating the head.

Aquatic mammals display a diversity of middle ear and otic morphologies that suggests the use of a variety of strategies for underwater sound detection. Cetaceans have attracted a great deal of attention, in part because of their vocalizations and echolocation behavior. Studies of hearing in cetaceans have emphasized the importance of specific routes of sound transmission to the inner ear. Each inner ear appears to be acoustically isolated by numerous sinuses extending from the middle ear cavity and nasopharynx and surrounding the periotic bone (fig. 6.33) (Fraser and Purves 1960). The sinuses are filled with air trapped in a lipid-mucus foam; underwater sound may be effectively reflected at this water-air interface, thereby limiting acoustic transmission to other routes. One such route could be along the external auditory meatus, which is narrow, usually convoluted (fig. 6.33), and often filled with mucus or fibrous material. Fraser and Purves (1960) claimed that effective sound transmission was restricted to the external auditory meatus, but a large body of evidence has demonstrated that fatty tissue (blubber) around the meatus acts as a major route for sound transmission (Reysenbach de Haan 1957; McCormick et al. 1970; Norris and Harvey 1974).

Norris (1969) provided an alternative hypothesis of sound transmission in the toothed whales (Odontoceti), suggesting that sound travels through the mandible rather than the lateral surface of the head and tympanum. The bone over the posterior surface of the mandible is exceptionally thin and could act as a window for sound to enter the intramandibular

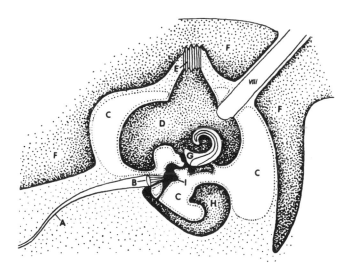

Fig. 6.33. Schematic diagram of the otic region of a toothed whale (suborder Odontoceti). In this dorso-ventral section, the convoluted external auditory meatus (A) passes from the head surface to the left. At its medial end is a tympanum (B) that attaches to the malleus (I) via a tympanic ligament. The malleus articulates with the other middle ear ossicles (incus and stapes) and is anchored to the tympanic bone (H). Note the enlarged, air-filled middle ear cavity (C) that extends to surround most of the periotic bone (D) encasing the inner ear (G) and that probably aids in directional sensitivity. The periotic is suspended from other cranial elements of the skull (F) by a ligament (E). VIII, auditory nerve. After Reysenbach de Hann (1957).

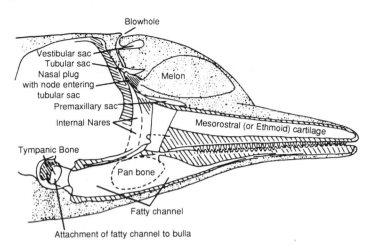

Fig. 6.34. The head of a dolphin (family Delphinidae) showing the mandibular fat channel which may function as a pathway for acoustic signals (especially at high frequencies above about 30 kHz). The pan bone is an area of very thin bone on the lateral surface of the mandible, and the fatty channel passes posteriorly to contact the tympanic bone. The latter is connected to the malleus (see fig. 6.33). From Norris (1969).

fat body (fig. 6.34). From there acoustic signals would be conducted posteriorly to the tympanic bone and, via a direct connection between the latter and the malleus (fig. 6.33), to the middle ear ossicles. Norris and Harvey (1974) found little attenuation of sound as it entered the mandible, and also observed that transmission was very dependent on angle of incidence, so such an arrangement could provide directional information. Work on dolphins (Bullock et al. 1968; McCormick et al. 1970) found that midbrain and cochlear responses to sound above 20 kHz increased in amplitude when the sound was presented over the posterior mandible compared to other head regions, although the responses were also high when sound was presented over the external auditory meatus. The present concensus is that sound transmission in odontocete cetaceans occurs along both meatal (including nearby fat tissues) and mandibular routes, and that the two routes are effective over different frequency ranges (Ketten 1992). The meatal route is most effective at lower frequencies up to about 30 kHz, and the mandibular route is most effective at higher frequencies. It is interesting to note that the mandibular route suggested by Norris (1969) is reminiscent of the mandibular-quadrate-stapedial pathway observed in many other tetrapods living in conditions in which acoustic energy can directly enter the body, such as aquatic salamanders and various fossorial reptiles.

Regardless of the pathway of acoustic signals to the ossicles, the cetacean ossicles themselves are unusual in both their massive size and their stiffness. The malleus and incus are very large, and the malleus is firmly anchored to the tympanic bone by an anterior process (fig. 6.33). The manubrium of the malleus is attached to a thick tympanic ligament that projects from a tympanum situated at the medial end of the external auditory meatus (fig. 6.33). The stapes is not exceptionally large, but is firmly attached to the margin of the oval window.

There have been several hypotheses of ossicular function in cetaceans. Fraser and Purves (1960) hypothesized that, in response to tympanic motion, the tympanic ligament would act to crank the manubrium and thereby produce ossicular motion. The increase in mass of the ossicles is suggested to act to counter the high pressures associated with underwater sound, and their stiffness may act to enhance high-frequency sound reception by countering the low-frequency bias produced by the increased ossicular mass (Reysenbach de Haan 1957). Work by Fleischer (1978) suggested that sound was absorbed mostly by the tympanic bone, and from there transmitted to the malleus and eventually to the inner ear via the ossicular chain. McCormick et al. (1970), however, presented evidence that the cetacean middle ear acts as an inertial system. Damping movement of the entire ossicular chain decreased auditory responses by as much as 18 dB, whereas removal of the malleus alone caused a decrease of only 4 dB. Therefore, absorbed sound energy may produce differential motion between the otic capsule and the independently suspended, massive ossicles, resulting in stimulatory fluid motion within the inner ear.

Pinniped mammals, which evolved aquatic habits independent of the cetacean lineage (Vaughan 1986), have evolved different strategies for underwater hearing. The amphibious seals and sea lions are faced with the problem of hearing both in air and in water, and to some degree their middle ears reflect this compromise. Repenning (1972) found that the harbor seal (*Phoca vulgaris*) was more sensitive to underwater sound than to aerial sound by about 15 dB. In comparison, *Homo sapiens,* which possesses a middle ear adapted for aerial hearing, loses about 30 dB of sensitivity when underwater. Unlike most cetaceans, the periotic and tympanic bones surrounding the middle ear cavity of pinnipeds are not suspended independently but are firmly anchored to the skull. Repenning (1972) argued that pinnipeds employ two strategies for underwater hearing, an inertial and a deformational mode. Repenning suggested that the phocid seals, which have massive, loosely anchored ossicles, employ the inertial mode. In contrast, the otariid and odobenid pinnipeds appear to employ the deformational mode. They possess greatly expanded mastoid processes that may selectively absorb sound and transmit it directly to the thin-walled (and therefore easily deformable) cochlear capsule. Repenning therefore argued that acoustic reception in these species was direct and bypassed the middle ear.

These last examples of aquatic hearing in pinniped mammals may be especially instructive. Repenning (1972) in effect argues that a tympanic middle ear configuration is not especially useful for underwater hearing. In those species with amphibious habits, a tympanic middle ear is retained for aerial hearing, although its sensitivity may be compromised by specializations for underwater hearing. Reviewing middle ear morphology in other aquatic tetrapods, this appears to be a promising perspective. In reptiles, the most thoroughly aquatic forms, such as the sea turtles and the extinct ichthyosaurs, have drastically reduced or absent tympanic ears. The thoroughly aquatic cetaceans have drastically modified tympanic ears and may use alternative pathways of acoustic transmission. Some pinnipeds have unique otic features that suggest that the tympanic middle ear is bypassed during underwater hearing, and other pinnipeds have middle ear elements that act as inertial elements rather than part of a transmission pathway. As in the case of fossorial tetrapods, nontympanic strategies tend to evolve in aquatic tetrapod lineages, and either the tympanic ear is lost or only certain elements, especially the auditory ossicles, are retained and incorporated into nontympanic receptive systems.

SUMMARY

In this chapter we have considered the evolution and function of diverse auxiliary components of the vertebrate ear. These structures have evolved to couple hair cells of the inner ear to pressure fluctuations or displacements associated with environmental sounds. Without them, hair cells are incapable of detecting even a tiny fraction of the broad range of frequencies and amplitudes present in sounds of natural origin. Since the hair cells used in auditory systems evolved from cells encapsulated in the skull as part of the vestibular system, the skull has been modified by, and has contributed to, the evolution of many of the auxiliary structures present in vertebrates.

The known modifications of the skull associated with hearing in fishes are, in most cases, subtle. Most consist of openings in the wall of the otic capsule for the passage of periotic systems coupling the hair cells to pressure-sensitive auxiliary structures or for the formation of low-impedance pathways coupling hair cells directly to water displacements. In some, however, the otic capsule is highly modified, as in the formation of the partially gas-filled bulla connected to the swim bladder in clupeids.

On the other hand, modifications of the skull associated with hearing in tetrapods are obvious. Most evident, and present in members of each tetrapod class, are modifications associated with the evolution of tympanic ears. Tympanic ears have evolved at least three times. Each has unique features, but all have major similarities. All make use of a periotic system coupling the auditory hair cells to the wall of the otic capsule at the fenestra ovalis, also a universal (though not necessarily homologous) feature of the skull in Recent tetrapods. All have an air-filled middle ear cavity lateral to the otic capsule. One wall of the cavity is bounded by a tympanic membrane. Spanning the cavity is a bone or set of bones connecting the fenestra ovalis to the membrane. The bones are derivatives of the splanchnocranial elements of the mandibular and hyoid arches. The tympanic membrane itself is suspended from modified elements of the skull. This suite of structures functions in transducing the pressure fluctuations of environmental sounds to displacements at the surface of the hair cells. The standard tympanic ear has been modified in several tetrapod lineages for sensitivity to ground vibrations, underwater sound, or low-frequency aerial sound, all of which may readily penetrate body tissues. A common trend in such lineages has been the evolution of nontympanic, inertially sensitive systems. Most of these systems employ massive ossicles retained from the tympanic ear, but occasionally new middle ear structures have evolved, as in the case of the amphibian opercularis system.

"Making do" is a constant theme in the evolution of structures associated with hearing in vertebrates. The modification of structures originally evolved for other purposes occurs repeatedly, starting with the use of vestibular hair cells. In addition, iterative use of the same structures also occurs, as in the use of the swim bladder as a pressure transducer in bony fishes, and the use of the stapes for displacement transfer in tetrapods.

APPENDIX

The points in figures 6.9, 6.10, and 6.14 were generated using the following equations from Seto (1971) for a monopole source and spherical spreading.

    a. Intensity: $I = W/4\pi r^2$

        where $W = 1 \times 10^{-6}$ Watts and r is the distance from the source in meters.

    b. Acoustic pressure: $P = \sqrt{2\rho c I}$

        where ρ is the density of the fluid (1,040 kg/m³ used for water and 1.21 kg/m³ for air) and c is the speed of sound (1,480 m/s used for water and 343 m/s for air)

c. Particle velocity: $v = P/\rho c \cos \theta$

where $\cos \theta = kr/\sqrt{1 + k^2 r^2}$, $k = 2\pi f/c$, and f is frequency.

d. Particle displacement: $u = v/\omega$

where $\omega = 2\pi f$

REFERENCES

Allin, E. F. 1986. The auditory apparatus of advanced mammal-like reptiles and early mammals. In *The Ecology and Biology of Mammal-like Reptiles*, N. Hotton, P. D. MacLean, J. J. Roth, and E. C. Roth, eds. Washington, D.C.: Smithsonian Institution Press, pp. 283–294.

Art, J. J., and R. Fettiplace. 1987. Variation of membrane properties in hair cells isolated from the turtle cochlea. Journal of Physiology 385: 207–242.

Ashmore, J. F. 1988. Hair cells. Scientific Progress, Oxford 72: 139–153.

Banner, A. 1967. Evidence of sensitivity to acoustic displacements in the lemon shark, *Negaprion brevirostris* (Poey). In *Lateral Line Detectors*, P. H. Cahn, ed. Bloomington: Indiana University Press, pp. 265–273.

Becker, R. P., and R. E. Lombard. 1977. Structural correlates of function in the "opercularis" muscle of amphibians. Cell and Tissue Research 175: 499–522.

Best, A. C. G., and J. A. B. Gray. 1980. Morphology of the utricular recess in the sprat. Journal of the Marine Biological Association of the United Kingdom 60: 703–715.

Blaxter, J. H. S., E. J. Denton, and J. A. B. Gray. 1981. Acousticolateralis system in clupeid fishes. In *Hearing and Sound Communication in Fishes*, W. N. Tavolga, A. N. Popper, and R. R. Fay, eds. New York: Springer-Verlag, pp. 40–59.

Bolt, J. R., and R. E. Lombard. 1985. Evolution of the amphibian tympanic ear and the origin of frogs. Biological Journal of the Linnean Society 24: 83–99.

Budelli, R., and O. Macadar. 1979. Statoacoustic properties of utricular afferents. Journal of Neurophysiology 42: 1479–1493.

Bullock, T. H., A. D. Grinnel, E. Ikezono, K. Kameda, Y. Katsuki, M. Nomoto, O. Sato, N. Suga, and K. Yanagisawa. 1968. Electrophysiological studies of the central auditory mechanisms in cetaceans. Zeitschrift für vergleichende Physiologie 59: 117–156.

Capranica, R. C. 1976. Morphology and physiology of the auditory system. In *Frog Neurobiology*, R. Llinas and W. Precht, eds. New York: Springer-Verlag, pp. 551–577.

Capranica, R. C., and A. Michelsen. 1988. Experimental verification that intertympanic coupling is the predominant source of directional sound sensitivity of the treefrog's ear. Abstracts of the Society of Neurosciences 322.

Carlström, D. 1963. A crystallographic study of vertebrate otoliths. Biological Bulletin 125: 441–463.

Cartmill, M. 1975. Strepsirhine basicranial structures and the affinities of the Cheirogaleidae. In *Phylogeny of the primates,* W. P. Luckett and F. S. Szalay, eds. New York: Plenum Press, pp. 313–356.

Coombs, S. 1981. Interspecific differences in hearing capabilities for select teleost species. In *Hearing and Sound Communication in Fishes,* W. N. Tavolga, A. N. Popper, and R. R. Fay, eds. New York: Springer-Verlag, pp. 174–177.

Coombs, S., and J. Janssen. 1990. Water flow detection by the mechanosensory lateral line. In *Comparative Perception,* W. C. Stebbins and M. Berkley, eds. New York: John Wiley and Sons, pp. 89–124.

Coombs, S., J. Janssen, and F. Webb. 1988. Diversity of lateral line systems: Evolutionary and functional considerations. In *Sensory Biology of Aquatic Animals,* J. Atema, R. R. Fay, A. N. Popper, and W. N. Tavolga, eds., New York: Springer-Verlag, pp. 553–593.

Corwin, J. T. 1977. Morphology of the macula neglecta in sharks of the genus *Carcharhinus.* Journal of Morphology 152: 341–362.

———. 1981. Audition in elasmobranchs. In *Hearing and Sound Communication in Fishes,* W. N. Tavolga, A. N. Popper, and R. R. Fay, eds. New York: Springer-Verlag, pp. 81–105.

Dijkgraaf, S. 1963. The functioning and significance of the lateral-line organs. Biological Reviews 38: 51–105.

Eggermont, J. J. 1988. Mechanisms of sound localization in anurans. In *The Evolution of the Amphibian Auditory System,* B. Fritzsch, M. J. Ryan, W. Wilczynski, T. E. Hetherington, and W. Walkowiak, eds. New York: John Wiley and Sons, pp. 307–336.

Enger, P. S. 1967. Hearing in herring. Comparative Biochemistry and Physiology 22: 527–538.

Fay, R. R. 1981. Coding of acoustic information in the eighth nerve. In *Hearing and Sound Communication in Fishes,* W. N. Tavolga, A. N. Popper, and R. R. Fay, eds. New York: Springer-Verlag, pp. 189–221.

———. 1984. The goldfish ear codes the axis of acoustic particle motion in three dimensions. Science 225: 951–954.

Fay, R. R., J. I. Kendall, A. N. Popper, and A. L. Tester. 1974. Vibration detection by the macula neglecta of sharks. Comparative Biochemistry and Physiology 47A: 1235–1240.

Fay, R. R., and A. N. Popper. 1980. Structure and function in teleost auditory systems. In *Comparative Studies of Hearing in Vertebrates,* A. N. Popper and R. R. Fay, eds. New York: Springer-Verlag, pp. 3–42.

Fleischer, G. 1978. Evolutionary principles of the mammalian middle ear. Advances in Anatomy, Embryology, and Cell Biology 55: 1–70.

Fraser, F. C., and P. E. Purves. 1960. Hearing in cetaceans. Bulletin of the British Museum of Natural History 7: 1–140.

Fritzsch, B. 1987. Inner ear of the coelacanth fish *Latimeria* has tetrapod affinities. Nature 327: 153–154.

Fritzsch, B., and M. H. Wake. 1988. The inner ear of gymnophione amphibians and its nerve supply: A comparative study of regressive events in a complex sensory system (Amphibia, Gymnophiona). Zoomorphology 108: 210–217.

Gans, C., and E. G. Wever. 1972. The ear and hearing in Amphisbaenia (Reptilia). Journal of Experimental Zoology 179: 17–34.

———. 1976. The ear and hearing in *Sphenodon punctatus*. Proceedings of the National Academy of Sciences 73: 4244–4246.

Gaudin, E. P. 1968. On the middle ear of birds. Acta oto-laryngologica 65: 316–326.

Hadžiselmovic, H., and M. Andelić. 1967. Contribution to the knowledge of the ear in the sea turtle. Acta anatomica 66: 460–477.

Hartline, P. H. 1971. Physiological basis for detection of sound and vibration in snakes. Journal of Experimental Biology 59: 349–371.

Hawkins, A. D. 1981. The hearing abilities of fish. In *Hearing and Sound Communication in Fishes*, W. N. Tavolga, A. N. Popper, and R. R. Fay, eds. New York: Springer-Verlag, pp. 81–105.

Hawkins, A. D., and D. N. MacLennan. 1976. An acoustic tank for hearing studies on fish. In *Aquaculture and Fisheries Science: Symposium on Sound Reception in Fish*, A. Shuif and A. D. Hawkins, eds. Amsterdam: Elsevier, pp. 149–169.

Henson, O. W. 1961. Some morphological and functional aspects of certain structures of the middle ear in bats and insectivores. Kansas University Science Bulletin 42: 151–255.

———. 1970. The ear and audition. In *Biology of Bats*, vol. 2, W. A. Wimsatt, ed. New York: Academic Press, pp. 181–262.

———. 1974. Comparative anatomy of the middle ear. In *Handbook of Sensory Physiology*, vol. 5, W. D. Keidel and W. D. Neff, eds. Berlin: Springer-Verlag, pp. 39–110.

Hetherington, T. E. 1987. Timing of development of the middle ear of Anura (Amphibia). Zoomorphologie 106: 289–300.

———. 1988. Biomechanics of vibration reception in the bullfrog, *Rana catesbeiana*. Journal of Comparative Physiology 163: 43–52.

———. 1989. Effect of the amphibian opercularis muscle on auditory responses. In *Progress in Zoology*, vol. 35, H. Splechtna and H. Hilgers, eds. Berlin: Springer-Verlag, pp. 356–359.

Hetherington, T. E., A. P. Jaslow, and R. E. Lombard. 1986. Comparative morphology of the amphibian opercularis muscle. I. General design features and functional interpretation. Journal of Morphology 190: 43–61.

Hetherington, T. E., and R. E. Lombard. 1982. Biophysics of underwater hearing in anuran amphibians. Journal of Experimental Biology 98: 49–66.

———. 1983. Electromyography of the opercularis muscle of the bullfrog *Rana catesbeiana*: An amphibian tonic muscle. Journal of Morphology 175: 17–26.

Hill, K. G., D. B. Lewis, M. E. Hutchings, and R. B. Coles. 1980. Directional hearing in the Japanese quail (*Coturnix c. japonica*). I. Acoustic properties of the auditory system. Journal of Experimental Biology 86: 131–151.

Hinchliffe, R., and A. Pye. 1969. Variations in the middle ear of the Mammalia. Journal of Zoology, London 157: 277–288.

Hudspeth, A. J., and D. P. Corey. 1977. Sensitivity, polarity, and conductance change in the response of vertebrate hair cells to controlled mechanical stimuli. Proceedings of the National Academy of Sciences 74: 2407–2411.

Hunt, R. M. 1974. The auditory bulla in Carnivora: An anatomical basis for reappraisal of carnivore evolution. Journal of Morphology 143: 21–76.

Jaslow, A. P., T. E. Hetherington, and R. E. Lombard. 1988. Structure and function of the amphibian middle ear. In *The Evolution of the Amphibian Auditory System*, B. Fritzsch, M. J. Ryan, W. Wilczynski, T. E. Hetherington, and W. Walkowiak, eds. New York: John Wiley and Sons, pp. 69–92.

Ketten, D. R. 1992. The marine mammal ear: specializations for aquatic audition and echo location. In *The Evolutionary Biology of Hearing*, D. B. Webster, R. R. Fay, and A. N. Popper, eds. New York: Springer-Verlag, pp. 717–750.

Khanna, S. M., and J. Tonndorf. 1972. Tympanic membrane vibration in cats studied by time-averaged holography. Journal of the Acoustic Society of America 51: 1904–1920.

Kingsbury, B. F., and H. D. Reed. 1909. The columella auris in Amphibia. Journal of Morphology 20: 549–628.

Kuhne, R., and B. Lewis. 1985. External and middle ears. In *Form and Function in Birds*, vol. 3, A. S. King and J. McLelland, eds. New York: Academic Press, pp. 227–272.

Lay, D. M. 1972. Hearing organs of gerbelline rodents. Journal of Morphology 138: 41–120.

Lewis, E. R., E. L. Leverenz, and W. S. Bailek. 1985. *The Vertebrate Inner Ear*. Boca Raton, Fla.: CRC Press.

Lombard, R. E., and J. R. Bolt. 1979. Evolution of the tetrapod ear: An analysis and reinterpretation. Biological Journal of the Linnean Society 11: 19–76.

———. 1988. Evolution of the stapes in Paleozoic tetrapods: Conservative and radical hypotheses. In *The Evolution of the Amphibian Auditory System*, B. Fritzsch, M. J. Ryan, W. Wilczynski, T. E. Hetherington, and W. Walkowiak, eds. New York: John Wiley and Sons, pp. 37–67.

Lombard, R. E., and I. R. Straughan. 1974. Functional aspects of anuran middle ear structures. Journal of Experimental Biology 61: 71–93.

McCormick, J. G., E. G. Wever, J. Palin, and S. H. Ridgway. 1970. Sound conduction in the dolphin ear. Journal of the Acoustical Society of America 48: 1418–1428.

McDowell, S. B. 1967. The extracolumella and tympanic cavity of the "earless" monitor lizard *Lanthanotus borneensis*. *Copeia:* 154–159.

Maisey, J. G. 1987. Notes on the structure and phylogeny of vertebrate otoliths. Copeia: 495–499.

Michelsen, A. 1971. The physiology of the locust ear. II. Acoustical properties of the intact ear. *Zeitschrift für vergleichende Physiologie* 71: 102–128.

Moffat, A. M., and R. C. Capranica. 1978. Middle ear sensitivity in anurans and reptiles measured by light scattering spectroscopy. Journal of Comparative Physiology A 127: 97–107.

Moore, W. J. 1981. *The Mammalian Skull*. Cambridge: Cambridge University Press.

Narins, P. M., G. Ehret, and J. Tautz. 1988. Accessory pathway for sound transfer in a neotropical frog. Proceedings of the National Academy of Sciences 85: 1508–1512.

Nelson, D. R. 1967. Hearing thresholds, frequency discrimination, and acoustic orientation in the lemon shark, *Negaprion brevirostris* (Poey). Bulletin of Marine Science 17: 741–768.

Norberg, R. A. 1978. Skull asymmetry, ear structure and function, and auditory localization in Tengmalm's owl *Aegolius funereus* (Linne). Philosophical Transactions of the Royal Society 282B: 325–410.

Norris, K. S. 1969. The echolocation of marine mammals. In *Biology of Marine Mammals,* H. T. Anderson, ed. New York: Academic Press, pp. 391–423.

Norris, K. S., and G. W. Harvey. 1974. Sound transmission in the porpoise head. Journal of the Acoustical Society of America 56: 659–664.

Northcutt, R. G. 1989. The phylogenetic distribution and innervation of craniate mechanoreceptive lateral lines. In *Neurobiology and Evolution of the Lateral Line System,* S. Coombs, P. Gorner, and H. Münz, eds. Berlin: Springer-Verlag, pp. 17–78.

Novacek, M. J. 1977. Aspects of the problem of variation, origin, and evolution of the eutherian auditory bulla. Mammal Review 7: 131–149.

Oeckinghaus, H., and J. Schwartzkopff. 1983. Electrical and acoustical activation of the middle ear muscle in a songbird. Journal of Comparative Physiology 150: 61–67.

Pinder, A. C., and A. R. Palmer. 1983. Mechanical properties of the frog ear: Vibration measurements under free and closed-field acoustic conditions. Proceedings of the Royal Society of London B 219: 371–396.

Repenning, C. A. 1972. Underwater hearing in seals: Functional morphology. In *Functional Anatomy of Marine Mammals,* vol. 1, R. J. Harrison, ed. New York: Academic Press, pp. 307–331.

Reysenbach de Haan, F. W. 1957. Hearing in whales. Acta oto-laryngologica 134 (suppl.): 1–114.

Romer, A. S. 1974. *Vertebrate Paleontology.* Chicago: University of Chicago Press.

Sand, O. 1981. The lateral line and sound reception. In *Hearing and Sound Communication in Fishes,* W. N. Tavolga, A. N. Popper, and R. R. Fay, eds. New York: Springer-Verlag, pp. 459–480.

Saunders, J. C., and B. M. Johnstone. 1972. A comparative analysis of middle ear function in non-mammalian vertebrates. Acta oto-laryngologica 73: 353–361.

Schuijf, A. 1981. Models of acoustic localization. In *Hearing and Sound Communication in Fishes,* W. N. Tavolga, A. N. Popper, and R. R. Fay, eds. New York: Springer-Verlag, pp. 268–310.

Schwartz, E. 1974. Lateral-line mechano-receptors in fishes and amphibians. In *Handbook of Sensory Physiology III/3,* A. Fessard, ed. New York: Springer-Verlag.

Schwartzkopff, J. 1957. Die Grossenverhaltnisse von Trommelfell, Columella-Fussplate und Schnecke bei Vogeln verschiedenen Gewichts. Zeitschrift für Morphologie und Okologie die Tierre 45: 365–378.

Seto, W. W. 1971. *Theory and Problems of Acoustics.* Schaum's Outline Series. New York: McGraw-Hill.

Tonndorf, J. 1972. Bone conduction. In *Foundation of Modern Auditory Theory,* vol. 2, J. V. Tobias, ed. New York: Academic Press, pp. 197–237.

Turner, R. G., A. A. Muraski, and D. W. Nielsen. 1981. Cilium length: Influence on neural tonotopic organization. Science 213: 1519.

Van Bergeijk, W. A. 1966. The evolution of vertebrate hearing. Contributions to Sensory Physiology 2: 1–49.

Vaughan, T. A. 1986. *Mammalogy*. Philadelphia: Saunders College Publishing.

Vlaming, M. S. M. G., A. M. H. J. Aertsen, and W. J. M. Epping. 1984. Directional hearing in the grassfrog (*Rana temporaria* L.). I. Mechanical vibrations of tympanic membrane. Hearing Research 14: 191–201.

Walkowiak, W. 1978. The coding of auditory signals in the torus semicircularis of the fire-bellied toad and grass frog: Responses to simple stimuli and to conspecific calls. Journal of Comparative Physiology 138: 131–148.

Webster, D. B., and M. Webster. 1975. Auditory systems of Heteromyidae: Functional morphology and evolution of the middle ear. Journal of Morphology 146: 343–376.

Wever, E. G. 1968. The ear of the chameleon: *Chamaeleo senegalensis* and *Chamaeleo quilensis*. Journal of Experimental Zoology 168: 423–436.

———. 1974. The evolution of vertebrate hearing. In *Handbook of Sensory Physiology*, vol. 5, W. O. Keidel and W. D. Neff, eds. Berlin: Springer-Verlag, pp. 39–110.

———. 1976. Origin and evolution of the ear of vertebrates. In *Evolution of Brain and Behavior in Vertebrates*, R. B. Masterson, M. E. Bitterman, C. G. B. Campbell, and N. Hotton, eds. Hillsdale, N.J.: Laurence Erlbaum Assoc., pp. 89–105.

———. 1979. *The Reptile Ear*. Princeton: Princeton University Press.

———. 1985. *The Amphibian Ear*. Princeton: Princeton University Press.

Wever, E. G., and J. A. Vernon. 1960. The problem of hearing in snakes. Journal of Auditory Research 1: 77–83.

Wever, E. G., and Y. L. Werner. 1970. The function of the middle ear in lizards: *Crotaphytus collaris* (Iguanidae). Journal of Experimental Zoology 175: 327–342.

Witschi, E. 1949. The larval ear of the frog and its transformation during metamorphosis. Zeitschrift für Naturforschung, Wiesbaden 4: 230–242.

7

Beams and Machines:
Modeling Approaches to the Analysis of
Skull Form and Function

DAVID B. WEISHAMPEL

INTRODUCTION

A GENERAL THEORY THAT RELATES the development, biomechanics, and evolution of the vertebrate skull is presently unavailable to functional morphologists, embryologists, and systematists. Indeed, it is very difficult to imagine what such a theory might look like. As a result, various methods have been undertaken to model isolated aspects of skull morphology. Most of these modeling approaches treat the skull as a collection of anatomical systems, each of which involves certain biomechanical problems and thus contributes to an overall network of cranial function.

By their very nature, these modeling approaches are pictures of, or statements about, cranial biomechanics. If reasonable, these models are based upon well-understood parameters from which predictions about the real world can ultimately be made. In turn, these predictions can be used to test the accuracy of the model and to make further statements about the topic at hand. Some of these subsequent statements may be empirical in nature or may be heuristic in that they may lead to interpretations that would have at first appeared counterintuitive. Examples of each are discussed in the text that follows.

Most often, functional morphologic modeling uses machine analogies to understand the operation of a particular anatomical system. Thus it is not surprising that many models of organismic form and function use actual physical models (e.g., Bock and Kummer 1968; Nobiling 1977; Demes et al. 1984; Demes 1984; Greaves, personal communication). Other approaches include graphical representation and mathematical computation (Kripp 1933a, c, d; DeMar and Barghusen 1973; Anker 1974; Lombard and Wake 1976, 1977; Wolff 1984; Thomason and Russell 1986), computer-based simulations (Elshoud 1980; Otten 1983, 1985; Weishampel 1983, 1984), or possibility thought experiments (Gingerich 1971; Hylander 1975). The application of any one of these methods depends on such things as the questions being asked, the techniques and time available, and the research preference of the investigator. However, all of the approaches should reciprocally enhance the others when used to explore the workings of and constraints on form and function.

By its very nature, modeling allows an investigator to ask not only which factors control and maintain the operation of a complex, but also how changes in the geometry of such a complex affect how the system works. This yin/yang parallelism inherent in the questions "How does the system work?" and "Why isn't it built differently and what might be the meaning of such differences?" provides the opportunity to investigate controls on the operation and evolution of the system, be they multiple evolutionary pathways, Darwinian optimizations, architectural constraints, or adaptive opportunities.

This chapter is intended as a review of some of the uses of modeling to understand the functional morphology of skulls. I have not attempted to provide exhaustive examples of modeling approaches. Those studies recounted here were chosen for the ways in which they approach their subjects. I have chosen those that are more or less limited to engineering principles and therefore to research on the statics, kinematics, and dynamics of certain aspects of skulls. Perhaps not surprisingly, most approaches pertain to the statics of biting and/or mastication. My choice reflects the prevailing use of beam and machine analogies for testing biomechanical units within the skull. Most relate to models of jaw mechanics in a specific group of animals, but some studies attempt to go beyond the immediate functional relevance of the model either to make comparisons with other groups of animals or to perturb the model in various ways, perhaps to look at an optimization of the system along some functional gradient.

STATICS: THE SKULL IN EQUILIBRIUM

Statics, the ability of the skull to transmit and ultimately absorb forces passing through it, has been investigated in a number of studies. For the most part, the approach has relied on engineering beam theory through either lever analogies or free-body analyses. Other examples use beam theory only implicitly in their discussion of static loadings, torques, and lever-arm mechanics in equilibrium conditions. The discussion below will concentrate first on a few examples of how elements of the facial skeleton and mandible can be modeled as statically loaded beams and then focus on models of masticatory equilibrium conditions in which components of the musculoskeletal system behave as a system of levers for force transmission.

The Facial Skeleton Modeled as a Beam

In his functional analysis of bill shape in birds, Bock (1966) used lever-arm mechanics to model the influences of various reaction forces on the shape of the upper bill when contacting upper and lower jaws are in equilibrium while biting and pecking. He did so by using both torque and trajectory analyses (fig. 7.1 a, b) to examine the relationship between external forces and the size, shape, and internal anatomy of the bill in crows (Corvidae), woodpeckers (Picidae), and cardinals (Fringillidae). The pattern of forces acting on the outside of the bill was determined by torque analysis, in which lever-arm mechanics provide information on local stress concentrations at the craniofacial hinge and quadratomandibular articulation. Trajectory analysis, in which internal compression and tension pathways were determined for a given load over a particular region, was then used to estimate the distribution of internal forces passing through the bill. Internal bony architecture, used as a test of the two methods, corresponds quite closely to the distribution of stresses that they predict.

In a second study, Bock and Kummer (1968) modeled the mechanics of the avian mandible as a structural girder or beam. In a reevaluation of Kripp's (1935d) study of the mandible modeled as a reinforced concrete girder, Bock and Kummer used photoelastic lucite models as surrogates for the mandibles of crow (Corvidae; fig. 7.1c, d). Using the same sort of trajectory analysis to derive stress patterns, the mandible appeared to behave as an I-beam in which the extensive bony regions of the dorsal and ventral edges of the ramus resisted dorso-ventrally disposed forces, yet remained flexible in the transverse plane.

Beam theory has also been used to model static biting in elasmobranchs. Nobiling (1977) used physical models, lever-arm mechanics, and aspects of cross-sectional architecture to model the mechanics of biting in the bullhead shark, *Heterodontus portusjacksoni* (fig. 7.2). He first estimated the loads applied by the jaw muscles on both the jaw joint and a variety of bite points (i.e., the dual support phase; see also Frank [1950] and Bramble [1978]). These loads were then used in conjunction with the cross-sectional architecture of the jaws to determine moments of resistance along various positions of the maxilla and mandible during biting. The magnitude and direction of these stresses were then compared with idealized stress patterns for beams and brackets drawn from engineering principles. Biting in *H. portusjacksoni* is best modeled as a beam resting on two supports rather than as a bracket resting on one support. Maximal bending moments are positioned at areas of muscle insertion, areas accompanied by strong ligamentous reinforcement of the perichondrium. The largest teeth, which are used for crushing bivalves and echinoids, are lo-

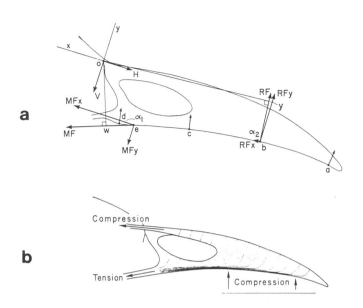

a

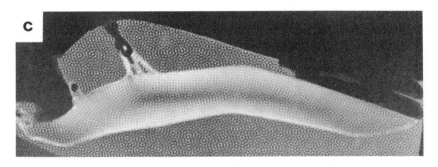

b

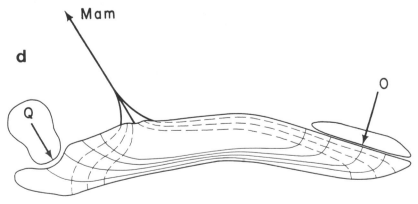

c

d

Fig. 7.1. *Opposite* A. Torque analysis of the upper bill of the crow (*Corvus brachyrhynchos*). a, b, c, d, additional resultant forces; H, compressional force at nasofrontal joint (O); MF, m. pterygoideus force; RF, resultant bite force; V, shear forces at nasofrontal joint. From Bock (1966), with permission. B. Trajectory analysis of the upper bill of *C. brachyrhynchos* indicating tensional trajectories (solid lines) and compressional trajectories (dotted lines). From Bock (1966), with permission. C. Photograph of plexiglass stressed by quadrate, mandibular adductor musculature, and object. D. Interpretation of photoelastic stress study. Mam, adductor musculature; O, object; Q, quadrate. From Bock and Kummer (1968), with permission.

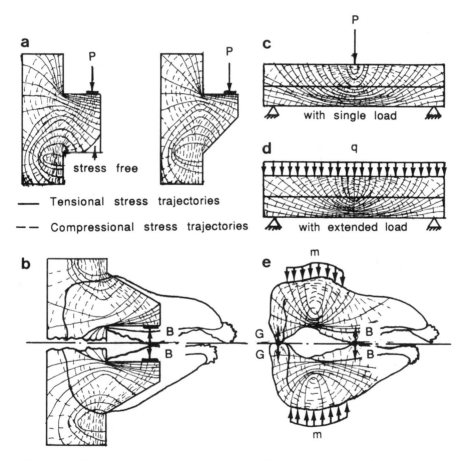

Fig. 7.2. a. The development of stress trajectories in a bracket or console. b. Bracket trajectories through the jaws of the bullhead shark *Heterodontus portusjacksoni*. c, d. Stress trajectories in a beam with two supports. e. Beam trajectories through the jaw apparatus in *H. portusjacksoni*. Solid lines, tensional trajectories; dashed lines, compressional trajectories. B, bite force; G, joint force; m, q, extended compressional force; P, single compressional force. From Nobiling (1977), with permission.

cated at the intersection of the line of action of the major jaw muscles and the maximal moment of resistance. In this position, muscles exert most of their force on the teeth, while causing only moderate compression at the jaw joint.

Jaw Joint and Mandible Loadings

In the same tradition of using physical models to understand force transmission and stress concentration, Demes et al. (1984) and Wolff (1982, 1984) used birefringent models of hominoid mandibles and mathematical models of beams of various configuration to explore the relationship of stress to strength in the mandible (fig. 7.3). Successive bending moments from a variety of bite positions were considered in lateral, transverse, and frontal projections. On the balancing side, bending moments from the adductor musculature acting around the temporomandibular joint compress

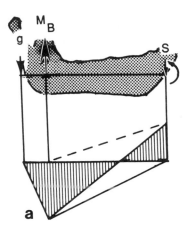

a

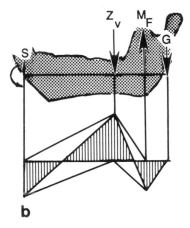

b

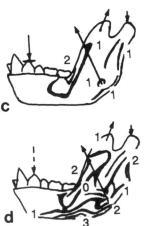

c

d

Fig. 7.3. a. Parasagittal bending moments of the gorilla mandible for the balancing-side jaw. b. Parasagittal bending moments of the working-side jaw. c. Isochromatic fringes on the working side of the gorilla mandible loaded at the first premolar. d. Isochromatic fringes on the balancing side of the mandible. Numbers indicate fringe orders. G, g, joint forces; M_B, M_F, muscle forces; S, symphyseal force; Z_v, vertical component of the bite force. From Demes et al. (1984), with permission.

the ventral margin and tense the dorsal margin of the lower jaw. As modeled, these moments are zero at the jaw joint, increase to their maximum and negative at the insertion site of the adductor musculature, and then decrease again to zero at the symphysis. A positive moment transmitted through the symphysis from the working side clockwise rotates the balancing-side mandible, thus creating reverse moments that compress the dorsal border and tense the ventral border. When superimposed, both sets of moments produce negative bending along the caudal region of the mandible and positive bending rostrally. On the working side, bending moments are zero at the glenoid, negative at the adductor insertion site, maximally positive at the bite point, and again zero at the symphysis. Rotational moments transmitted across the symphysis from the balancing mandible produce negative bending moments of the mandibular body. The pattern of superimposed moments includes alternating negative (at the symphysis and insertion site) and positive (bite point) bending moments. The asymmetry of modeled bending moments between the balancing- and working-side mandibles is reflected only in part in the photoelastic experiments. Stress concentrations on both lower jaws are concentrated in the middle portions of the mandibular body near the area of muscle insertion on both jaws, where bending moments are at their maximum. However, the balancing side always has higher fringe orders than the working side. This situation is surprising in that bending moments derived from mathematical modeling are concentrated more on the working-side mandible, particularly within the region of the bite point.

The largest components of masticatory stress are perpendicular to the occlusal surface, but additional, smaller stress components are found in the transverse plane. Transverse bending moments on the balancing side tend to compress the lingual surface of the mandibular body as well as tense its buccal surface within the molar region and reverse this relationship approaching the symphysis. Therefore total bending stress occurs along an inclined twisted plane. On the working side, tension occurs along the outer and lower surface of the mandible beneath the molars and last premolars; the bending plane is inwardly inclined. Rostrally, the dorsal and lateral borders of the mandible are under tension and the bending plane now has an outward inclination. Again, the bending plane assumes an inclined and twisted orientation.

By way of testing the implications of modeled bending moments, Demes et al. (1984) examined cross sections of actual mandibles. In these, the greatest diameters are indeed coincident with the inclination of the major bending plane and hence with the highest resistance to bending on the working-side mandible. Of more relevance to the mathematical and birefringent models are the in vivo strain gauge studies by Hylander and colleagues (Hylander 1984, 1985; Hylander and Crompton 1986; Hylander et al. 1987) of mandibular stress-strain relationships in galagos (*Galago crassicaudatus*) and macaques (*Macaca fascicularis*). During the power stroke, the body of the working-side mandible is principally twisted and sheared in the sagittal plane, in contrast to the modeling of Demes and colleagues. However, some bending moments within the first molar region are discernible and it is possible that these reflect to a small degree the positive bending moments in the same region predicted by the model. These sagittal bending moments produce tension on the dorsal margin of the mandibular body, while the ventral margin is loaded in compression. During twisting, on the other hand, medial rotation of the ventral margin of the mandible is incurred immediately at the level of the bite, while an outward rotation is present at the caudal end of the mandible. On the balancing side, a large degree of sagittal bending is revealed by Hylander's strain-gauge studies. Such bending results in compression of the lower mandibular border and tension on the dorsal border. In addition, the mandibular body is again longitudinally twisted, but such twisting is effected at its most rostral-to-caudal extremes. Rostrally, the ventral margin is rotated medially, while caudally it is twisted laterally. The symphysis also experiences dorso-ventral shear and bending during the power stroke as a result of lateral bending of the mandibular bodies in the transverse plane. Such bending is similar to that predicted by Demes et al. (1984) and Wolff (1984) and is due to the laterally directed components of both bite and adductor muscle forces and produces maximal stresses on the lingual aspect of the symphysis.

Skull Torsion

A number of important studies have used beam theory to model the skull under torsion. Russell and Thomason (this volume) discuss some of these, including their work on torsional biomechanics of the rostrum in the American opossum *Didelphis virginiana* and its relevance to the evolution of the mammalian secondary palate (see also Thomason and Russell 1986). I turn instead to Greaves's (1985b) model of the skull as an idealized cylinder. In this work, Greaves analyzed the biomechanical significance of the mammalian postorbital bar as a torsion-resisting helical strut (fig. 7.4). Asymmetrical loading of this ideal cylinder through unilateral chewing will tend to twist the braincase relative to the more rostral tooth-bearing part of the skull along the zone of potential weakness between the orbits. These maximal compressive and tensile shear stresses lie along 45° helices on a cylinder that is loaded in torsion. In animals with very large masseter and pterygoid muscles, torsional effects are even further exaggerated. The lines of action of the masseter and pterygoid muscles are oriented at high angles to the long axis of the skull, providing large components of force that twist the skull segments against one another. The postorbital bars in these forms

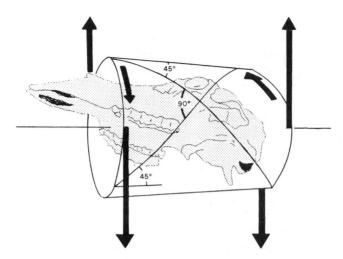

Fig. 7.4. The skull of the deer *Odocoileus* with superimposed transparent cylinder. Vertical arrows at each end of the cylinder represent forces rotating each end of the cylinder in the direction of the curved arrows. Helical lines indicate orientation of maximum compressive and tensile stresses under torsion. From Greaves (1985b), with permission.

follow the predicted three-dimensional spatial orientation required to re-sist these torsional forces. In contrast, when the temporalis musculature dominates (as in carnivores), the effects of torsion about the long axis of the skull are usually less drastic because this muscle acts at a lower angle to the skull axis. The model therefore predicts that the bar should com-monly be absent in these animals, and it is.

In addition to these biomechanical differences in the distribution of the postorbital bar among mammals, the model also predicts that the post-orbital bar should be grossly loaded in compression on the chewing side and in tension on the balancing side. Experimental studies of the postor-bital bar in vervet monkeys (*Cercopithecus aethiops*) show that the post-orbital bar loadings are not nearly as simple as suggested by Greaves's model (Oyen, personal communication). Data from strain gauges mounted on the surface of the postorbital bar indicate that tensional stresses are present on both balancing and working sides of the skull, in contrast to the prediction of the model. Whether these tensional loads reflect the stress-strain regime for the entire bar or just the regional phenomenon of surface bone properties remains an open question.

Models of Masticatory Statics

In the tradition of studies of the reconstruction of mandibular adductor muscles and the force vectors imparted by them (viz., Maynard Smith and Savage 1959; Crompton 1963a, b, 1972; Barghusen 1968, 1972; Barghusen and Hopson 1970; Kemp 1972a, b), DeMar and Barghusen (1973) provided a two-dimensional mathematical model of the lever-arm mechanics of jaw adduction in synapsids prior to the origin of mammals (fig. 7.5). In particular, they modeled the various means by which the relative moment arm of the adductor musculature can be maximized. DeMar and Barghusen identified two possibilities: (1) increasing the distance from the jaw joint to the base of the coronoid process and (2) raising the coronoid process with concomitant caudal inclination of the line of action of the temporalis without undue sacrifice of the mechanical advantage of the muscle. In essence, the former pathway consists in moving the origin and insertion of external adductor jaw musculature forward relative to the position of the jaw joint, while the latter requires the area of muscle origin to move caudally while the line of action is rotated so as to act in a caudal direction. The authors examined the morphological consequences of both options to evaluate the degree to which nonmammalian synapsids might map these two pathways.

Among these synapsid taxa, few have exploited the first pathway for increasing adductor lever-arm mechanics by increasing the distance between the jaw joint and the principal muscle attachment. Most utilized the second pathway by which jaw adductors maximize their effect: changes in the lever-arm mechanics through modification of the size and position of the coronoid process. These changes are thought to reflect a shift toward predation on relatively large prey, in which the load applied to the lower jaw (presumably rostrally) by the weight and forward struggles of the prey is large. However, with the development of masseteric musculature (in particular the superficial muscle division) in animals like *Thrinaxodon* and *Trirachodon,* the biomechanical milieu is radically reorganized over more primitive conditions. Qualitative functional changes (rostro-dorsal muscle pull, initiation of puncture crushing) aside, DeMar and Barghusen suggested that with the evolution of the superficial masseter, bite-point forces increased principally as a consequence of its large moment arm around the jaw joint. The concomitant rise in the position of the jaw articulation fur-

---

Fig. 7.5. *Opposite* a–f. Evolution of the external adductor musculature in cynodont reptiles. a, d. A procynosuchid. b, e. *Thrinaxodon.* c, f. *Trirachodon.* g. Relationship between changes in the coronoid height and the movement arm acting around the jaw joint. Dev M Mass, developing masseter; MAMIPt, pteryoideus. M Mass P, deep masseter; M Mass S, superficial masseter; M Temp, temporalis; Δm, changes in the moment arm of the adductor musculature acting around the jaw joint; ΔX, changes in the distance of the insertion of the adductor musculature from the jaw articulation. From DeMar and Barghusen (1973), with permission.

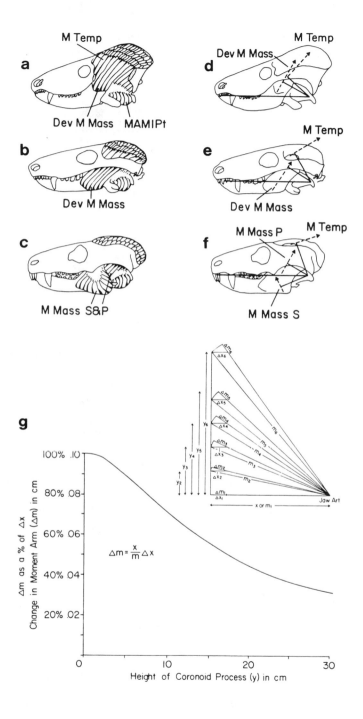

a — M Temp, Dev M Mass, MAMlPt

b — Dev M Mass

c — M Mass S&P

d — M Temp, Dev M Mass

e — M Temp, Dev M Mass

f — M Mass P, M Temp, M Mass S

g

Change in Moment Arm (Δm) in cm
Δm as a % of Δx

$$\Delta m = \frac{x}{m} \Delta x$$

Height of Coronoid Process (y) in cm

ther increased the moment arm of the superficial masseter by extending the distance of the jaw joint from the line of action of the muscle.

The Bifulcral Model

Bramble's (1978) bifulcral model of tetrapod jaw mechanics treats the bite point as a distinct and independent fulcrum equal in status to the jaw articulation or joint fulcrum (fig. 7.6; see also Frank [1950] and Nobiling [1977]). This two-dimensional bifulcral approach allows all of the mechanical forces to be evaluated in terms of purely rotational and purely translational components relative to both fulcra. Translation (fig. 7.6b) can occur only along the bifulcral axis that passes between the jaw joint and bite point and is expressed in positive (i.e., in the caudal direction) and negative (i.e., toward the rostrum) values. Rotation occurs normal to the bifulcral axis. Under the bifulcral model, both positive and negative vertical joint loadings can be achieved through rotation about the bite point (fig. 7.6e). Moreover, depending on the position of the bite point, a given muscle force vector can provide different jaw joint loadings. Positive joint forces are incurred when the force vector passes forward of the bite point; negative loading is produced when the vector passes behind the bite point (fig. 7.6f). The intervening neutral point represents the position where all muscle force is delivered directly to the bite point with no loading at the jaw joint. Such a mechanical arrangement allows the mandible to act purely as a link (Gingerich 1971; see below). Pairs of muscles acting on the mandible (e.g., the temporalis and masseter) will produce opposing rotational- and translational-forces components via their secondary moments acting around the bite point (fig. 7.6g). The resolution of these positive and negative forces at the jaw joint depends on the position of the bite point and the balance of interacting muscle forces. In particular, an equilibrium point, the multimuscle equivalent of a single-muscle neutral point, is achieved where secondary moments about the bite point cancel one another. In such cases, bite force is sacrificed in order to maintain zero loading at the jaw joint.

Bramble used the bifulcral model to examine diversity among tetrapod jaw joint structure and function, in particular with respect to the origin of the mammalian feeding complex. Thus, the bifulcral model predicts that the quadrate will act as a strutlike element resisting positive rotational loads *and* positive and negative translational loads in the jaw joint of amphibians, reptiles, and birds. In contrast, the squamosal-dentary joint in mammals will resist both negative rotational loads and a mixture of translational loads in those mammals (i.e., carnivores) and nonmammalian synapsids that are temporalis-dominated.

When secondary moments about the bite point are included in an

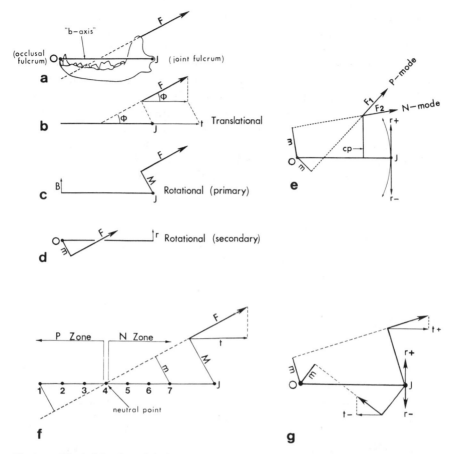

Fig. 7.6. The bifulcral model of jaw mechanics. a. Adductor musculature (F) acting on jaw joint (J) and bite point (O). b. Translation at the jaw joint through contraction of the adductor musculature. c. Primary rotational moment (M) about the jaw joint and producing a bite force (B). d. Secondary rotational moment (m) provided by the adductor musculature acting around the bite point and producing an upward rotational force at the jaw joint (r). e. Relationship between adductor muscle vectors and rotational moments about the bite point. P-mode muscle forces produce upward or positive rotation of the mandibular condyle into the glenoid, while N-mode forces rotate the condyle downward out of the glenoid (negative rotations). f. Determination of the positive and negative bite-point zones and neutral point relative to the muscle force vector. g. Intermuscular competition as interpreted from secondary moments about the bite point. The upper muscle vector represents pull of the temporalis, while the lower vector pertains to the superficial masseter. Note that secondary rotational forces at the jaw joint are opposite one another. Other abbreviations: cp, coronoid process; r +, positive rotational force; r −, negative rotational force; t +, positive translational force; t −, negative translational force; 1–7, bite points. From Bramble (1978), with permission.

analysis of the origin of mammalian jaw mechanics, Bramble noted only a modest elevation of bite force and a *decrease* in prehension of large prey through the same series used by DeMar and Barghusen (1973). These differences between Bramble (1978) and DeMar and Barghusen (1973) result from a consideration of the bite point as a fulcrum. From the point of view of the bite point, the effects of changes in the lines of action of the temporalis musculature and the development of the coronoid process alter both the positive and negative rotational forces at the jaw joint. Secondly, the superficial masseter muscle acts to offset negative joint forces in addition to increasing bite force. Not surprisingly, the masseter is found only among those advanced cynodonts with negatively loaded jaw joints.

Working-Side, Balancing-Side Models

Using three-dimensional aspects of lever-arm mechanics, Greaves published a series of papers on mammalian jaw systems (Greaves 1978, 1980, 1983, 1985a) in which the positions of the working-side jaw joint, the balancing-side joint, and the bite point define the geometry of the lever arm (fig. 7.7). In his initial study of ungulate jaw mechanics, Greaves (1978) discussed the distribution of muscle resultants (single-bite forces resulting from symmetrical, bilateral contraction of adductor muscles) acting within the triangular field demarcated by the balancing-side and working-side joints and by the bite point (fig. 7.7b). Within these boundaries, the mesial limit of the tooth row is predicted to be found where the mechanical advantage of the lever arm passing from the effective fulcrum to mesial teeth decreases. The distal limit of the tooth row is predicted to be no farther than the muscle resultant, since a more distal position would tend to rotate the working-side jaw joint out of articulation (see also Druzinsky and Greaves 1979). In Greaves's model, nonparallel tooth rows are seen as a means of shortening the resistance lever arms and hence increasing the force at the mesial teeth. In a similar study, Greaves (1980) analyzed the biomechanics of the high glenoid in ungulate mammals (fig. 7.7a). As before, vectors provided by the bilaterally and symmetrically contracting adductor musculature are projected from the occlusal plane of the working-side dentition; the balancing-side jaw joint acts as the fulcrum, as is required by the three-point model. Given these constraints, Greaves in effect asked what might be the geometry of the jaws for muscles to act most efficiently relative to the working-side occlusal plane. In order to bring the teeth together, the muscle forces must be perpendicular to the occlusal plane, which itself is also perpendicular to the lever from the balancing-side joint to the bite point. This happens when the plane defined by the occlusal surface of the working-side mandible intersects the balancing-side condyle. With the balancing-side glenoid positioned within the plane of the working-side occlusal surface, the ipsilateral masseter and

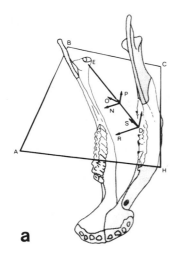

a

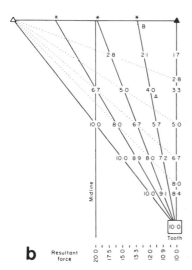

b

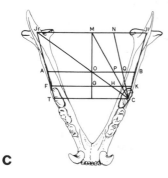

c

Fig. 7.7 a. Dorsolateral view of the lower jaw of an artiodactyl including the occlusal plane (ABCH) of the left tooth row intersecting the balancing-side jaw joint (E) on the right. Arrow O represents the line of pull of the medial pterygoid muscle on the working side and/or the masseter on the balancing side. Arrow S is in approximately the direction of the line of action of the medial pterygoid on the balancing side and the masseter on the working side. Arrows P and T are perpendicular to the plane ABCH and perpendicular to the lever that extends from E to D. Arrows R and N indicate the direction of the muscle force components in the occlusal plane and perpendicular to the lever that extends from E to D. From Greaves (1980), with permission. b. Selected positions within the triangle of support of the muscle resultant perpendicular to the plane of the page. Numbers indicate force applied at the tooth when the muscle resultant is positioned at the point. The effective joint (*) is the point at which an appropriate force could replace both joints and is located in each instance along the line joining the two joints. A force of 10 units is assumed to be applied by the muscles on the working side. The amount of force (0–10 units) on the balancing side determines the position and magnitude of the muscle resultant. The tooth force increases as the muscle resultant moves rostrally and as it moves medially. Note that positions of the muscle resultant that produce the same tooth force are connected by dotted lines. A-B: the lever when 10 units of force are delivered by the working side and 2 units are applied by the balancing side to produce 4 units of bite force. △, balancing-side joint; ▲, working-side joint; *, effective joint. From Greaves (1978), with permission. c. Dorsal view of the lower jaw of the carnivore *Felis catus*. Jr, right joint; Jl, left joint; C, carnassial tooth. Line MG is the midline and AB lies 60% of the way from the joints to the carnassial teeth. The plane JrJlC is defined by the position of the condyles and the carnassial notch. From Greaves (1985a), with permission.

contralateral medial pterygoid musculature will always pull medially when the working-side teeth are in occlusion. To a lesser degree but consistent with the orientation of the working-side occlusal plane and the balancing-side jaw joint, the contralateral masseter and ipsilateral medial pterygoid also can impart a medial movement to the working-side jaw. Thus, Greaves's modeling indicates that the height of the glenoid is directly related to the orientation of the occlusal surface of the dentition, ultimately controlling the forces and movements associated with masticatory biomechanics.

In two later papers, Greaves (1983, 1985a) used his three-point model to analyze the lever-arm mechanics of carnassial biting (fig. 7.7c). Again, the positions of the jaw joints and the carnassial are the sole contact points between the skull and lower jaw during carnassial biting and provide limits to the positions of the muscle resultant. If this resultant lies rostral to the lever arm operating from the balancing-side point to the carnassial, then the working-side joint will disarticulate. If the resultant is positioned far caudal (i.e., near the jaw joints), the muscles will apply large forces to these joints and very little between occluding teeth. Greaves's model also identifies an inherent compromise in carnivore skull biomechanics. The position of the muscle resultant has an effect not only on carnassial bite force, but also on gape angle; the two are in fact nearly inversely related. Thus, the widest gape is coupled with maximum bite force when the resultant force of the muscles is located 60% of the way from the joint to the carnassial tooth (see fig. 7.7c). There appears to be no possibility of otherwise altering the relationship between gape and bite force in the carnivore carnassial system, unless it is through increasing body size or altering muscle architecture.

The Mandible as Link

Instead of the more common perspective of lever-arm force transmission, Gingerich (1971) modeled the mandible as a two-dimensional link between muscle and bite forces (fig. 7.8a–d). He argued that the caudal fibers of the temporalis muscle produce caudal translation of the jaw, such that muscle forces are directly aligned with, and hence converted absolutely into, the bite forces, with no reaction force at the jaw joint. The functional significance of such caudal translation of the jaw is to bring these two opposing forces (muscle force, bite force) into alignment; such movement is termed orthal retraction. In reviewing nonlever models of jaw mechanics, Hylander (1975, 1978) tested Gingerich's link model using a variety of data, including those from electromyography of the adductor musculature and strain-gauge studies of the direction of forces during incisal biting in humans (see also Walker 1976). When analyzed from the perspective of forces acting on the mandible at the bite point, working-side joint, and balancing-side joint, reaction forces must act on both balancing

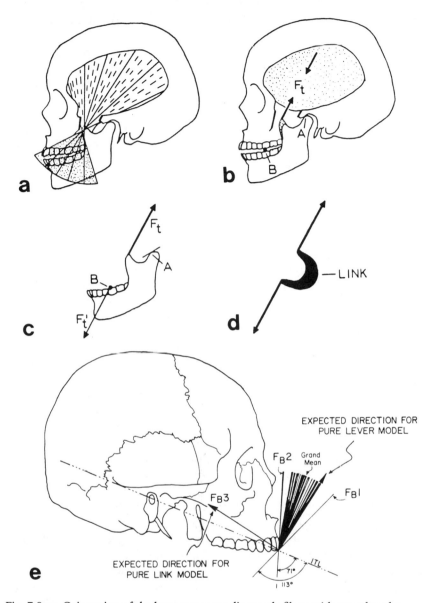

Fig. 7.8. a. Orientation of the human temporalis muscle fibers with regard to the tooth row. b. Origin and insertion of the temporalis muscle and location of bite point. c. Two-dimensional diagram of the forces acting on the mandible. d. Diagrammatic representation of the mandible as a link between muscle and bite forces. e. Diagram of Hylander's (1978) incisal force vector data and positions of expected vectors from a pure lever model and pure link model of mandibular mechanics. Note that the observed directions can be explained as a combination of both lever and link models of mandibular function. A, jaw joint; B, bite point; F_B^1, maximum muscle force vector from Hylander (1978) in comparison with F_B^3; F_B^2, minimum muscle force vector from Hylander (1978) in comparison with F_B^3; F_B^3, direction of bite force when mandible functions purely as a link; F_t, muscle force; F_t', bite force; ITL, incisor-tragus reference line. (a–d) from Gingerich (1971), with permission; (e) from Gingerich (1979), with permission.

and working condyles. Such a pattern of loading refutes the major premise of the two-dimensional link model of Gingerich (1971). In a later work, Gingerich (1979) reviewed Hylander's (1978) data and noted that although incisal loadings are grouped relatively near the force vector predicted by a pure lever-arm model, most are inclined slightly toward the direction predicted by a pure link model (fig. 7.8e). From these deviations, Gingerich concluded that human incisal biting must be a combination of lever and link mechanics, although the lever component clearly predominates.

KINEMATICS: THE SKULL AS SOURCE OF MOVEMENT

Because of the inherent mobility of the skulls of many vertebrates, these skulls have often been modeled as a network of movable segments. Such a machine-for-movement approach (kinematics) has been invoked principally for those vertebrates known or thought to have some degree of intracranial mobility (e.g., cranial kinesis, streptostyly; including elasmobranchs, teleosts, lizards, snakes, and birds).

Kinematic analysis is primarily concerned with patterns of displacement of one or more components of a mechanism, with attending dynamics. Displacement refers to the positional change of a rigid body (link) relative to another body through the transmission of motion across a joint or joints. If the displacement of any link within the network is specified, the corresponding spatial displacement of any other link and the coordinates of any point on the link can be calculated. Motion at a joint is considered either translational (i.e., linear) or rotational (angular) depending primarily on the configuration of the joint surface. The nature of link-joint networks provides for the transfer and control of motion by one body to another and it is for this reason that kinematics provides a useful modeling approach to the study of motion in vertebrate skulls.

Bühler (1977) abstracted the vertebrate jaw system as kinematic chains or networks; these appear to fall into three basic groups of linkage systems. First, there are those mechanisms in which the lower jaws are the only mobile elements relative to the skull. Subsumed in this category are two-link kinematic chains with movement between fused mandibles and the skull (bats, anthropoid primates, horses), three-link chains with movement between unfused mandibles and the skull (insectivores, ruminants, prosimian primates), and five-link chains with fusion of the upper jaw and cranium (some anurans). Second, there are those mechanisms in which the palatoquadrate bars participate in the formation of mobile suspensoria between the neurocranium and lower jaw. By far the most diverse, these systems incorporate the suspensoria as movable elements. Thus they include four-link chains (many birds, some tetraodontiform teleosts), five-link chains (most lizards, many osteichthyans), six-link chains (owls), seven-link chains (varanid lizards, many teleosts), eight-link chains (diverse avian groups), and nine-link chains (snakes). Finally, there are those mechanisms in which two palatoquadrate arches are movable relative to the neurocranium and are rostrally connected to each other. Kinematically, these reduce to four-link chains with mobile upper and lower jaw units (elasmobranchs and *Acipenser*).

Avian Intracranial Mobility

Among the earliest to use kinematic principles to analyze cranial movement was Kripp (1933a, c, d, 1935a; see also Zusi, this volume). His studies relied strictly on graphic approaches to kinematics. Kripp's major works concentrated on the upper-jaw mechanism in birds from the perspective of three-dimensional kinematics (fig. 7.9), although a brief diversion considered jaw mechanics in the hadrosaurid dinosaur *Edmontosaurus* (Kripp 1933b). By modeling the avian skull as a three-dimensional linkage network of bones, joints, and ligaments, Kripp graphically manipulated the quadrate, maxilla, mandible, and postorbital ligament, and determined the combination of conditions that must be met kinematically for upper-jaw elevation to occur. Essentially, forward rotation of the quadrate is coupled by way of the postorbital ligament (tightened by mandibular depression via the depressor mandibulae muscle) with consequent upward motion of the premaxilla. Long-axis rotation of the

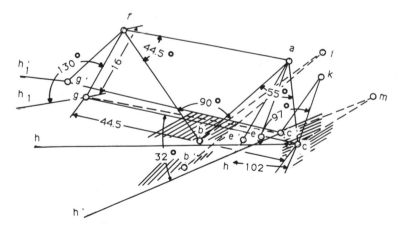

Fig. 7.9. Graphic kinematic analysis of jaw opening to 32° in the raven. a–e, postorbital ligament; b–i, adductor musculature; c, quadrate-mandibular joint; f, craniofacial joint; g, bending zone within the maxilla; h, tip of bill; k, quadrate-squamosal joint; mn, m. depressor mandibulae. From Kripp (1933a).

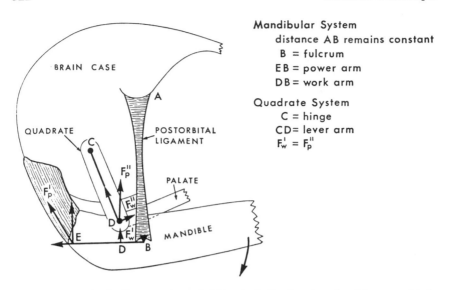

Fig. 7.10. Free-body diagram of coupled kinesis, indicating the role of the postorbital ligament and the quadrate in coupling mandibular movement to elevation of the upper jaw. A–B, postorbital ligament; C, quadrate-squamosal joint; D, quadrate-mandibular joint; E, attachment site of m. depressor mandibulae; F'_p, m. depressor mandibulae muscle force; F'_w, resultant force of mandibular system; F''_w, resultant force of the quadrate system; F''_p, resultant force of the mandibular system acting on the quadrate system. From Bock (1964), with permission.

quadrate is analyzed as a means of widening the intermandibular space (with concomitant bending of the mandibular rami). Using such a kinematic framework, Kripp went on to compare the quadrate-squamosal articulation in various related species to construct a sequence of increasing specializations in jaw mechanics in storks (Ciconiidae), herons (Ardeidae), and cormorants (Phalacrocoracidae).

Like Kripp's work, Bock's (1974) two-dimensional kinematic model of the avian skull is based on an analysis of the size, shape, and position of the bony elements, the configuration of articular surfaces, the position of ligaments, and the position and size of cranial muscles (fig. 7.10; see also Zusi, this volume). Skull elements are considered rigid links, while articular surfaces and ligaments are thought to constrain movement. Again, like other kinematic analyses, muscle vectors are considered input factors. According to Bock, birds have either uncoupled or coupled kinesis. In the former, found in birds lacking a postorbital ligament and an unspecialized jaw articulation, the two jaws have completely independent actions; that is, there is no kinematic linkage or coupling between lower and upper jaw elements. However, in birds that have a postorbital or lacrimomandibular ligament, or an interlocking quadrate-articular hinge, the upper and lower jaws are coupled mechanically in such a way that movements of both are partly interdependent. Depression of the lower jaw elevates the upper jaw through the latter's linkage with the craniomandibular ligament system, the jugal bar, and the palatal skeleton, ultimately driven by parasagittal rotation of the quadrate (see also Kripp 1933a, c, d, 1935a, and discussion above). Bock viewed uncoupled kinesis as the more primitive of the two conditions among birds that possess such systems. Uncoupled kinesis is thought to increase gaping ability, improve the line of sight, prompt faster closing of the jaws, and absorb shocks better than can akinetic skulls. All of these functions apply equally well to the more derived coupled kinesis, which itself also maintains the mandible in closed position against gravity or when carrying an object in the beak. Thus the two modeled systems are very similar in their functional/biological contexts.

Quadric-Crank Model in Lizards

Two-dimensional kinematic models similar to that outlined by Bock (1964) for birds have been applied by Frazzetta (1962, 1983) in studies of intracranial mobility in lizards (see also Rieppel 1978, 1979). Based on skull geometry, position of ligaments, and input muscle vectors, lizard intracranial movement was modeled as a quadric-crank, four-bar linkage mechanism (fig. 7.11). All movable articulations were treated as uniaxial pinned joints; no effort was made to include information on constraints on skull movement imposed by joint surface morphology. In simple terms, the quadric-crank model specifies that mandibular depression is accompanied by protraction and elevation of the muzzle. As the jaws open, the quadrate rotates forward at its joint with the squamosal, while the skull roof is depressed along a rotational axis between itself and the occiput (the metakinetic joint). Coupled with these movements, the palatomaxillary segment is lifted and protracted (via the mesokinetic joint). The lifting and protracting forces provided to the palate come from the levator and protractor pterygoideus musculature, parts of the constrictor dorsalis group. This palatomaxillary movement is transmitted to the muzzle unit (premaxillae, maxillae, nasals, among other elements), which is then elevated along the zone of flexibility at or around the nasofrontal joint. As the lower jaws are adducted, the quadrate and pterygoid withdraw from their more protracted position and the muzzle unit is lowered.

Experimental data, in the form of high-speed cinematography, cineradiography, and strain-gauge approaches, have been used to test different aspects of Frazzetta's quadric-crank four-bar mechanism. First, in some lizards (e.g., *Amphibolurus*), the skull roof appears to be elevated rather

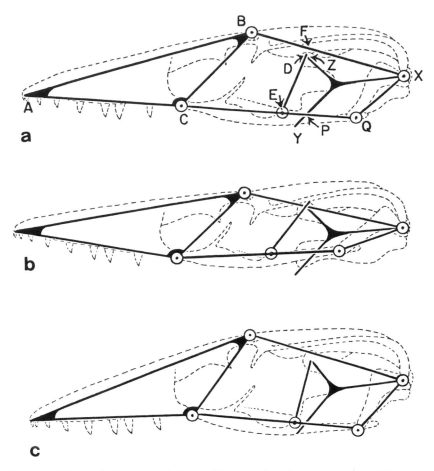

Fig. 7.11. Kinematic diagrams of the quadric-crank four-bar mechanism in *Varanus*. a. Mechanism at rest. b. Protracted condition. c. Retracted conditions. Triangle ABC, muzzle unit; line BX, parietal unit; CQ, basal unit; DE, epipterygoid unit; QX, quadrate unit; XYZ, occipital unit. From Frazzetta (1962), with permission.

than depressed as the lower jaws are depressed, contrary to predictions from Frazzetta's model (Throckmorton and Clarke 1981). In others, quadrate rotation appears to be independent of the elevation of the muzzle unit rather than an integral part of such movement (Smith 1980, 1982), even though it is true that the quadrate swings forward as the mouth is opened and backward as it closes (Frazzetta 1983). Most revealing, strain-gauge data at the nasofrontal joint appear to contradict Frazzetta's model of upper-jaw mobility (Smith and Hylander 1985). Strain in this region in

Varanus exanthematicus differs in both magnitude and direction from that expected at this site using a quadrate-driven four-bar model. As a result, Smith and Hylander concluded that intracranial mobility in lizards does not include an actively moving palatal unit and that quadrate-related jaw movement is not coupled with other skull elements to increase gape or actively control upper-jaw movement. If they have been sampled from appropriate ecological and behavioral contexts, these experimental data appear to falsify some or all of the biomechanical aspects of the quadric-crank model of intracranial mobility among lizards.

Hyobranchial Kinematics

In his study of the stickleback fish *Gasterosteus aculeatus,* Anker (1974) used data from the muscle-skeleton-ligament system to successively "construct" the head of this animal. Such data are principally derived from serial sections and used to generate quantitative graphic kinematic models of cranial, palatal, and mandibular movements (fig. 7.12). These three-dimensional models were then used to make predictions about the ways in which mandibular, hyoidal, palatal, hypaxial, and epaxial muscles produce movement of the oral, buccal, and branchial cavities. These movements are then tested against kinds and degrees of movement in living individuals of the species. Not surprisingly, the more parts of the complex ligamentous system that are introduced into the model, the better the model approaches actual movement in the living fish. Barel et al. (1977) extended Anker's work to include kinematic linkages of mandibular depression in a variety of teleost fishes. Their model relies on two superimposed four-bar systems that are configured for depression of the mandible (which they term a hyoid system or an opercular system, depending on the musculature driving the four-bar mechanism). During opening of the mouth, the hyoid system acts as a force transmitter to the mandible to a greater degree than the opercular system, principally through contraction of the sternohyoid muscle. In contrast, the opercular system is capable of transmitting jaw-opening velocity to a greater degree than the hyoid system, through contraction of the opercular levator musculature.

Along similar lines, Lombard and Wake (1976, 1977) provided a three-dimensional model of movement of the hyobranchial skeleton during prey capture in plethodontid salamanders (fig. 7.13). Prey capture involves rapid and accurate projection of the tongue; once affixed to the tip of the tongue, the prey item is then withdrawn into the mouth. The configuration of the hyobranchial skeleton (fig. 7.13a), articular morphology, and associated musculature comprise the raw data upon which the model is based. Tongue projection modeling consists in the mechanical folding of the hyobranchial skeleton of the tongue. In particular (fig. 7.13b), the paired

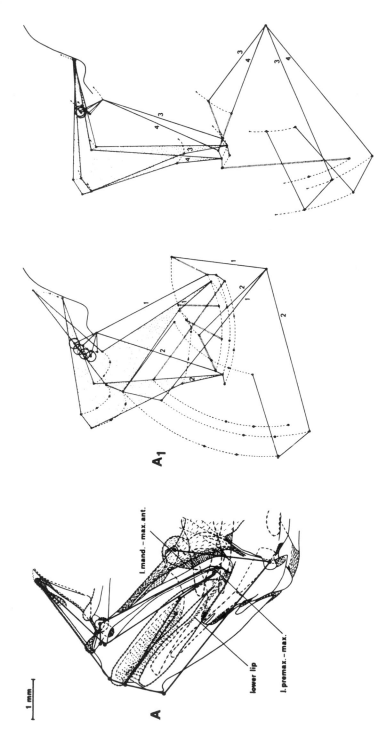

Fig. 7.12. Diagram of the kinematics of mouth opening in the stickleback *Gasterosteus aculeatus*. l. mand.-max. ant., rostral (i.e., anterior) mandible-maxillary ligament; l. premax.-max., fibrous connection between the caudal parts of the premaxilla and maxilla; 1–4, four phases of jaw opening. From Anker (1974), with permission.

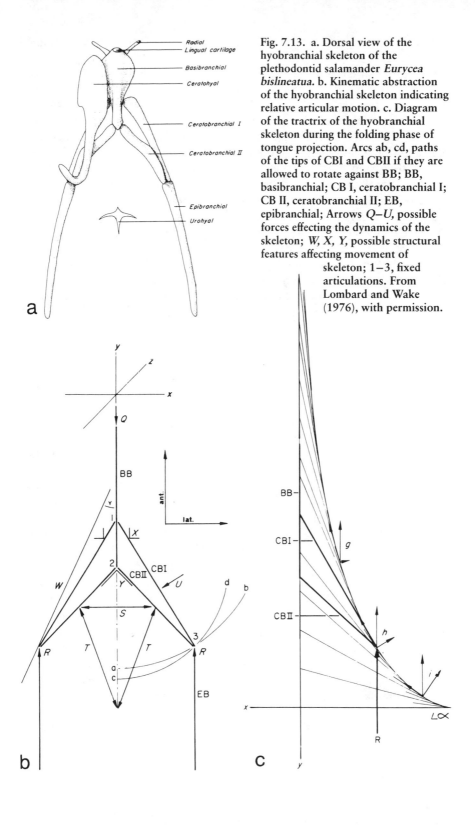

Fig. 7.13. a. Dorsal view of the hyobranchial skeleton of the plethodontid salamander *Eurycea bislineatua*. b. Kinematic abstraction of the hyobranchial skeleton indicating relative articular motion. c. Diagram of the tractrix of the hyobranchial skeleton during the folding phase of tongue projection. Arcs ab, cd, paths of the tips of CBI and CBII if they are allowed to rotate against BB; BB, basibranchial; CB I, ceratobranchial I; CB II, ceratobranchial II; EB, epibranchial; Arrows *Q–U*, possible forces effecting the dynamics of the skeleton; *W, X, Y*, possible structural features affecting movement of skeleton; 1–3, fixed articulations. From Lombard and Wake (1976), with permission.

ceratobranchial elements of the hyoid rotate to a collapsed or folded position on the midline. Such movement acts as a crank for the projection of the midline basibranchial element forward and with it projection of the tongue out of the mouth. The kinematics of tongue projection specify (1) that the three-dimensional interactions of skeletal element position, size, and shape, and joint mobility permit the kinds of rotations and translations suggested by the model, and (2) that the effector musculature is capable of rotating the ceratobranchials into and out of their folded positions. Given these constraints, the hyoid skeleton can be folded to project the basibranchial along a track or tractrix that ever increases the distance of the basibranchial from its unfolded position (fig. 7.13c). From this model, predictions were made about the shape of the tractrix, the distance and speed of projection, and directional versatility, all ultimately based on known plethodontid hyobranchial anatomy. These predictions were tested against known projection styles among plethodontids and in each case found to be accurate within the constraints of the model.

Pleurokinesis

Three-dimensional kinematics has only rarely been used to model jaw systems in vertebrates known only from the fossil record. Weishampel (1983, 1984; see also Norman and Weishampel 1985) used these techniques as a means to test a variety of models of jaw mechanisms in ornithopod dinosaurs (fig. 7.14). The skulls of these animals were treated as multilink chewing machines designed to comminute plant matter. In this way, it was possible to compare the many jaw systems that had been proposed in the literature. These range from simple jaw closure to complex movement of the quadrate and longitudinal rotation of the lower jaws, with many middle-ground mechanisms intercalated between. As a consequence, the potential for movement at these and other sites exponentially multiplies the complexity of analyses, especially over many taxa. To solve this problem, computer modeling was used to examine the various combinations of intracranial mobility suggested for ornithopod skulls.

In these kinematic analyses, each ornithopod skull was decomposed into sites of potential mobility among skull elements specified by a given mechanism, all of which pertain to the facial and mandibular skeleton and their relationship to the neurocranium. Sites of mobility were located in three-dimensional space and the kind of mobility (hinge joints, spheroidal joints, planar joints, etc.) was assessed. A given suite of mobility constituted a model for a given jaw mechanism. Each model was then manipulated to simulate chewing apropos the mechanism being analyzed.

The kinematic abstraction and manipulation of ornithopod skulls produced wide-ranging possibilities of functional complexes. Without information to the contrary, each represents a possible feeding system. Tooth wear was deemed the critical data base for testing each model. Information on potential tooth wear was extracted for each kinematic analysis; that is, each mechanism was evaluated for the way wear would have been inscribed on the dentition during the power stroke phase of the masticatory cycle. These predictions about tooth wear from a modeled mechanism were then tested against tooth wear on actual ornithopod dentitions (fig. 7.14a–f).

Tooth wear parameters were best predicted by two jaw mechanics models. The first involves the development of hingelike rotation of the maxillae and associated elements against the premaxillae and skull roof (fig. 7.14g), a feature that the majority of ornithopods (Hypsilophodontidae and Iguanodontia) appear to have possessed. This kind of intracranial mobility, termed pleurokinesis (Norman 1984), produces a transverse power stroke during chewing (as indicated by tooth wear) through the lateral rotation of the maxillae in concert with continued adduction of the lower jaws.

Among remaining ornithopods, pleurokinesis is absent in Heterodontosauridae. However, in this group, transverse chewing is achieved by a slight rotational mobility of the lower jaws that is facilitated by modified symphyseal joints at the front of the lower jaws (see also Crompton and Attridge 1986; Norman and Weishampel 1991). This system seems to be restricted solely to these basal ornithopods.

Both the pleurokinetic and heterodontosaurid jaw systems appear to parallel the development of anisognathy (altering the width between lower jaws to accommodate a unilateral transverse power stroke) in tranversely chewing ungulates. At the level of occlusion, all of these systems are very similar, although their mechanical basis involves distinctly different modifications of the facial skeleton. These facial reorganizations comprise the limits on evolutionary pathways to achieve a transverse power stroke. These three pathways all begin from a more primitive isognathous jaw frame capable solely of bilateral occlusion. A transverse power stroke in mammals is achieved biomechanically through the evolution of anisognathy. In heterodontosaurids, the same stroke is brought about by the evolution of longitudinal rotation of the lower jaws. Finally, in hypsilophodontids and iguanodontians, it is pleurokinesis that allows transverse chewing to take place. In each case, independently acquired modifications of the facial skeleton released these animals from the mechanical constraints imposed by a rigid skull and bilateral occlusion (Norman and Weishampel 1985). Such a release may have even provided the raw materials for trophic diversification under the realm of vertebrate herbivory (Norman and Weishampel 1985; Weishampel and Norman 1989).

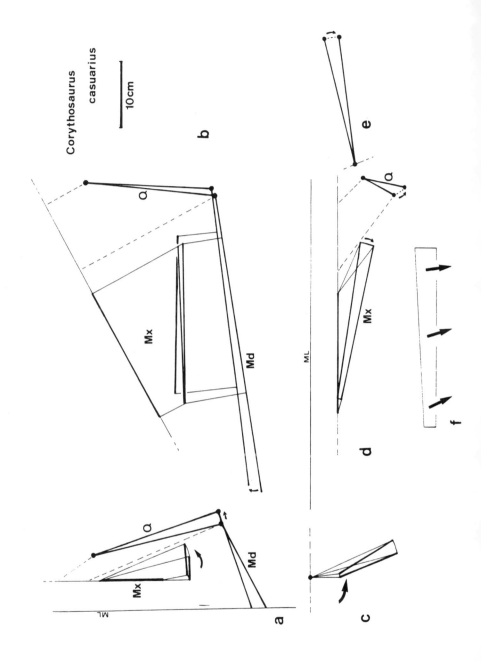

Corythosaurus
casuarius

10cm

a

b

c

d

e

f

α

Mx

Md

ML

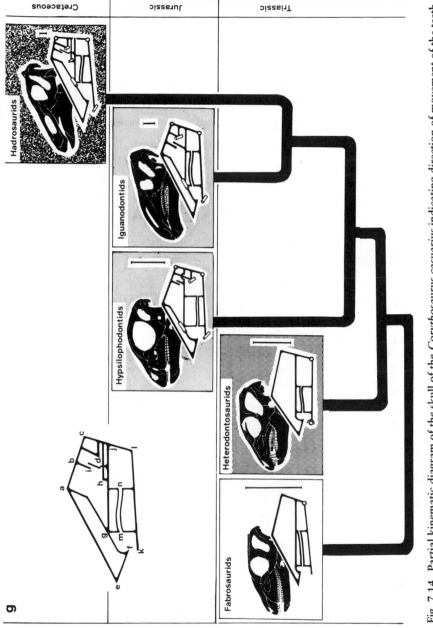

Fig. 7.14. Partial kinematic diagram of the skull of the *Corythosaurus casuarius* indicating direction of movement of the teeth during the power stroke. a. Rostral view. b. Lateral view. c. View along the premaxilla-maxilla articulation. d. Dorsal view. e. View encompassing rotation of the quadrate. f. Occlusal view with arrows indicating direction of the power stroke. g. Summary of the distribution of pleurokinesis (found in hypsilophodontids, iguanodonts, and hadrosaurids) among ornithopods. Md, mandible; ML, midline of skull; Mx, maxilla; Q, quadrate. From Weishampel (1984), with permission.

DYNAMICS: THE SKULL AS MACHINE

The ultimate mechanistic approach to the skull is machine modeling. Intrinsic in these models is the dynamism of forces and movements of the various cranial and mandibular elements. Dynamics models take displacement pathways and integrate with them moments of forces acting about one or more joints making up the mechanism. In doing so, it is possible to evaluate the dynamic performance of the system (e.g., input-output work ratios, energy-to-work transformations). Because of the inherent complexity of assessing instantaneous forces along paths of movement, particularly in three-dimensional space, there are very few detailed studies of the dynamics of vertebrate skull mechanisms. Three examples are discussed here, the first pertaining to modeling the oral cavity and gill apparatus in tadpoles as a buccal pump, the second involving the dynamics of jaw protrusion and premaxillary biting in cichlid fishes, and the last reporting on some preliminary studies of the jaw system in rats.

The Buccal Pump of Tadpoles

The operation of the buccal apparatus in tadpoles has been modeled as a piston-style pump (fig. 7.15; Wassersug and Hoff 1979). Morphologically, the buccal cavity is shaped like an inverted, truncated, right-triangular pyramid. The floor of the buccal cavity, supported by the ceratohyal and hypobranchial plate (fig. 7.15a), forms a triangle. The paired ceratohyal cartilages articulate with the single midline copula and with paired hypobranchial cartilages caudally. The intervening articulations act as fulcra about which the ceratohyals rotate when the depressor muscles contract (e.g., the lateral margin of each ceratohyal is elevated, the medial margin is depressed). Rotation of the ceratohyals acts to depress the floor of the buccal cavity, expand the cavity, and decrease buccal pressure (fig. 7.15b).

Fig. 7.15. *Opposite* a. Dorsal view of the buccal apparatus in the *Rana pipiens* tadpole. b. Buccal pump model as seen in rostral oblique view. The hatched bent triangular plate represents the ceratohyal cartilage. The triangle with height C and base A represents the floor of the buccal cavity. D represents the muscular process of the palatoquadrate and fulcrum of the ceratohyal. H represents the depressor musculature. Other abbreviations: B, transverse breadth of the ceratohyal; B–C, horizontal distance of the tip of the lateral process of the ceratohyal from the base of the processus muscularis of the palatoquadrate; E, depressed distance of the lateral process of the ceratohyal; F–H, length of the depressor musculature at contraction; G, elevated distance of the medial process of the ceratohyal; α, rotation of the medial process of the ceratohyal; β, rotation of the lateral process of the ceratohyal; δ, dorsal angle between the lateral process of the ceratohyal and the horizontal; From Wassersug and Hoff (1979), with permission.

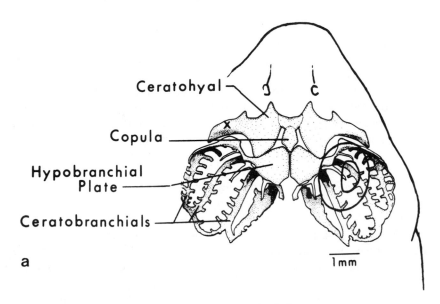

Ceratohyal

Copula

Hypobranchial Plate

Ceratobranchials

a

1mm

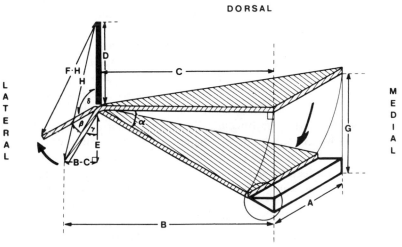

DORSAL

LATERAL

MEDIAL

b

VENTRAL

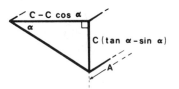

C − C cos α

C (tan α − sin α)

A

The ceratohyals are returned to their original position via contraction of the interhyoideus muscles attached to their ventral surface.

On the basis of relative proportions of the supporting elements, the positions of fulcra, associated lever-arm mechanics, and specified amounts of contraction of the depressor musculature, the buccal pump model can be used to evaluate changes in (1) amount of deflection of the buccal floor (related to ceratohyal rotation; termed stroke), (2) mechanical advantage of the pump, and (3) buccal volume (related to buccal floor area; termed bore) in anuran species. Wassersug and Hoff calculated these parameters in 40 species drawn from 11 anuran families in order to correlate them with the three major feeding ecologies found in the group. Macrophagous carnivores (e.g., *Scaphiopus bombifrons, S. holbrooki*) have ceratohyals with a long lateral margin. Thus, they have high mechanical advantage. Combined with a large bore, the buccal pump mechanism delivers a large buccal volume. Midwater microphagous suspension feeders (e.g., *Xenopus laevis, Hypopachus barberi*) have a low mechanical advantage, but achieve a large buccal volume by having a high stroke. Finally, benthic larvae (e.g., *Heleophryne natalensis*) have a high mechanical advantage, but only a modest buccal volume. These are the features expected of larvae that adhere to the substrate and feed on encrusting algae.

Given the correspondence between modeled function and feeding ecology among anuran larvae, Wassersug and Hoff used the parameters on which their model is based to predict the feeding strategies of a dozen anuran larvae whose feeding biology is not known particularly well. Of these, seven species have relatively low lever-arm ratios, high rotation for the ceratohyals, and large buccal volumes, together strongly suggesting that these forms are microphagous suspension feeders. Another three have high mechanical advantage, but reduced buccal volume, suggesting that they are benthic feeders. The remainder have little specialization of the buccal system, suggesting that they feed in a generalized fashion.

Cichlid Jaws

The dynamics of the jaw movement in the cichlid fish *Haplochromis elegans* was computer modeled by Elshoud (1980) and Otten (1983, 1985). The complex model of the cichlid jaw mechanism contains 20 elements comprising the head skeleton, cranial musculature, and associated ligaments. Thirty-one connections maintain the integrity of these links in a close-ended kinematic network (fig. 7.16a). Data come from sectioned specimens. The three-dimensional kinematics and dynamics studies focused on two aspects: (1) modeling the effects of growth on the kinematics of jaw protrusion and force equilibria during premaxillary biting, and (2) altering the design of the kinematic network to produce an optimal configuration along a functional gradient in both young and old individu-

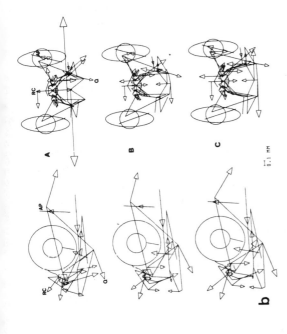

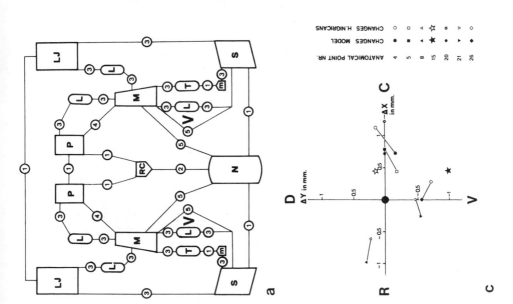

Fig. 7.16. a. Kinematic abstraction of the skull and mandible of *Haplochromis elegans*. L, ligament; LJ, lower jaw; M, maxilla; m, adductor mandibulae muscle A1; N, neurocranium; P, premaxilla; RC, rostral cartilage. S, suspensorium; T, tendon. V indicates connection via 5 or 3-L-3, but not both. Numbers indicate degrees of freedom at a given joint. b. Successive stages of mouth opening and suspensorial abduction in the first free-swimming stage of *H. elegans*. Graphics from computer modeling. The left illustrations are left lateral views; the right are rostral views. Upper pair of graphics shows mouth almost closed and suspensorium adducted; middle pair shows mouth opened and suspensorium adducted; lower pair shows mouth opened and suspensorium abducted. c. Displacement of seven anatomical points relative to adult *H. elegans* (filled symbols) using iterative perturbation analysis for maximizing premaxillary bite force. Comparisons are made with the positions of the same points in the hard biter *H. nigricans* (open symbols). Note disagreement of the displacement number 15 (caudo-ventral shift of the insertion of the adductor musculature of the upper jaw onto the maxilla) indicated by large star. C, caudal; D, dorsal; R, rostral; V, ventral. From Otten (1983), with permission.

als. This perturbation analysis (i.e., the systematic reorganization or alteration of a given mechanism to perform in an improved way) is based on iteratively moving the three-dimensional coordinates of the joints within the mechanism with a minimum of positional changes. In the growth studies, the jaw mechanism of young *H. elegans* (from the first free-swimming stage) were compared with those of adult individuals in an attempt to identify scaling effects of premaxillary biting (fig. 7.16b). The proportions of the head skeleton differ widely between early and late ontogenetic stages, yet the ratio of adductor muscle force to biting force remains approximately the same. From perturbation analyses of adult individuals, anatomical positions most sensitive to achieving a high bite force were chosen for the young stage and compared with their actual positions. Many of the proportional changes in the kinematic network are considered favorable for hard biting in the free-swimming stage, but others are seriously compromised by the position of the relatively large eye in these young individuals (Otten 1983).

Perturbation analysis can also identify anatomical "hot spots," those positions for which even a small displacement will yield a significant increase in a functional attribute. Such a perturbation analysis was carried out for premaxillary bite force in adult *H. elegans*. Seven points were identified as hot spots in terms of maximizing premaxillary bite force (fig. 7.16c) and the "improved" version of *H. elegans* was then compared with *H. nigricans,* a species known for more powerful premaxillary biting. Resemblance between the two species is very close (six out of seven displacements are approximately the same). Because of the discordance of the seventh point (position of the insertion of the adductor musculature of the upper jaw on the maxilla) between the improved *H. elegans* and *H. nigricans,* Otten (1985) invoked a positional compromise in the latter species between biting force and gape, vision, and respiration at this site in the construction of the jaw mechanism. Hence, perturbation analysis, with its creation of altered and improved versions of a given mechanism, is capable of detecting compromises with, and constraints on, other functional complexes within the skull.

A Dynamic Model of Mammalian Mastication

A hierarchical model of the dynamics of mammalian mastication, presented by Otten (1987; see also Otten et al. 1986), consists of several superimposed submodels or units. Termed a myocybernetic approach, it begins with a model of static muscle fiber contraction relating force to fiber length and based on sarcomere information. It then abstracts to a model of static contraction of whole skeletal muscle, relating muscle force to muscle length and based on muscle morphometry and the preceding static fiber model. A dynamic skeletal muscle model, relating muscle force to

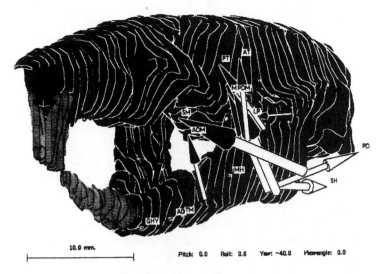

Fig. 7.17. Reconstruction of the skull and lower jaw of the rat using Otten's (1987) myocybernetic model of mastication. Skull outline based on sectioned skull material. The arrows indicate the maximal active force vectors of the jaw and hyoid muscles used in the model. There are 13 muscles at one side of the head. AD, rostral (i.e., anterior) belly of the digastric; ADM, rostral (i.e., anterior) deep masseter; AT, rostral (i.e., anterior) temporal; GHY, geniohyoid; LP, lateral pterygoid; MH, mylohyoid; MP, medial pterygoid; PD, caudal (i.e., posterior) belly of the digastric; PDM, caudal (i.e., posterior) deep masseter; PT, caudal (i.e., posterior) temporal; SH, sternohyoid; SM, superficial masseter; TM, transversus mandibularis. From Otten (1987), with permission.

muscle length, contraction velocity, and stimulation rate is superimposed upon the previous static muscle model. Kinematic modeling of the rat jaw system relates possible movements of the jaw system to the morphometrics of the bones, joints, and connective tissue, and includes information from lower levels in the modeling hierarchy. Finally, Otten's three-dimensional model of skull dynamics incorporates the kinematics and muscle dynamics of prior modeling stages to analyze and display the morphometrics of the jaw system in terms of force vectors, positions, and movements of the jaw system (fig. 7.17). Tailored to the jaw system of the rat, the myocybernetic model is used to calculate muscle forces based on electromyographic and muscle morphometric data; trajectories of the lower jaw and hyoid are then predicted on the basis of these forces. The overall similarity of predicted forces and trajectories with those observed experimentally suggests that the myocybernetic model can provide a robust approach to relating the details of muscle dynamics to cranial kinematics in mammalian mastication.

DISCUSSION

Modeling studies have generally focused on the statics of tooth and jaw-joint loadings, particularly among mammals. Multilink kinematic approaches have centered primarily on those vertebrates in which the skull elements are highly mobile, such as teleost fishes, squamates, and birds. Only a few recent studies have attempted to model skull dynamics per se, including work on buccal ventilation in tadpoles, fish jaw mechanics, and mammalian mastication. Any one of these three approaches may be particularly relevant to the specific questions at hand and they may of course be used in concert to better express the functional environment of certain cranial structures.

Surprisingly, many modeling approaches suffer from too little testing. Perhaps because of inherent problems in deriving suitable tests (e.g., technology may be unavailable), the ebb and flow of research funds, or possibly the putative schism between theoretical and experimental studies, many modeling efforts stand totally without relation to experimental testing. Those methods that have been brought to bear on theoretical models include both strain-gauge analysis relevant to static and dynamic modeling, and high-speed cinematography and cinefluorography for kinematic studies. Many of these are directly relevant as tests of the details and diversity of Frazzetta's (1962) quadric-crank, four-bar jaw mechanism in lizards (Smith 1982; Smith and Hylander 1985), Greaves's (1978 et seq.) studies of the three-dimensional geometry and static loadings of the working- and balancing-side jaw joints and bite points among mammals (Hylander 1977 et seq.; Weijs 1981), and Greaves's (1985b) modeling of torsional loads within the facial skeleton (Kakudo and Amano 1968; Buckland-Wright 1978; Behrents et al. 1978; see also discussion in Russell and Thomason, this volume). Other modeling approaches have yet to see this kind of attention. Clearly what is needed to probe the content, accuracy, and plausibility of the model is a good deal more testing.

Given that modeling approaches yield both accurate and heuristic information about the operation of vertebrate skulls, these same methods are useful in establishing boundary conditions of skull form beyond which a particular mechanical configuration breaks down. Both Greaves (1978, 1983, 1985a) and Otten (1983, 1985) used their jaw mechanics models to enumerate suboptimal or mechanically disadvantageous jaw constructions for both mammals and fishes, thereby establishing some of the boundary conditions for a given functional complex. In the same vein, skull modeling makes it possible to invoke optimality theory for a particular functional gradient by theoretically reorganizing the mechanical configuration of the skull. Otten's (1983, 1985) studies of the skull of *Haplochromis* use perturbation analysis to posit more optimal skull constructions with regard to premaxillary biting. Most important, these *Haplochromis* studies reveal the topological aspects of the combination of growth and mechanics, so often neglected in modeling studies.

Part of the nature of theoretical models is that they make possible the identification of interactive constraints on form imposed by the different anatomical systems housed by the skull and by history, architecture, and adaptation. Only a few modeling studies go beyond the usual aspects of jaw mechanics, but they have received very little attention. Otten's (1983) study of the cichlid jaw system during growth and Bramble's (1978) study of the bifulcral lever-arm mechanics and the origin of the mammalian jaw system stand out as particularly good examples of the ways that geometric compromises between different cranial systems dictate less than optimal conditions for each of the systems. Obviously, further studies of the balance among competing functional complexes within the skull will allow the proper evaluation of optimality for any one of these complexes and hence a more realistic approach to general cranial structure and function.

Couched in these modeling approaches is the implicit notion that we are trying to provide not only a necessary but also a sufficient explanation of skull form and function via the parameters that make the model work. Since it is always possible to erect new models ad infinitum to explain the differences in animal design in a functional way, the degree to which any of these models approach reality must be seen in conjunction with other evolutionary effects on biological form. Hence Dobzhansky's (1973) admonishment that "nothing makes sense in biology except in the light of evolution" necessitates that all morphological models be tailored to their particular evolutionary-ecological context. By this, I mean the range and variation of the problem(s) that the functional complex is presumably addressing. These modeling approaches should account not only for their adaptive aspects, as they most commonly do, but also their historical and architectural relationships as well. The invention of "new" organisms with differing skull mechanics creates a suite of theoretically possible or potentially available skull configurations. From such a universe of theoretical arrangements, it then becomes possible to decipher the realized biomechanical configurations deployed in morphological space, as well as through time. The possibility of producing potential biomechanical configurations may yet allow these altered versions to be used as null hypotheses against which architectural, historical, and adaptive constraints on skull form can be tested (Konstruktions-Morphologie: Seilacher 1970; Reif 1975, 1981; Thomas 1979; Reif et al. 1985).

ACKNOWLEDGMENTS

I thank M. F. Teaford, L. M. Witmer, and W.-E. Reif for critically reading this manuscript and offering many helpful suggestions. I also thank O. Oyen for information on his strain-gauge studies of the postorbital bar in vervet monkeys, and J. Hanken and B. K. Hall for inviting me to contribute this paper and for their helpful comments on it.

REFERENCES

Anker, G. C. 1974. Morphology and kinetics of the head of the stickleback, *Gasterosteus aculeatus*. Transactions of the Zoological Society of London 32: 311–416.

Barel, C. D. N., J. W. van der Meulen, and H. Berkhoudt. 1977. Kinematischer Transmissionskoeffizient und Vierstangensystem als Funktionsparameter und Formmodell für Mandibulare Depressionsapparate bei Teleostiern. Anatomisches Anzeiger 142: 21–31.

Barghusen, H. R. 1968. The lower jaw of cynodonts (Reptilia, Therapsida) and the evolutionary origin of mammal-like adductor jaw musculature. Postilla 116: 1–49.

———. 1972. The origin of the mammalian jaw apparatus. In *Morphology of the Maxillo-Mandibular Apparatus*, G.-H. Schumacher, ed. Leipzig: V. E. B. Georg Thieme, pp. 26–32.

Barghusen, H. R., and J. A. Hopson. 1970. Dentary-squamosal joint and the origin of mammals. Science 168: 573–575.

Behrents, R. G., D. S. Carlson, and T. Abdelnour. 1978. *In vivo* analysis of bone strain about the sagittal suture in *Macaca mulatta* during masticatory movement. Journal of Dental Research 57: 904–908.

Bock, W. J. 1964. Kinetics of the avian skull. Journal of Morphology 114: 1–42.

———. 1966. An approach to the functional analysis of bill shape. Auk 83: 10–51.

Bock, W. J., and B. Kummer. 1968. The avian mandible as a structural girder. Journal of Biomechanics 1: 89–96.

Bramble, D. M. 1978. Origin of the mammalian feeding complex: Models and mechanisms. Paleobiology 4: 271–301.

Buckland-Wright, J. C. 1978. Bone structure and patterns of force transmission in the cat skull (*Felis catus*). Journal of Morphology 155: 35–62.

Bühler, P. 1977. Comparative kinematics of the vertebrate jaw frame. Fortschritte für Zoologie 24: 123–138.

Crompton, A. W. 1963a. The evolution of the mammalian jaw. Evolution 17: 431–439.

———. 1963b. On the lower jaw of *Diarthrognathus* and the origin of the mammalian lower jaw. Proceedings of the Zoological Society of London, ser. B 108: 735–761.

————. 1972. The evolution of the jaw articulation in cynodonts. In *Studies in Vertebrate Evolution*, K. A. Joysey and T. S. Kemp, eds. Edinburgh: Oliver and Boyde, pp. 231–251.

Crompton, A. W., and J. Attridge. 1986. Masticatory apparatus of the larger herbivores during Late Triassic and Early Jurassic times. In *The Beginning of the Age of Dinosaurs*, K. Padian, ed. New York: Cambridge University Press, pp. 223–236.

DeMar, R., and H. R. Barghusen. 1973. Mechanics and the evolution of the synapsid jaw. Evolution 26: 622–637.

Demes, B. 1984. Mechanical stresses at the primate skull base caused by the temporomandibular joint force. In *Food Acquisition and Processing in Primates*, D. J. Chivers, B. A. Wood, and A. Bilsborough, eds. New York: Plenum Press, pp. 407–413.

————. 1985. Biomechanics of the primate skull base. In *Functional Morphology in Vertebrates*, H.-R. Duncker and G. Fleischer, eds. Fortschritte für Zoologie 30: 139–151.

Demes, B., H. Preuschoft, and J. E. A. Wolff. 1984. Stress-strength relationships in the mandibles of hominoids. In *Food Acquisition and Processing in Primates*, D. J. Chivers, B. A. Wood, and A. Bilsborough, eds. New York: Plenum Press, pp. 369–390.

Dobzhansky, T. 1973. Nothing in biology makes sense except in the light of evolution. American Biology Teacher 35: 125–129.

Druzinsky, R. E., and W. S. Greaves. 1979. A model to explain the posterior limit of the bite point in reptiles. Journal of Morphology 160: 165–168.

Elshoud, G. C. A. 1980. APL and functional morphology. In *APL 80*, G. A. van der Linden, ed. New York: North-Holland Publ. Co. (Elsevier), pp. 175–181.

Frank, L. 1950. Muscular influence on occlusion as shown by x-rays of the condyle. Dental Digest 56: 484–488.

Frazzetta, T. H. 1962. A functional consideration of cranial kinesis in lizards. Journal of Morphology 111: 287–319.

————. 1983. Adaptation and function of cranial kinesis in reptiles: A time-motion analysis of feeding in alligator lizards. In *Advances in Herpetology and Evolutionary Biology*, A. G. J. Rhodin and K. Miyata, eds. Cambridge: Harvard University Museum of Comparative Zoology, pp. 222–244.

Gingerich, P. D. 1971. Functional significance of mandibular translation in vertebrate jaw mechanics. Postilla 152: 1–10.

————. 1979. The human mandible: Lever, link, or both? American Journal of Physical Anthropology 51: 135–138.

Greaves, W. S. 1978. The jaw lever system in ungulates: A new model. Journal of Zoology, London 184: 271–285.

————. 1980. The mammalian jaw mechanism—the high glenoid cavity. American Naturalist 116: 432–440.

————. 1983. A functional analysis of carnassial biting. Biological Journal of the Linnean Society 20: 353–363.

————. 1985a. The generalized carnivore jaw. Zoological Journal of the Linnean Society 85: 267–274.

———. 1985b. The mammalian postorbital bar as a torsion-resisting helical strut. Journal of Zoology, London, A 207: 125–136.

Hylander, W. L. 1975. The human mandible: Lever or link? American Journal of Physical Anthropology 43: 227–242.

———. 1977. *In vivo* bone strain in the mandible of *Galago crassicaudatus.* American Journal of Physical Anthropology 46: 309–326.

———. 1978. Incisal bite force direction in humans and the functional significance of mammalian mandibular translation. American Journal of Physical Anthropology 48: 1–7.

———. 1984. Stress and strain in the mandibular symphysis of primates: A test of competing hypotheses. American Journal of Physical Anthropology 64: 1–46.

———. 1985. Mandibular function and biomechanical stress and scaling. American Zoologist 25: 315–330.

Hylander, W. L., and A. W. Crompton. 1986. Jaw movements and patterns of mandibular bone strain during mastication in the monkey *Macaca fascicularis.* Archives of Oral Biology 31: 841–848.

Hylander, W. L., K. R. Johnson, and A. W. Crompton. 1987. Loading patterns and jaw movements during mastication in *Macaca fascicularis:* A bone-strain, electromyographic, and cineradiographic analysis. American Journal of Physical Anthropology 72: 287–314.

Kakudo, Y., and N. Amano. 1968. Strain in the rabbit and dog maxillomandibular bones during biting and mastication. Journal of Dental Research 47: 496.

Kemp, T. S. 1972a. The jaw articulation and musculature of the whaitsiid Therocephalia. In *Studies in Vertebrate Evolution,* K. A. Joysey and T. S. Kemp, eds. Edinburgh: Oliver and Boyde, pp. 213–230.

———. 1972b. Whaitsiid Therocephalia and the origin of cynodonts. Philosophical Transactions of the Royal Society of London B 264: 857–911.

Kripp, D. von. 1933a. Beiträge zur mechanischen Analyse des Schnabelmechanismus. Morphologisches Jahrbuch 72: 541–566.

———. 1933b. Die Kaubewegung und Lebensweise von *Edmontosaurus* spec. auf Grund der mechanisch-konstruktiven Analyse. Palaeobiologica 5: 409–421.

———. 1933c. Der Oberschnabel-Mechanismus der Vögel. Morphologisches Jahrbuch 71: 469–544.

———. 1933d. Die Spezialisationreihe der Störche, Reiher und Kormorane von konstruktiven und biotechnischen Standpunkt. Morphologisches Jahrbuch 72: 60–92.

———. 1935a. Die mechanische Analyse der Schnabelkrümmung und ihre Bedeutung für die Anpassungsforschung. Morphologisches Jahrbuch 76: 448–494.

———. 1935b. Die Unterkeifer der Vögel als Eisenbetonträgerkonstruktion. Morphologisches Jahrbuch 76: 659–662.

Lombard, R. E., and D. B. Wake. 1976. Tongue evolution in the lungless salamanders, family Plethodontidae. I. Introduction, theory and a general model of dynamics. Journal of Morphology 148: 265–286.

———. 1977. Tongue evolution in the lungless salamanders, family Plethodontidae. II. Function and evolutionary diversity. Journal of Morphology 153: 39–80.

Maynard Smith, J., and R. J. G. Savage. 1959. The mechanics of mammalian jaws. School Scientific Review 141: 289–301.

Nobiling, G. 1977. Die Biomechanik des Kieferapparates beim Stierkopfhai (*Heterodontus portusjacksoni* = *Heterodontus philippi*). Advances in Anatomy, Embryology, and Cell Biology 52: 1–52.

Norman, D.B. 1984. On the cranial morphology and evolution of ornithopod dinosaurs. Symposium of the Zoological Society of London 52: 521–547.

Norman, D. B., and D. B. Weishampel. 1985. Ornithopod feeding mechanisms: Their bearing on the evolution of herbivory. American Naturalist 125: 151–164.

———. 1991. Feeding mechanisms in some small herbivorous dinosaurs: Processes and patterns. In *Biomechanics in Evolution*, J. M. V. Rayner and R. J. Wootton, eds. Cambridge: Cambridge University Press, pp. 161–182.

Otten, E. 1983. The jaw mechanism during growth of a generalized *Haplochromis* species: *H. elegans* Trewavas 1933 (Pisces, Cichlidae). Netherlands Journal of Zoology 33: 55–98.

———. 1985. Proportions of the jaw mechanism of cichlid fishes: Changes and their meaning. In *Architecture in Living Structure*, G. A. Zweers and P. Dullemeijer, eds. Dordrecht, The Netherlands: Martinus Nijhoff/Dr. W. Junk Publishers, pp. 207–217.

———. 1987. A myocybernetic model of the jaw system of the rat. Journal of Neuroscience Methods 21: 287–302.

Otten, E., J. Ijkema-Paasen, and J. D. Van Willigen. 1986. A computer reconstruction technique for biomechanical analyses of jaw mechanisms. Journal of Dental Research 65: 846.

Reif, W.-E. 1975. Lenkende und limiierende Faktoren in der Evolution. Acta biothereoretica 24: 136–162.

———. 1981. Konzepte und Methoden der Funktionsmorphologie. In: *Funktionsmorphologie*, W.-E. Reif, ed. Munich: Paläontologisches Gesellschaft, pp. 11–24.

Reif, W.-E., R. D. K. Thomas, and M. S. Fischer. 1985. Constructional morphology: The analysis of constraints in evolution. Acta biotheoretica 34: 233–248.

Rieppel, O. 1978. Streptostyly and muscle function in lizards. Experientia 34: 776–777.

———. 1979. A functional interpretation of the varanid dentition (Reptilia, Lacertilia, Varanidae). Gegenbaurs Morphologisches Jahrbuch 125: 797–817.

Seilacher, A. 1970. Arbeitskonzept zur Konstruktionsmorphologie. Lethaia 3: 393–395.

Smith, K. K. 1980. Mechanical significance of streptostyly in lizards. Nature 283: 778–779.

———. 1982. An electromyographic study of the function of the jaw adducting muscles in *Varanus exanthematicus* (Varanidae). Journal of Morphology 173: 137–158.

Smith, K. K., and W. L. Hylander. 1985. Strain gauge measurement of mesokinetic movement in the lizard *Varanus exanthematicus*. Journal of Experimental Biology 114: 53–70.

Thomas, R. D. K. 1979. Constructional morphology. In *The Encyclopedia of Paleontology*, R. W. Fairbridge and D. Jablonski, eds. Stroudsburg, Pa.: Dowden, Hutchinson and Ross, pp. 482–487.

Thomason, J. J., and A. P. Russell. 1986. Mechanical factors in the evolution of the mammalian secondary palate: A theoretical analysis. Journal of Morphology 189: 199–213.

Throckmorton, G. S., and L. K. Clarke. 1981. Intracranial joint movements in the agamid lizard *Amphibolurus barbatus*. Journal of Experimental Zoology 216: 25–35.

Walker, A. 1976. Functional anatomy of oral tissues: Mastication and deglutition. In *Textbook of Oral Anatomy*, J. H. Shaw, E. A. Sweeney, C. C. Cappuccino, and S. M. Meller, eds. Philadelphia: W. B. Saunders, pp. 277–296.

Wassersug, R. J., and K. Hoff. 1979. A comparative study of the buccal pumping mechanism of tadpoles. Biological Journal of the Linnean Society 12: 225–259.

Weijs, W. 1981. Mechanical loading of the human jaw joint during unilateral biting. Acta morphologica neerlando-scandinavica 19: 261–262.

Weishampel, D. B. 1983. Hadrosaurid jaw mechanics. Acta palaeontologia polonica 28: 271–280.

———. 1984. Evolution of jaw mechanisms in ornithopod dinosaurs. Advances in Anatomy, Embryology, and Cell Biology 87: 1–110.

Weishampel, D. B., and D. B. Norman. 1989. Vertebrate herbivory in the Mesozoic: Jaws, plants, and evolutionary metrics. Geological Society of America Special Paper 238: 87–100.

Wolff, J. E. A. 1982. Die funktionelle Gestalt der menschlichen Unterkiefersymphyse. Munich: Minerva-Verlag.

———. 1984. A theoretical approach to solve the chin problem. In *Food Acquisition and Processing in Primates*, D. J. Chivers, B. A. Wood, and A. Bilsborough, eds. New York: Plenum Press, pp. 391–405.

8

Mechanical Analysis of the Mammalian Head Skeleton

ANTHONY P. RUSSELL AND JEFFREY J. THOMASON

INTRODUCTION

THE COMPOUND AND COMPLEX HEAD SKELETON of vertebrates (Gans and Northcutt 1983; de Beer 1985) has, primitively, three distinct functional roles—food gathering and processing, maintenance of respiratory flow, and the protection of various soft tissues of the head, especially the central nervous system and special sense organs. All of these involve the resistance of stresses imposed upon the skeletal elements. In lower vertebrates the three functional roles may, to some extent, be separated, with the splanchnocranium, neurocranium, and dermatocranium being linked, but not firmly united, into a composite structure. In the tetrapods, however, there is a greater structural unification, and in the amniotes the responsibility of respiratory flow has shifted from the buccal force pump to the thoracic suction pump. This unification is especially marked in the Mammalia, where all three developmental components of the head skeleton are fully integrated in the adult state. The basic emphasis of this chapter will be on the mechanical properties of the mammalian head skeleton, especially in the context of feeding. Much of the work so far has been devoted to the mechanics of the lower jaw, and relatively few contributions have concentrated on the cranium proper. We attempt to redress this imbalance, but in certain instances, such as the documentation of bone strain, we must still rely chiefly on data available for the analysis of the lower jaw.

This chapter has two main components. In the first we establish the context for mechanical analysis of the adult head skeleton in mammals by considering the functional units of the head skeleton in tetrapods in general, the forces influencing cranial form, and feeding mechanisms. In the second section we examine some approaches to the mechanical analysis of the mammalian head skeleton. The topics range from a wide-ranging categorization and analysis of the form/function relationship in the skull throughout the mammals to our own work on the acquisition of a secondary palate. The highlighted works are linked in that they almost all involve an application of some aspect of the principles of beam theory (see Weishampel, this volume) which have formed the basis for much of mechanical engineering for the past century. However, they only scratch the surface of what is possible, and of what is needed from such studies before a full appreciation of the relationships between mechanical form and function in the head skeletons of individual mammalian species can be obtained. To close, we speculate on future possibilities for research, indicating methods and directions which may provide answers to questions of structural adaptation in the mammalian head skeleton.

THE BACKGROUND TO MECHANICAL ANALYSES

The basic kinematics of aquatic feeding in lower vertebrates have been outlined by Lauder (1985). Here, much of the emphasis has been on the integration of food-gathering and respiratory current-generating systems. Although some studies of bone strain have been made (Lauder and Lanyon 1980), mechanical analyses of the material properties of the skeletal components have not yet, in general, been carried out.

For the lower terrestrial tetrapods a survey similar to that of Lauder (1985) was carried out by Bramble and Wake (1985). Differences in head design between aquatic and terrestrial feeders were outlined (Bramble and Wake 1985, table 13-1), with particular emphasis being placed on the hyolingual complex. The principal components of a generalized feeding cycle were outlined, with stages of ingestion, mechanical reduction (if any), and food transport to the esophagus identified. While these stages depend upon integrated movements of the head skeleton, little information concerning the mechanics of these units is available. Information processing in the governance of these activities has been summarized by Lucas et al. (1986). Maximum movements are variously limited by the shape of the articular surfaces, the ligaments, the muscles, and tooth shape and form, but final control is exercised through the central nervous system. Analysis of the form/function relationships of the head skeleton addresses the question of how skulls are built to resist the loads imposed upon them by muscles or by externally imposed forces.

Investigations of the feeding mechanisms of mammals have concentrated on the morphology and function of the jaw apparatus in relation to broad dietary habits (Hiiemae and Crompton 1985). Such studies have paved the way for a more complete understanding of the mechanics of the head skeleton and the relationship between form and function. For mammals, the forces generated during mastication and the reaction forces resulting from these are dictated by such factors as the form of the jaw-closing muscles, the unilateral breakdown of food, the degree of lateral movement of the lower jaw, and the accurate occlusion of the cheek teeth (Crompton and Parker 1978). Food breakage occurs during the power stroke, as the force generated by the adductor muscles is applied through the teeth to the material between them (Hiiemae and Crompton 1985). It is such activities that are important in the ontogeny and evolution (Gingerich 1979) of head skeleton form. As with other skeletal units (Lanyon 1987), those of the skull respond to forces imposed upon them by soft tissues (van der Klaauw 1963; Moore 1965, 1980).

Normal cranial growth is a result of the synchronous coordinated activities of skeletogenesis, sutural growth, and continuous appositional growth and resorptive remodeling in response to induced loading (Sarnat 1971). Thus, craniofacial skeletal form is not merely a framework onto which the soft tissues are disposed, but is a reflection of their activities. Different diets may result in different surface topography and internal architecture of bone as a direct result of plastic bone response to induced loading (Bouvier and Hylander 1981). Hence, epigenetic mechanical factors play an important role in molding the form and internal architecture of the head skeleton (Dullemeijer 1985; Herring 1985; Bouvier 1986; Schoof et al. 1986; Schumacher et al. 1986).

Such interactions mean that an understanding of the biological significance of skull form is facilitated by a consideration of the head skeleton not only in terms of its developmental components (neurocranium, splanchnocranium, and dermatocranium), but also in terms of definable functional components. For mammals these are the braincase, rostrum, and lower jaw (Radinsky 1970). Jaw muscle action and the forces so generated are important for an appreciation of rostral morphology, and the form of the braincase is affected not only by brain and sense organ dimensions but also by the relationship of the braincase to the rostrum and the functional demands of the jaws and jaw-closing muscles (Moss and Young 1960; Weijs et al. 1987).

During the last fifteen years considerable effort has been devoted to gaining a greater understanding of the functional aspects of the mammalian masticatory apparatus (Hylander 1986). Much of this attention has focused on the power stroke of mastication, with data being accumulated on the activity patterns of the jaw-closing muscles and the loading patterns of the teeth. To this end data have been acquired through a variety of techniques such as the use of bite-force transducers, strain gauges, piezo-electric crystals, electromyography, and cineradiography.

There are developmental indications that the functional components of the mammalian head skeleton are recognizable units. Growth of the rostral region is dependent upon a variety of relationships and is easily disturbed (Urbanus 1985). Craniofacial growth is partially controlled by the forward growth of the cartilaginous nasal septum (Griffioen and Smit-

Vis 1985), and this provides the basis of rostral form. The pattern of brain growth exerts control over the braincase and optic and otic capsules (Park and Nowosielski-Slepowron 1983), and the soft tissues external to the braincase are also important molding influences (Griffioen and Smit-Vis 1985). The formation of the secondary palate is also of significance in bringing about correct proportioning and regional subdivision of the head skeleton (Smiley et al. 1971; Dahl et al. 1982; Krogman et al. 1982). As with all interacting systems, however, aspects of facial growth are significant for normal secondary palate morphogenesis (Wragg 1971). Computer-assisted tomography and magnetic resonance techniques have been significant in providing the basis for a fuller understanding of the three-dimensional growth of the craniofacial complex (De Lussanet de la Sablonière and Van Der Stelt 1985), but have not yet been widely applied.

Ontogenetic allometric studies have indicated how skull form is influenced by differential growth and paedomorphic effects. In dogs, for example, puppies have wide, rounded braincases, large orbits, and broad palates, while the average adult dog has a long, narrow rostrum and a tapered braincase. Differential growth is responsible for this change, as it is in the change of form of pig skulls (Wayne 1986). Conversely, the head skeletons of kittens and cats differ in size but not shape, indicating different developmental relationships between the functional cranial components.

A variety of developmental, interactive processes are, therefore, involved in the molding of the rostrum, braincase, and lower jaw as gross mechanical units (Flint and Ede 1978). These processes are important in the establishment of the relationship between the various mechanically definable regions of the skull (Tucker 1954a).

As well as form-building aspects of the ontogeny of head skeleton development, there are time-based changes in the material properties of the bony tissue of the skull that are related to functional demands. A study of the lower jaw of the dog has revealed that the bone of which it is made is essentially isotropic (Ashman et al. 1985). By means of ultrasonic techniques to measure the elastic properties of various bones, it was found that canine mandibular bone has a value of less than half the modulus of elasticity of canine femoral bone. There are, then, regional differences in the mechanical properties of bony tissue that are probably related to the functional demands placed upon them, although appropriate functionally related comparative studies have not yet been carried out.

The Mechanical Role of Sutures, Joints, and Kineses

As the head skeleton is made up of a mosaic of individual elements, and as the functioning of the masticatory apparatus depends upon lever mechanics, a brief consideration of the sutures and joints of the head skeleton will be given before the mechanical analysis of the skull as a whole is discussed.

The cranium (and the lower jaw in all vertebrates except mammals) is composed not of a single unit but of intricately shaped components that must maintain specific relationships to each other. The junctions at which the components of the head skeleton come together are sutures, and their varying form reflects the types of mechanical stresses to which they are subjected. In certain regions these sutural junctions may be significantly mobile, in which case they are able to contribute to kinetic movements, while in other regions they are firmly united and transmit stress without major displacement. The joints between the lower jaw and the cranium are also mechanically significant, as they permit the major role of the jaws to be accomplished. Thus, while it is possible to consider the mechanics of the head skeleton, especially that of mammals, by modeling it as a largely static structure, the nature of the sutures and other cranial joints, and the ways they are affected by induced loading, will play a greater role in mechanical studies in the future.

Sutures resist the separation of bones but may allow relative motion between them (Moss and Young 1960). Their location is determined by the relative growth of adjacent bones (Chierici 1977), and their form is largely determined by the type of loading they experience. Beveled and interdigitated sutures have been derived from simpler, butt-ended articulations through evolutionary modification (Moss and Young 1960; Nanda and Hickory 1984). Once growth has ceased, sutural fusion may occur in areas where this is mechanically appropriate.

Kemp (1972) and Moore (1980) considered how the sutures along the lower and upper edges of the lower jaw of Whaitsiid mammal-like reptiles reflect differing functional demands. Those of the lower edge are designed to resist compressive loading, while those of the upper edge must cope with tensile loading during biting. With the reorientation of the direction of pull of the jaw-closing muscles in the transition from mammal-like reptile to mammal (Crompton and Parker 1978), vertical and horizontal stresses imposed on the lower jaw tended to be canceled out, leaving the region of dentary-postdentary contact only lightly stressed. Alterations in the mechanical loading of this region of the lower jaw were contributory factors in permitting the transformation of certain of these postdentary elements into middle ear bones (Allin 1975).

Where particularly strong bonds between cranial elements are required, complex serrate sutures representing fractal curves may develop to enhance contact patterns (Long 1985). Such highly convoluted curves (fig. 8.1) are apparently important in animals bearing heavy cranial ornamentation such as antlers and horns. On occasion such sutures are subjected to high degrees of stress when the cranial ornaments are used in combat bouts. Even just the burden of carrying such heavy cranial ornamentation may be contributory to the development of such serrate sutures.

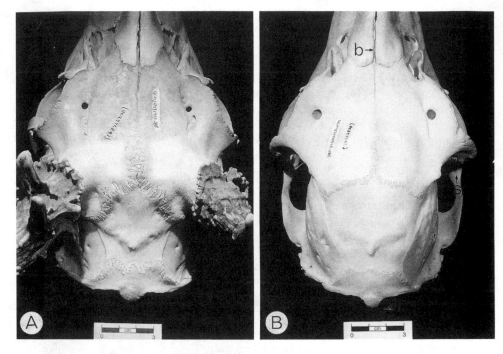

Fig. 8.1. The intricate serrate fractal sutures of the frontoparietal region of the skull
of the mule deer. In the male (A) the antlers impart a high loading to the frontals,
parietals, and occipitals both in the terms of their static weight and during combat
when they are dynamically loaded. In the female (B) the antlers are absent and there is
less intricacy of the serrate fractal sutures. Note also the presence of butt joints (b)
between the nasal bones, typical of joints that withstand compression but little
shearing or bending; and scarf joints (s) between the jugal and squamosal, typical of
joints where the entire area of contact is evenly stressed by most loads.

Positionally such fractal sutures are most complex closest to the sites of
maximum stress.

Some studies have been carried out that have attempted to measure
the stresses developed at sutures during normal functioning of the head
skeleton. Behrents et al. (1978) conducted an in vivo strain-gauge analysis
of strain at the sagittal suture in macaques. Their results indicated that
tensile bone strain is transmitted along the cranial vault to the parasagittal
region and that this is sufficient to bring about measurable separation of
the sagittal suture. Thus, tensile loading imposed by the pull of the masticatory muscles may influence sutural form in this region. Increasing bite
force was found to be directly correlated with increasing strain across the
suture. Behrents et al. (1978) concluded that such sutures behave as viso-
elastic tissues that are able to release the strain gradually upon cessation of

the stimulus. Such properties of sutures probably have implications for patterns of cranial growth, the timing of suture closure, and the evolution of skull form (Alberius and Selvik 1986; Alberius et al. 1986; Alberius and Isberg 1987).

The temporomandibular joint (TMJ) has been another area of focus with respect to mechanical properties (see Weishampel, this volume). Its form is known to vary greatly with the specific mode of feeding employed (Smith and Savage 1959), and it is an articulation to which forces are transmitted during normal dental function (Hinton 1981). It is known to undergo adaptive remodeling in response to imposed loads.

In reptiles the jaw-closing muscles insert closer to the jaw joint than they do to the bite point, and the vertical forces channeled through the jaw joint are quite high (Crompton and Parker 1978) compared with the forces generated at the teeth (fig. 8.2A). The jaw-closing muscles of reptiles do not form muscular slings and the jaw joint must thus withstand powerful medial and vertical forces even in straight orthal biting. The jaw joint is thus relatively massive when compared to that of mammals, where the jaw-closing muscles have become rearranged and reoriented such that the forces acting through the jaw joint are much reduced (Crompton and Parker 1978) while those acting at the teeth are increased (fig. 8.2B). The main components of the forces produced by the jaw-closing muscles now meet above the cheek teeth and can be balanced around the meeting point, leading to a restructuring of the rostrum (Thomason and Russell 1986) and a change in proportions of the three functional regions of the head skeleton. Such factors have been important in permitting the expansion of the mammalian braincase (Demes 1984; see below). With the lower jaw held in muscular slings (fig. 8.2C), jaw movements became more precisely controllable, occlusion more exact, and effective mastication feasible.

Within the array of TMJ form that has developed in mammals, translational functions have become important in many forms. This gives the potential for the lower jaw to act both as a lever (Picq et al. 1987) and a link (Gingerich 1979; Weishampel, this volume), the direction of bite force determining which of these will predominate (fig. 8.2D, E). This gives the lower jaw of certain mammals increased degrees of freedom and permits a variety of masticatory movements, as seen in omnivores and herbivores but not in carnivores. The relative loading of the jaw joint will influence the design of the head skeleton in this region. The magnitude of the reaction force at the TMJ varies with respect to the positional location of the bite force (Pruim et al. 1980), and with the direction of the bite force (primarily mediolateral or primarily vertical) (Smith et al. 1986). With mediolateral displacements, TMJ loading is high and markedly asymmetrical (Smith et al. 1986; Faulkner et al. 1987), while with vertical bite forces condylar loading is more symmetrical (Smith et al. 1986). Such data are the result

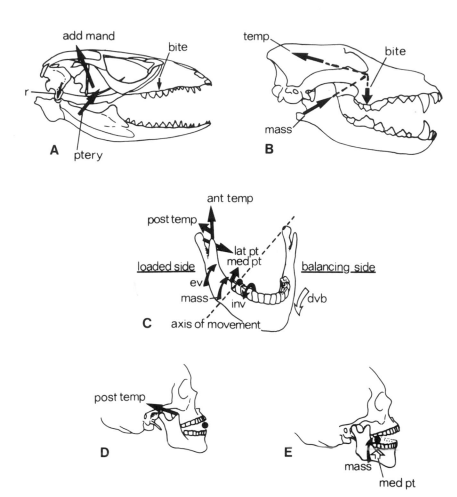

Fig. 8.2. Aspects of jaw mechanics. A. In reptiles the jaw joint acts as the fulcrum of a third-class lever. The jaw-closing muscles (add mand = adductor mandibulae; ptery = pterygoideus) are inserted closer to the jaw joint than to the bite point. The vertical forces passing through the jaw joint induce reaction forces (r) that are probably of greater magnitude than the bite force (bite). The jaw-closing muscles attach to the medial face of the lower jaw and do not form muscular slings. B. In mammals each side of the lower jaw is held in a muscular sling; the masseter (mass) and temporalis (temp) insert on its lateral face, while the pterygoideus inserts on its medial face. The positioning and arrangement of the jaw-closing muscles with respect to each other, the jaw joint, and the bite point keep the jaw joint relatively unloaded and transfer a greater proportion of the force to the bite point. C. The action of the major muscles of the mandible during molar biting in the human. The axis of movement passes through the condyle on the balancing side and the molar on the loaded side, at the bite point. The condyle of the loaded side slides down and forward and is relatively unloaded, while that of the balancing side slides up and back and is more heavily loaded. On the balancing side the mandibular corpus is primarily dorso-

of numerical analyses of models based upon the human lower jaw, but their implications are pertinent to the study of other mammals with different dietary habits and TMJ morphologies. The theoretical numerical analyses of Smith et al. (1986) are in general agreement with the direct strain-gauge data for TMJ loading obtained by Hylander (1979). Similar theoretical analyses of TMJ loading have been carried out by Throckmorton (1985).

Cranial kinesis has been reported for all tetrapod classes except the mammals. Two basic categories have been recognized—metakinesis, permitting displacement between the dermatocranium and the underlying neocranium, and mesokinesis, permitting relative movement between adjacent components of the dermatocranium (Bramble and Wake 1985). Mesokinetic joints are modified syndesmoses (sutures), while metakinetic joints are synovial. Smith and Hylander (1985) and Condon (1987) detail many of the aspects of cranial kineses in lizards, and other chapters in this volume deal more explicitly with this phenomenon in general. Suffice it to say here that the Mammalia exhibits a great reduction in kinetic properties of the skull, and the mechanics of the skull thus are significantly affected by its essential akinesis.

Crompton (1955) sought to provide an explanation for the disappearance of kinetism in the transition from mammal-like reptile to mammal. When compared to the head skeleton of scaloposaurid mammal-like reptiles, that of mammals had greater rigidity and brain protection. The skull of scaloposaurids was metakinetic and the kinetism acted as a shock absorber when a hard bite was delivered (Crompton 1955). Brain size was limited by the functional demands of mesokinetism, and only when mesokinetism could be dispensed with would it be possible for the two involved

---

ventrally bent (dvb), resulting in tensile stresses at the alveoli and compressive stresses along its lower border. On the working side the mandibular corpus is primarily twisted about its long axis, muscle forces tending to evert (ev) the lower border and invert the alveolar process, while the twisting moment associated with the bite force has the opposite effect (inv). Muscle abbreviations: ant temp, anterior temporalis; lat pt, lateral pterygoideus; mass, masseter; med pt, medial pterygoideus; post temp, posterior temporalis. D. In incisal biting the posterior temporalis acts parallel to the plane of sliding of the TMJ. The mandibular condyle can translate parallel to the line of action of this muscle and the mandible functions mechanically as a link. E. In molar biting the masseter and medial pterygoideus muscles function perpendicular to the plane of sliding of the TMJ. The mandicular condyle is not free to translate parallel to the line of action of these muscles as it abuts the articular eminence. In this case the mandible functions as a lever. Abbreviations for (D) and (E) are the same as those for (C). (A) and (B) are based upon concepts presented by Crompton and Parker (1978); (C) is based upon Hylander (1981) and Shipman et al. (1985); (D) and (E) are after Shipman et al. (1985).

components of the skull to fuse. Reduction of the canines and of bite force in derived scaloposaurids permitted this fusion to occur, and with the ensuing rigidity the braincase was able to increase in size. Along with this went changes in jaw-closing musculature and jaw joint constriction, leading to a reorganization of head skeleton design. Mammals are now able to inflict powerful bites without the need for kinetism as a shock absorber. The mammalian skull is a unitary structure and braincase size is no longer absolutely limited by the reactions from bite force.

Considerations of Bite Force

An area of investigation that is becoming increasingly important in the understanding of the mechanical design of the mammalian head skeleton is the quantification of bite forces and their relationship to stress distribution. Much of the recording of bite forces has been carried out on primates, but other mammals are now beginning to be investigated. The consideration of strain analysis in relation to bite force has generally focused on the lower jaw, but again investigations of correlation between bite force and bone strain are beginning to be carried out for cranial bones (see below).

Human dental investigative techniques have been influential in the development of methods of assessing isometric bite forces (Linderholm and Wenström 1970; Ringqvist 1973; Proffit and Fields 1983; Proffit et al. 1983). For experimental animals other than humans, bite force transducers employing strain gauges have been pioneered by Dechow and Carlson (1983). Force recording has been combined with muscle stimulation in order to investigate the reproducibility of the results (Dechow and Carlson 1983) and to attempt to estimate peak bite force (Thomason et al. 1990).

The relationship between myoelectric activity of the jaw-closing muscles and bite force has been investigated using both surface electrodes and subdermally implanted electrodes (Haraldson et al. 1985; Hylander et al. 1987). To complement these approaches, new methods of determining muscle cross-sectional area via computer-assisted tomography are now available (Weijs and Hillen 1985). So far such techniques have been employed only for human subjects, but they will be of significance in the determination of potential maximal force output in mammals in general. Of nonhuman subjects, including reptiles (Sinclair and Alexander 1987), assessments of muscle mass, cross-sectional area, and fiber length, for gaining estimates of maximal muscle force output, still rely on more traditional dissection and morphometric techniques. The force vectors of the jaw-closing muscles and the actions of these muscles in different combinations are important in the assessment of stress patterns generated in the bones.

The relationships between bite force, muscle force output, and patterns of stress in the head skeleton have been assessed by applying combinations of the above-mentioned techniques, and a series of papers dealing with the macaque mandible exemplifies this. Hylander (1981) documented the pattern of stress and strain in this element by way of strain-gauge analysis. Patterns of deformation in both the power stroke and during opening of the mouth were recorded, and data were obtained from both the loaded and the balancing side. Both bending and twisting deformations were recorded, the mandible undergoing continuous deformation in a cyclic pattern as the process of mastication continued. The upper jaw is not subjected to such continuous distortion, as it is a site of absorption of reaction forces but generally is not directly affected by muscle pull (except in the case of certain rodents; Tucker 1955a).

Patterns of bone strain in the macaque mandible were then used as a means of estimating masticatory bite force (Hylander 1986). Bone strain patterns along the working side of the mandible were found to be a good indicator of bite force generated in the power stroke. Strain-gauge data were also employed by Hylander and Crompton (1986) to determine strain patterns in the mandible in different phases of the chewing cycle. Hylander et al. (1987) then added cineradiography to the strain-gauge and electromyographic techniques, an approach that allowed movement at the TMJ to be monitored and its translational and rotary movements to be correlated with its loading. Data were again recorded for the loaded and balancing side.

Such combined investigative techniques have been particularly important in gaining an understanding of the mechanics of the mammalian mandible, the mobile component of the head skeleton during mastication. Similar approaches will be of importance in the continuing investigation of the mechanical properties of the skull, but in this case the data must be interpreted in the context of the physical parameters outlined by Tucker (1954a), Buckland-Wright (1978), Demes (1982), and Thomason and Russell (1986).

THE MECHANICAL ANALYSIS OF THE MAMMALIAN HEAD SKELETON: APPLICATIONS OF BEAM THEORY

Although the relationship between form and function in the mammalian head skeleton has long been realized, the demonstration of this relationship has seldom been addressed from a mechanical viewpoint. In this section we outline the development of mechanical analyses of the mammalian skull. Early authors such as Becht (1953) and Tucker (1954a–e,

1955a–d) attempted comprehensive treatments of the class. Tucker's work is a stepping-off point for two, apparently divergent, later lines of study. On the one hand is Buckland-Wright's (1978) study of stress distribution and bone architecture in the skull of the cat. On the other are the beam-theory analyses of the primate cranium (Demes 1982; Preuschoft et al. 1985a; see also Weishampel, this volume) and our own investigations of the rostrum in the opossum (Thomason and Russell 1986). All of these works, from Tucker's onward, are applications of different aspects of beam theory (see Weishampel, this volume) which, therefore, forms a link between them.

Overall Considerations of Form: Becht and Tucker

The foundations for mechanical studies were laid by Becht (1953), who examined the head skeleton, teeth, and masticatory muscles in an array of mammals of diverse dietary habits. Morphological and cinematographic investigations were combined and the basic mechanical demands on each skull type were set forth. He concluded that for carnivores the important factors, from a mechanical viewpoint, are structures that permit rapid and efficient grasping of prey by the canines, and dismemberment of the prey by the cheek teeth. The roller-type jaw joint was identified as important in limiting transverse movement of the lower jaw and in promoting orthal closure. In contrast, the TMJ of rodents was found to be gutter-shaped and designed to permit anteroposterior shifting of the lower jaw. Gnawing takes place with the lower jaw in the protracted position, and mastication when it is retracted. Guiding ridges on the cheek teeth control lateromedial masticatory movements. Ungulates were also found to have a transverse component in mastication, with the TMJs operating with partly sliding and partly hingelike movements. In this case the condyle of the lower jaw is primarily horizontal and markedly lateromedially widened. The occlusal planes of the cheek teeth were found to be reciprocally inclined.

The relative proportions of the jaw-closing muscles were compared in these types (Becht 1953) and the relative position of the dental batteries with respect to jaw joint position were noted. The latter was documented in the context of the relative force generated by each muscle. All of these basic points were reiterated by Smith and Savage (1959).

From these rather modest beginnings grew a perceptive yet much overlooked series of papers by Tucker (1954a–e, 1955a–d). In this collection of essentially theoretical studies, the relationships between masticatory activities and their mechanical consequences for the mammalian head skeleton were explored. The basic parameters of stress loading of the head skeleton were outlined (Tucker 1954a), with primary stresses being recognized at the muscle attachment sites, secondary stresses at the TMJs, and tertiary stresses in the upper and lower jaws, occurring as a result of reaction forces from items being bitten between the teeth (fig. 8.3A). Tucker (1954a) recognized that the resistance of food against the force that originates from the masticatory muscles creates stresses that radiate into the surrounding bone. Such stresses were proposed to occur in defined areas of the mandible and maxilla, and Tucker (1954a) set up his analysis of the mammalian head skeleton to attempt to document the stress-resisting tracts. He indicated that stresses of mastication may be circumscribed or dispersed, and that their pattern influences skull structure. Circumscribed stresses were outlined as those limited to a relatively small area, but of relatively great magnitude. Dispersed stresses, conversely, result when contacting surfaces of the maxilla and mandible are markedly enlarged, and the load is spread.

The skeletal elements were then considered in a mechanical context, with the maxilla and mandible described as beams (Tucker 1954a). Dispersed stresses were stated to be diffuse enough to be resisted locally, while circumscribed stresses were those whose magnitude necessitated transmission to distant regions of the skull for effective resistance. This led to a concept that tracts exist in the head skeleton for the transmission of circumscribed stresses, and that the rostral beam is thus supported at distant points. Such concepts enabled Tucker (1954a) to propose a series of tracts and nodes in the mammalian head skeleton that delineate the directions and magnitudes of stresses induced by normal activities. These morphological characteristics were related to the form and moment arms of the three jaw-closing muscles.

These concepts allowed Tucker (1954b) to classify mammalian skulls by function. At the ends of his continuum of functional types were those designed to resist the extremes of circumscribed and dispersed stresses, respectively. Stress transmission was seen by Tucker (1954b) as a function of the entire skull. An arch between the sites of the secondary and tertiary stresses (TMJ and upper tooth row) was proposed to be the most common structure involved in stress transmission. This was recognized as the principal cranial arch, which may be short or long. Where transmission of stress between these two points is poor, resulting in shearing stresses, the cranial arch is flat. Thus, Tucker's (1954b) three principal functional skull types were breviarcuate, longoarcuate, and planoarcuate (fig. 8.3).

The arch of the breviarcuate skull spans from the region of the carnassial tooth to the TMJ, and incorporates the postorbital process of the frontal (fig. 8.3B). Tensions in the skull floor were said to be transmitted through the perpendicular lamina of the palatine (Tucker 1954b). The principal arch of the longoarcuate skull spans from the TMJ to the premaxilla (fig. 8.3D), while the planoarcuate skull lacks any distinctly shaped cranial arches (Tucker 1954b). The major site of stress concentration in the breviarcuate skull was stated to be at the carnassial, during

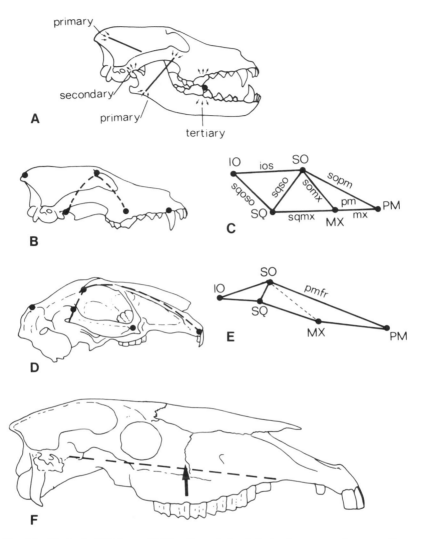

Fig. 8.3. Tucker's (1954a–e; 1955a–d) analysis of the basic aspects of mammalian skull form in relation to diet. A. Location of the stresses generated in the head skeleton as a result of biting, exemplified here by the breviarcuate skull of the dog. Primary stresses are induced by the pull on the head skeleton by the jaw muscles. Secondary stresses occur as a result of reaction forces at the TMJ. Tertiary stresses arise in the jaws and facial skeleton as a result of the reaction forces of items being bitten. B. Basic features of the breviarcuate skull as exemplified by the dog. The heavy dashed line represents the location of the principal mechanical arch of the skull. The black dots represent the nodes identified in C. C. Triangulation of the breviarcuate skull, with the nodes (uppercase letters) and tracts (lowercase letters) identified. Nodes: IO, interparieto-occipital; MX, maxillary; PM, premaxillary; SO, supraorbital; SQ, squamosal. Tracts: ios, interparieto-occipito-supraorbital; pmmx,

dismembering of food, and here the zygomatic arch also becomes an important transmissive structure. In the longoarcuate skull the chief stresses were stated to arise during gnawing (Tucker 1954b), and in the planoarcuate skull these occur during crushing along the extensive cheek tooth battery. In neither the longoarcuate nor the planoarcuate conditions did Tucker (1954b) consider the zygomatic arch to be an important transmissive structure.

The major example Tucker (1954c) presented for the analysis of the breviarcuate skull was that of the dog, with the major stress-bearing regions determined to lie at the canines, carnassials, and TMJ. The skull was modeled as three triangles, with bony tracts defining each of these (fig. 8.3B,C). At the TMJ, canine, and carnassial, stresses are imposed by the upward drive of the mandible and the resistance of items between the jaws, while at the sagittal crest and postorbital processes they are created by the masticatory muscles. In connection with the postorbital processes the masseter muscles set up stresses in the zygomatic arch and these are transmitted to the postorbital processes by the postorbital ligament (Tucker 1954c). In situations where the temporalis is the dominant muscle, as it is in carnivores (Turnbull 1970), the torsional effect of mastication (the tendency to twist the rostrum on the braincase) is relatively small and the postorbital bar is absent (Greaves 1985), allowing the postorbital ligament to act as a tensile structure transmitting the forces imposed by the masseter. The masseter also sets up tensile stresses that radiate to the carnassial and TMJ region along the zygomatic arch.

In the breviarcuate skull the action of the masseter tends to attempt to fracture the cranium through the middle triangle (Tucker 1954c), but these reactions are resisted by the perpendicular lamina of the palatine, under tension, and by the sphenoid. The stress-resisting tracts bear no particular relationship to individual bones, and in the breviarcuate skull the important tracts are the maxillo-premaxillary, premaxillo-supraorbital,

---

premaxillo-maxillary; somx, supraorbito-maxillary; sopm, supraorbito-premaxillary; sqmx, squamoso-maxillary; sqoso, squamoso-occipito-supraorbital; sqso, squamoso-supraorbital. D. The longoarcuate skull of the rabbit. The heavy dashed line represents the principal mechanical arch of the skull. E. Triangulation of the longoarcuate skull with the nodes (uppercase letters) and tracts (lowercase letters) identified. Nodes and tracts are essentially the same as those for the breviarcuate skull, but their disposition is altered. The long processes of the premaxillae reach the frontals, leading to the recognition of the premaxillo-frontal tract (pmfr). The supraorbito-maxillary tract does not constitute part of the principal arch of the skull. F. The planoarcuate skull of the horse. The heavy dashed line represents the flattened principal cranial arch. Masticatory forces are not generally transferred to the braincase region but are instead channeled vertically through the face (arrow).

supraorbito-squamosal, interparieto-occipito-squamosal, and occipito-interparieto-supraorbital (fig. 8.3C).

More extreme forms of the breviarcuate skull were then considered (Tucker 1954d), with the domestic cat being the major subject of investigation. Here the rostrum is shortened and the focused stresses are more concentrated. Structural changes associated with this are a strengthening of the squamosal-jugal joint and differentiation of internal bone architecture. Strains and vectors in the breviarcuate skull were considered (Tucker 1954e), with emphasis upon the asymmetrical use of the canines and carnassials.

The longoarcuate skull was then similarly analyzed (Tucker 1955a), with examples taken from rabbits and rodents. Here the development of the premaxilla was emphasized, with stresses being transmitted through the supraorbito-maxillary tract via the elongated frontal processes of the premaxilla (fig. 8.3D, E). Stresses are reduced in the maxillae of the rabbit and this was associated with their typical fenestration. This point was also recognized by Moss and Feliciano (1977), investigating the ontogeny of fenestration. They demonstrated that artificial loading of the vertical plate of the maxilla of the rabbit could induce the formation of compact bone in the area that is normally fenestrated. In rodents parts of the masticatory musculature may be anteriorly translocated onto the rostrum (Turnbull 1970), placing the vertical plate of the maxilla under tensile loading and resulting in the toothless premaxillo-maxillary tract lacking the fenestrations of the rabbit (Tucker 1955a).

In the longoarcuate skull the maxillary and supraorbital regions are not subjected to lateral stresses at the alveolar processes of the maxillae, the palatine processes are reduced, and stresses are instead concentrated in a premaxillary-frontal tract (fig. 8.3E). In rodents the zygomatic arch and frontal create another node, the preorbital, which provides the opportunity for the masseter to migrate onto the rostrum (Tucker 1955a), exempting the zygomatic arch from much of its imposed stress.

The attributes of the planoarcuate skull were outlined by Tucker (1955b), using equids as his chief example. Here the most significant changes are seen in the orbit, supraorbital node, and zygomatic arch. In this type of skull the morphology of the alveolar processes of the maxillae is closely connected with the dispersal of stresses. In these regions there is an increase of bony mass (fig. 8.3F). Transmissive tracts are not well developed and the transference of stresses from the rostrum back to the braincase is not marked. In both ungulates and primates the braincase is largely free of reactive masticatory stresses (Tucker 1955b). The absorption of such stresses in the rostral region may have been a significant contributory factor in such events as massive expansion of the braincase in anthropoid primates and the development of cranial combative ornamentation in artiodactyls. Reaction forces from the teeth create a vector that is directed dorsally and affects the roof of the nasal cavity. The nasals tend to have a lateral and a dorsal face and stresses are directed around this angle (Tucker 1955b). The strong nasal septum counteracts dislocation. Greaves (1985) considered the role of the postorbital bar in the planoarcuate skull (primates and artiodactyls) and discussed it as a torsion-resisting helical strut, but did not refer to the analytical studies of Tucker (1955b).

In summary, Tucker (1955c) concluded that the masticatory mechanism is an important morphogenetic influence on all mammalian skulls, particularly those subjected to circumscribed stresses. The form of both the rostrum and braincase is greatly influenced by these stresses. To demonstrate the existence of the proposed transmissive tracts, Tucker (1955d) undertook a radiographic examination of a variety of skull types and noted the marked increase of bone density about the nodes and tracts. Other areas of high density were observed to occur at the foramen magnum, indicating that high stress due to the support of the skull on the neck may be an important mechanical molding factor in this region.

Despite these perceptive and thought-provoking analyses of mammalian skull form in relation to mechanical stress, Tucker's contributions have gone largely unnoticed until relatively recently. Indeed, important works on the morphology of the mammalian masticatory apparatus (Freeman 1979) and the structure and function of the head skeleton (Moore 1980; Greaves 1985) fail to mention Tucker's work. His work is an intuitive application of engineering principles, supported by radiographic observations of material distribution in cranial skeletons. It is important because it attempts to relate the diversity of cranial form in mammals to the mechanical requirements of the many feeding mechanisms within the group. The major weakness is in the necessarily qualitative treatment of the magnitude of the stresses involved and the manner of their distribution. This is not a criticism of Tucker's methods. It is still logistically difficult to assess the distribution of stresses within the cranial skeleton even with the technological advances in the last 30 years. Endo (1965) recorded bone strain from human skulls in vitro, but it was not until Buckland-Wright's (1978) study of the cat that quantified in vivo experimental data were available to verify the procedure. In the next sections we describe two approaches to quantifying the mechanical properties of the mammalian head skeleton. However, we are still far from providing the breadth of data required to validate or refute the full scope of Tucker's hypothesis.

Stress Distribution and Bone Structure: Buckland-Wright

The most significant tests of Tucker's (1954a–e, 1955a–d) concepts of the design of the mammalian head skeleton have come from Buckland-Wright (1978). He examined the patterns of stress transmission in the cat skull, beginning with a radiographic examination of the nodes and tracts as initially outlined by Tucker (1955d). Having verified the existence of these features, Buckland-Wright (1978) embarked upon an analysis of force transmission through these during the process of jaw closure. A variety of techniques were employed in order to measure the direction and magnitude of these forces. Optically analyzable resin coatings were applied to dried skulls under simulated conditions of loading in order to appreciate more fully the location of the tracts. Strain-gauges were then applied to specific regions of the skull, both in dried specimens under simulated loading and in anesthetized cats whose jaw-closing muscles were electrically stimulated in order to simulate loading conditions in life. Muscles were stimulated in different combinations in order to examine variations in strain produced by different muscle sets (fig. 8.4A, B).

Deformations produced by the masseter were found to be greater than those produced by the temporalis. During biting, compressive forces were found to predominate in the facial bones (fig. 8.4B, C) and small movements to occur between these bones. The movement at the sutures was proposed by Buckland-Wright (1978) to be a mechanism to avoid overstressing the facial bones. This re-emphasizes the importance of the study of the role of sutures in the mechanical properties of the skull.

Buckland-Wright (1978) found the TMJ to be a load-bearing joint. In general, he found that the forces generated during biting are resisted within the head skeleton by forces of an opposite nature generated within the system, the incompressible nature of bone, and the effect of the soft tissues. As predicted by Tucker (1954d), the pattern of stress distribution in the cat skull was found to be essentially the same whether the resistance is located at the canines or carnassials.

As a result of his findings, Buckland-Wright proposed a theory of structural continua to describe the relationship of structure to stress distribution in cranial bones. In fact, he presented this theory as an alternative to the trajectoral theory of bone architecture of Wolff (1892), but it has attracted little attention in the literature on bone remodeling. However, the theory does categorize the relationship between the architecture of individual bones in the cat cranium and the stresses transmitted through those bones. Structural continua are defined as zones in the bone that exhibit a high degree of structural orientation and an increased density of osseous structures. In compact bone these are areas delineated by approximately parallel vascular canals, and they are contiguous with the trabeculae in the spongiosa. Structural continua are aligned along the direction of internal force, whether tensile or compressive, and in a given area there are an equal number of continua and directions of force. The tensile and compressive continua do not necessarily bear an orthogonal relationship to one another (as would be predicted by the trajectoral theory), but each

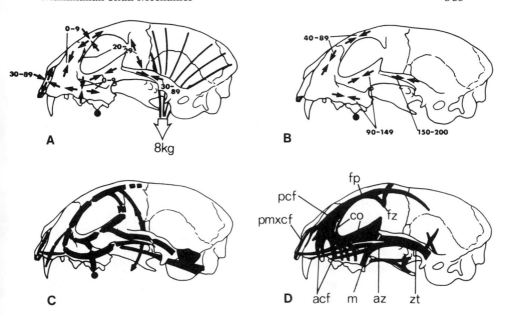

Fig. 8.4. Buckland-Wright's (1978) analysis of the facial skeleton of the cat. A. Type and magnitude of strain in the facial skeleton of dried cat skulls when loaded with 8 kg from cords representing the temporalis and masseter muscles, with the support at the carnassials. Diverging arrows represent tensile strains, converging arrows represent compressive strain. The figures represent mean deformation in microstrain. B. Distribution, type, and magnitude of strain in the facial skeleton of anesthetized cats during tetanic stimulation of the temporalis and masseter muscles, with a brace placed between the carnassials. Converging arrows indicate compressive strain, diverging arrows indicate tensile strain. The figures represent mean deformation in microstrain. C. Pattern of force transmission in the cat skull when a resistance is placed between the carnassials. Divergent arrows represent a tensile force and convergent arrows a compressive force. The width of the arrows represents the relative magnitude of the forces. The arrow from the lower surface of the zygomatic arch represents the ventral rotation of the jugal as a result of the pull exerted by the masseter. D. Arrangement of some of the structural continua in the skull of the cat. Abbreviations for continua; acf, alveolo-canino-frontal; az, alveolo-zygomatic; co, circumorbital; fp, fronto-parietal; fz, fronto-zygomatic; m, masseteric; pcf, principal canino-frontal; pmxcf, premaxillo-canino-frontal; zt, zygomatico-temporal.

is aligned in the optimum direction for force transmission to a region of resistance by thicker bone, by an opposite force generated within the system, or by soft tissues (fig. 8.4D). There is a functional continuum of stresses across sutural junctions and the entire head skeleton is implicated in the presence of these continua (Buckland-Wright 1978). The demonstration of structural continua in the cranial skeletons of genera other than *Felis* would represent an outgrowth and affirmation of Tucker's (1954–1955) observations.

The Cranial Skeleton as a Cantilever Beam

So far we have discussed the relationship between the form of the head skeleton in different mammals and the requirements of distributing the stresses of mastication. Tucker and Buckland-Wright were both concerned with the heterogeneity of bone architecture and the identification of stress-distributing tracts. They demonstrated the high degree of optimization of architecture to load bearing. Another approach is to ignore the architecture and to analyze the mechanical properties conferred by the general shape of structural form of the head skeleton. To date, the most productive structural analyses have been based on the principles of beam theory. This theory was central to mechanical and civil engineering until the advent of the computer made available more detailed numerical solutions of structural problems (e.g., finite-element analysis, which we discuss below). Ideally, internal architecture and shape should be considered in combination, but methodological complexity has so far been prohibitive. Beam theory gives at best a first approximation to the solution of mechanical issues where biological materials and structures are involved (see Weishampel, this volume). Finite-element methods have the most promise for integrating the analysis of shape and architecture in future studies, but in biological situations these methods are also beset with logistical problems that are not faced by engineers (Huiskes and Chao 1983).

Most of the discussion in the next sections is based on our published and unpublished work on the opossum, and on papers from the Functional Morphology Research Group at the Ruhr University in Germany. Members of this group are investigating form versus mechanical function in the mammalian skull, with emphasis on that of primates, as part of a general program of mechanical analysis of the vertebrate skeleton. They are interested in the mechanical effects of changes in shape and in interpreting the functional design of primate skulls using theoretical applications of beam theory (Demes 1982, 1984; Preuschoft et al. 1985, 1986).

Theoretical and Methodological Background. The main structural properties are strength (the force required to break the structure), and stiffness (the amount by which it deflects under a given force). They are analogous to, and partly dependent upon, the material strength and stiffness, and have different values for bending, torsion, and shear. Structural properties of the skull have largely been analyzed by considering it to be a cantilever beam—one that is free at one end and fixed or supported at the other. An infrequent alternative is to treat it as a shell—a tubular or spheroid structure in which the thickness of the walls is small compared with its diameter (Demes 1984).

Relatively few quantitative structural analyses have been performed to date, some theoretical, some empirical. The theoretical analyses use the formulas of beam theory (summarized in Roark and Young 1975) which quantify the effects of shape on the mechanical properties of the structure. A drawback in applying these formulas to analyze the head skeleton is that the mechanical properties of the constituent materials are assumed to be constant. The difference in stiffness and strength between sutures and the adjacent bone is not taken into account. In addition, the relevant equations have assumptions in their derivation and conditions for their use which cannot be precisely met in treating the head skeleton as a cantilever (Thomason and Russell 1986). Solely on the basis of these assumptions, caution must be exercised in interpreting the results of such studies. It is inappropriate to calculate absolute magnitudes of strength and stiffness of skulls. However, it is possible to quantify values that are in proportion to the strength and stiffness, and some relative quantities, such as the variation in strength along the length of the skull, are probably represented quite accurately.

The data required for a theoretical analysis are the loading regimes to which the skull is normally subjected, and a quantification of the shape of the skull.

The loading regimes may include forces from muscles, reaction forces from objects being bitten, and forces due to the inertia and weight of the skull. These forces act directly on the structure to cause shearing stresses. For example, imagine a vertical plane at the junction of rostrum and neurocranium. A force acting vertically on any or all of the teeth tends to make the rostrum slide off the front of the neurocranium, causing shear stresses in the material on either side of our imaginary vertical plane. Forces can also exert turning moments which load the structure in bending or in torsion. Bilateral and unilateral bites are respective examples of such forces. Inertial forces caused by rapid accelerations of the head also load the skull in bending, but in a manner different from the forces of biting (fig. 8.5). Bending can occur in more than one plane. Bilateral bites bend the skull dorsally; shaking the head from side to side with a prey item in the mouth bends it laterally. Clearly, it is important to know the magnitudes of each type of force that may act on a given skull. While bite forces can be directly measured, the corresponding muscle forces are harder to derive, and inertial forces have to be estimated (Demes 1982).

The data required to quantify the shape of the structure include linear dimensions form points of loading to points of support, and geometrical parameters of cross sections such as the area and second moment of area. The advent of the CAT scanner has obviated the necessity of physically sectioning specimens (Conroy and Vannier 1984; Preuschoft et al. 1985),

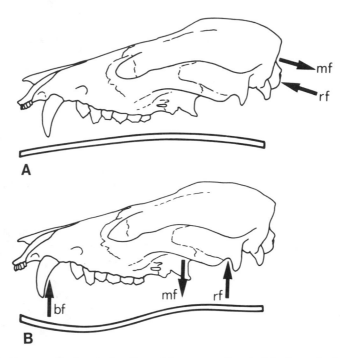

Fig. 8.5. Factors affecting the bending of the mammalian skull in the sagittal plane, with the skull modeled as a beam. A. The weight force of the skull results in bending moments which cause the beam to deflect along its length (mf, muscle force induced by the muscles supporting the head; rf, reaction forces at the occipital condyles). B. Bite forces result in a superimposition of additional bending moments on those of weight force. The lower jaw is driven toward the upper jaw and the bite force (bf) results in upward deflection of the rostrum, while the reaction forces (rf) at the TMJ and the muscle forces (mf) induced by the jaw-closing muscles result in deflections in the braincase region. After Demes (1982).

and digitizer/computer combinations facilitate the numerical integration of areas and second moments (Demes 1982; Thomason and Russell 1986; Phillips and Kaplan 1987).

On the assumption of constant material properties, the shape data can be combined to give estimates of the strength and stiffness of the whole skull in bending and torsion, or the variation in these properties and in the shear strength along its length. The cross-sectional area of any section indicates its strength against shear stresses in the plane of the section. The second moment of area, in combination with various linear measurements, can be used to indicate the strength and stiffness of the section to bending forces. Another geometrical measurement, similar to the second moment of area, indicates the resistance to torsion. Integrals of the second moment along the length of the skull are proportional to the total strength or stiffness. One of the most powerful uses of this analysis is to assess the effects of changes in shape, which can be accomplished simply by graphically altering the tracings or photographs of the sections through the skull.

One experimental method of assessing structural properties is simply to support the head skeleton as a cantilever and record how much it deforms under known loads (to evaluate its stiffness) and the force at which it breaks (to evaluate its strength). This method is almost free of the assumptions in the previous theoretical one, but is itself constrained by the fact that the methods of supporting and loading the head skeleton in vitro may not accurately reflect the in vivo situation. In addition, it is difficult to use fresh material for such experiments because of the problems of mounting and attaching recording sensors to fresh bone. Cleaned, dried skulls are considerably easier to use, but the properties of bone material are known to change when dried. The sutures also become relatively inflexible. Consequently, as was the case with the theoretical methods, dried material is appropriate only for assessing relative values of strength and stiffness. We have used this method to assess the structural effects of removing the nasal septum, vomer, and secondary palate as a means of inferring the contribution of these elements to the strength and stiffness of the whole rostrum.

The strain-gauge methods used by Buckland-Wright (1978) and Endo (1965) are of limited value in assessing the structural properties of the whole skull (or even of functional segments of it such as the rostrum), for two main reasons. The first is that they provide data on the deformation or strain experienced locally by the small area of bone to which the gauge is attached, and only the surface strain is recorded. Thus a large number of gauges is needed to document strain patterns over the whole skull, and this is necessary to infer general structural properties. This is a logistic problem which can be overcome, especially if gauges are used in combination with some other techniques, such as the application of a thin layer of photoelastic material to a large area of bone. Reflected polarized light shows the distribution of lines of equal strain across the covered area. These lines can be quantified by noting which ones intersect with gauge sites, at which strain levels are known.

The second disadvantage of strain gauges is that the elastic moduli (stiffnesses) of the underlying bone must be known before stresses corresponding to the recorded strains can be calculated. Data on the elastic moduli of craniofacial bone, and the manner in which these vary throughout the skull, are difficult to obtain and few are yet available. Ashman et al. (1985) have recorded them for the canine mandible using ultrasound. We have used strain data to augment structural analysis of the rostrum in the opossum, in which the primary methods were to record deformation and strength of the whole structure.

The above methods of theoretical or experimental application of beam theory analyze the mechanical performance of the structure under consideration. To reiterate, the beam formulas are sensitive to the effects of shape. The strength and stiffness of the materials of which the structure is made are relevant but of secondary importance (in that they must be assumed to be constant). Despite some limitations in trying to apply beam theory to the study of mechanically complex structures, this approach can provide answers to questions of functional design that were previously unapproachable. The methods can be and have been used to examine the mechanical significance of differences or evolutionary changes in shape (Demes 1982; Preuschoft et al. 1985, 1986; Thomason and Russell 1986), to interpret the optimization of functional design in individual skull types (Preuschoft et al. 1985, 1986), to assess the strength of canine teeth (Van Valkenburgh and Ruff 1987), and to study the dynamics of tooth displacement under loading (Behrend 1978).

The Rostrum of Long-Faced Mammals. The variation in form of the head skeleton is extremely broad in mammals, and was so among their therapsid ancestors. However, a recurring form, which may be considered primitive for both groups, is one in which the rostrum comprises almost half the length of the skull, tapering more or less evenly from posterior to anterior. The cross-sectional shape of this type of rostrum often approximates to a semicircle or a rounded square with flanges at each lateral margin, which are the alveolar processes of the maxillae (bearing the teeth). The semicircle or square is divided vertically by the nasal septum, with the vomer at its ventral border, and the conchae intrude on the nasal space. The skull of the North American opossum, *Didelphis virginiana,* is a good example of this general shape, despite anatomical peculiarities such as the palatal vacuities. The rostrum in such long-faced mammals can be readily envisaged as a cantilever and is the cranial unit most amenable to structural analysis as a beam. It projects free of the neurocranium (which supports it at the "base" of the cantilever). It has no major muscular attachments, and is loaded primarily through the teeth. Forces acting through the teeth can be represented as point loads or loads distributed along the length of the beam, as necessary. In contrast, the posterior half of the skull has many features that confound structural analysis. The most restrictive is that the forces acting on the neurocranium and zygomatic arches from the jaw adducting musculature cannot be readily assessed or reconstructed, and have an undoubtedly complex distribution. The compound structure of the neurocranium and zygomatic arches adds to the difficulties, but would be less of an obstacle were the loading more readily determinable. In short-faced mammals, our own skull representing an extreme form, analysis of the rostrum is itself impeded because very little of it projects forward of the neurocranium or zygomatic region.

One reason, therefore, for taking the rostrum of long-faced mammals as a starting point is because it is easiest to analyze. A more important reason is that we might expect closer structural optimization on beam principles, analogous to the architectural optimization documented by Buckland-Wright (1978), in this type of rostrum than in any other unit of the mammalian head skeleton, simply because of its beamlike form and usage. Clearly the rostrum is under ontogenetic and anatomical constraints which are likely to affect its mechanical behavior—it has to provide rooting for the teeth and enclose the volume of the nasal cavity, for example. However, if functional design on mechanical principles is to be documentable in the mammalian skull, it is in the rostrum of long-faced mammals that such design should be most evident.

Preuschoft et al. (1985, 1986) argued for a strong correspondence between form and mechanical function in long rostra, but their results show that much variation exists. They started with the hypothesis that the most probable optimizing criterion for such a structure was for it to be equally strong along its length under any usual loading regime applied through the teeth. In other words, the peak stress acting in any section through the rostrum would be independent of its position along the length. They demonstrated qualitatively that the rostral profile of a baboon was curved in similar fashion to that predicted for a beam designed on equal-strength criteria, with the main loads being applied at the canines. However, their quantitative analysis of several skulls of varying rostral length (dog, baboon, pig, with gavial and crocodile as examples of extremely long-snouted skulls) indicated that, as is usual in biology, situations do not rest on single criteria. (They also included a gorilla and chimpanzee as short-faced animals. We discuss these in the section on the primate skull below).

Only in the case of shear was the equal-strength criterion even approximated. Vertical shear stresses are produced by forces of biting on any tooth. Since the maximum force of any tooth is, in theory, inversely proportional to the out-lever of the jaw muscles (i.e., the distance from TMJ to bite point), bite forces may be expected to increase parabolically from anterior to posterior. Resistance to shear stresses so produced is directly proportional to the cross-sectional area of bone, which also increased parabolically toward the rear of each rostrum studied by Preuschoft et al. (1985, 1986). They estimated and compared stress values at three points on the rostrum (front, middle, back) to determine how closely the equal-stress criterion was met. For the pig, the difference between the maximum and minimum of the three stress estimates was only 8%, but it was 35–36% for the baboon and dog.

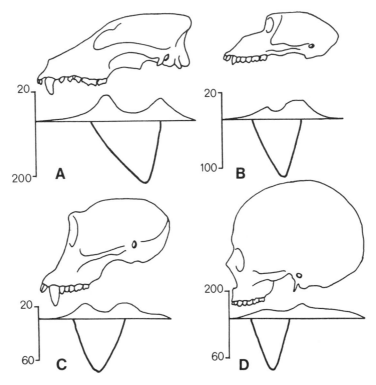

Fig. 8.6. The skulls of a (A) dog, (B) baboon, (C) chimpanzee, and (D) human show the incongruence between bending strength and a common loading regime (forces due to a 30 kP bite on the molars). The resistance to bending along the length of each skull is indicated above the axis on each graph (in cm³); the distribution of bending moments (in kP.cm) is below the axis. Notice that the peaks above each axis are not coincident with those below, and note the relatively high ratio of bending resistance to moments for the human skull. After Demes (1982).

The resistance to bending loads does not vary along the rostrum in proportion to the variation in bending moments, which indicates that the rostrum is not optimized for bending. When analyzing bending, Preuschoft et al. (1985, 1986) considered only forces applied near the anterior end of the rostrum, as we did for the opossum (Thomason and Russell 1986). This is because bending stresses depend on the distance between load point and the section under consideration. The following remarks hold for both dorso-ventral and latero-medial bending. For an anteriorly placed force, the bending moment increases linearly for sections taken progressively more posteriorly. However, the bending strength increased faster than linearly for the baboon and dog, as a consequence of the widening and deepening of the rostrum posteriorly. (Figure 8.6A illustrates this parabolic increase for the dog's rostrum.) Thus, stresses due to bending appear to decrease posteriorly in these animals. The pig and the two reptiles varied from this pattern in that the stress estimates were higher in the middle of the rostrum than at each end. Our results for the opossum appear to fall into this latter category (Thomason and Russell 1986). We analyzed the strength at two rather than three sections, and found the most posterior to be considerably weaker and less stiff than the anterior one. We attributed this to the thickening of the bony walls of the anterior section to accommodate the large roots of the canines.

The pattern of variation within and among skulls for torsion is similar to that for bending. Torsional strength in the baboon increases posteriorly, while it is greatest at the midpoint of the rostrum in the pig, and higher just behind the canine than at the second molar in the opossum.

The apparent departure of rostral shape from a mechanical optimum has two possible explanations. The first is that optimizing criteria other than equal strength apply to the rostrum, though it is difficult to imagine a criterion that fits with the above observations and which may have some biological relevance. The second possibility, which is more plausible, is that the other constraints on rostral form, already mentioned, override general structural factors. This is, of course, seen in others parts of the skeleton; the triangular cross-sectional shape of the adult tibia results from muscular pressure rather than by "design" (Lanyon and Bourne 1979). A seemingly trivial constraint is that the rostrum must be as wide and deep at its posterior end as the neurocranium with which it is confluent. Thus, the volumetric demands of the brain may determine posterior dimensions of the rostrum, and hence its structural properties toward its base. Anchoring the teeth is an example of a factor which has its primary effect on the material of the alveolus, with important secondary consequences on the structural properties of the whole rostral unit.

The Short-Faced Skull of Primates. From the skulls of extant primates it is possible to choose a structural series to approximate the evolution from a long-faced ancestor to the extremely short, high skull of humans. As we might expect, there is no greater degree of optimization toward beam behavior in any short-faced primate than in the long rostra we have been discussing. The rostra of chimpanzee and gorilla are similar to that of baboon and dog; shear stresses vary little and bending stresses decrease posteriorly (Preuschoft et al. 1985, 1986). When the whole skulls of a dog, baboon, chimpanzee, and human were analyzed in bending (Demes 1982; see also Weishampel, this volume), the shorter skulls were found to be disproportionately stronger (fig. 8.6). In none of the skulls did the peaks in bending strength correspond to the peak bending moments they might normally experience (fig. 8.6). For the dog and baboon the peaks in bending strength occurred where the zygomatic arches attach to the main body of the cranium, owing to an increased thickness of bone at these points. This is another example of local strengthening, in this case to provide firm attachment for the arches, enhancing the general structural properties of the whole skull.

The human skull is certainly stronger than necessary for the bending forces it experiences. The expansion of the neurocranium is a more important determinant of its adult form. The thickness and diploic construction of the calvarial bones are related to another mechanical factor, the resistance of impact, and the resultant bending strength of the whole skull is a consequence of these other functional demands. However, the stresses of mastication, to which the skull is subjected more frequently than impacts, do appear to have a closer relationship to form. Demes (1984) made resin models approximating to the lower half of the human neurocranium. Each model was coated with a photoelastic resin and was loaded unilaterally at one TMJ. The strain distributions indicated that areas in which the bone is thin (e.g., the orbital floor) or is perforated by numerous nerves and vessels are not strained in this type of loading. The highest strain levels were in the temporal region above the loaded TMJ, indicating that bending occurred in the wall of the calvarium itself. The outer surface was loaded in tension, the inner in compression. This loading within the wall of the neurocranium suggests that it may behave mechanically more like a shell than a beam. Demes (1984) further suggested that the action of the temporalis muscles may counteract the loading pattern from the TMJ force, reducing stress levels close to zero. This correlates with Endo's (1965) in vitro analysis of strain distribution and supports Tucker's (1954b) proposition that the stresses of mastication are largely confined to the face in the planoarcuate skull.

The general conclusion that may be drawn from beam analyses of the mammalian rostrum and skull is that structural properties appear to be much less important than other constraints. An important category of constraints are those which primarily affect local strength but which have marked secondary consequences on structural properties. For example, the increased thickness of bone around the teeth and at the base of the zygomatic arch appears to strengthen the skull as a whole.

The Evolution of the Secondary Palate. We are interested in the mechanical significance of the changes in the facial skeleton from mammal-like reptiles to mammals (Thomason and Russell 1986). Although the anatomical and ecological diversity of the mammal-like reptiles is at least equal to that of living mammals (Kemp 1982; Hotton et al. 1986), specimens do exit which indicate the possible course of evolution of the secondary palate and associated craniofacial structures. A secondary palate developed early in the cynodonts (e.g., *Procynosuchus*), before marked reduction in the post-dentary bones of the lower jaw, and simultaneously with flaring of the zygomatic arches. The significance of these two features is that the force of biting may have been quite high in the animals which originally acquired the secondary palate, as suggested by Greaves (1988). The palate appears to have formed as longitudinal shelves which approach the midline along most of their anteroposterior length (rather than being initially complete at the front and migrating backward). We have proposed that the palate has a mechanical function in extant mammals, and that palatal evolution may have been a means of strengthening the rostrum as biting force increased, and we have both theoretical and experimental data which support the hypothesis.

In a preliminary study, we assessed the effects of removing the secondary palate from the rostrum of the opossum on the structural strength and stiffness in torsion and bending for loads applied to the canines (Thomason and Russell 1986). We evaluated the contribution of two separate sections through the rostrum to its overall properties. Then we repeated the analysis but omitted segments of the secondary palate, thereby quantifying the change in properties. As noted above, the beam theory formulas are particularly suitable for this type of procedure. To model the process of acquisition of the secondary palate we presented the results as the change in structural properties as the palate was added to the rostrum, rather than removed. Formatted this way, the results showed that the increase in torsional strength and stiffness was greater than the increase in bone area from the situation without the palate to a complete section. The increase in bending properties paralleled the increase in bone area, but the tooth-bearing maxillae were braced by the addition of the horizontal shelves to their medial aspects. Thus the mechanical advantages of having a secondary palate appear to have been greater than the energetic disadvantages of forming and carrying around an extra bony shelf in the skull. In addition, the final closure of the intermaxillary suture theoretically resulted in a major jump in torsional properties. On closure, the strength in pure torsion was predicted to jump to between 3 and 14 times, and stiffness, 19 to 85 times the values before the palate was added.

Our conclusion, that increase in torsional properties could have provided selective advantage for palatal formation, must be regarded as tentative, because the analysis was based on several unavoidable assumptions. In addition to the general assumption discussed in the "Theoretical Background" section, we could not take into account the nasal septum (which runs as a brace between the dorsal and ventral aspects of the rostrum) and the vomer (which braces the secondary palate against the bisicranium). These problems were largely overcome in a recent series of experiments in which we mounted the neurocranium of opossum skulls in resin and physically loaded the rostrum as a cantilever. All the assumptions made in the theoretical test can be accounted for, with the exception of those pertaining to material properties; the skulls were dry. Drying does affect material properties, particularly stiffness (Currey 1984), but this drawback was overcome because we estimated the factor of change in structural properties on palatal removal, rather than absolute values. If the effect of drying is a constant multiplying factor on material properties in all directions, then the relative change in structural properties should be the same as it would be for the living rostrum.

Loads were applied by inverting each skull and suspending weights of varying magnitude from the canines or second premolars, first bilaterally, then unilaterally. A "physiologically" correct range of forces was determined a priori by allowing a size range of living opossums to bite on a force transducer. The forces used on the dried skulls were well within this range, peaking at 100–120 N compared with peaks approaching 500 N for the bite forces of large male opossums in vivo (Thomason et al. 1990).

The pattern of testing each skull approximated to the procedure of the theoretical study: it was loaded first with and then without the secondary palate. An important advantage over the theoretical study was that we were able to assess the contribution of the nasal septum and vomer in addition to the palate. The changes in stiffness and strength of the rostrum were assessed for dorso-ventral bending and torsional loads applied to the canines and separately to the second premolars. To date we have more data for stiffness.

Changes in structural stiffness in bending and torsion were recorded by measuring deflection of the free anterior end of the rostrum with transducers (deflection is inversely proportional to structural stiffness). The transducers were connected between the zygomatic arch and base of the canine on each side, ensuring recording deflections of the rostrum only. Five skulls were each tested in the order: (a) whole, (b) turbinates and nasal septum removed, (c) vomer severed, (d) palate split, (e) palate completely removed. Stages b and c tested for the strengthening effect of nasal septum and vomer. Stages a, d, and e correspond to stages in the theoretical study above and to the bars in figure 8.7, which shows the results for bending on five skulls (A to E). The pattern of change was similar for torsion. All the represented deflections were obtained under a bending force of 50 Newtons applied symmetrically to both canines. (For torsion the force was applied to one canine.) The results in figure 8.7 are normalized to the lowest value, i.e., when the palate is completely removed (stage e), so the leftmost bar in each block of three has a value of 1. The middle bar represents the palatal shelves split in the midline (stage d), and the right bar is for the complete rostrum (stage a).

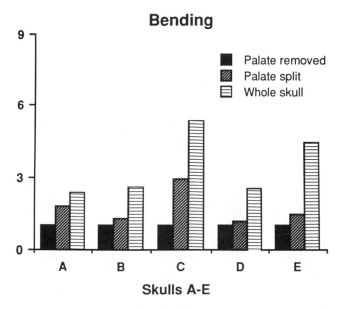

Fig. 8.7. The stiffness of five skulls (A–E) plotted as the inverse of deflection under an applied load of 50 N. Each skull was first loaded whole, then with a saw-cut along the midpalatal suture, and finally, with the secondary palate totally excised. Values are normalized to the lowest value in each case, which occurred when the secondary palate was completely removed. Thus the ordinate shows the factor of effective increase in stiffness if the palate were added to the skull.

The increase in stiffness between stages d and e is by a factor between 1.2 and 3.1 (for both bending and torsion). This range is close to the predicted values of 1.2 to 2.4. There is a further increase on closure (stage a) by 2.4 to 8.3 of the initial values, which is an order of magnitude less than predicted.

Figure 8.7 demonstrates the importance of the palate to the structural integrity of the rostrum in *Didelphis*. It also demonstrates the degree of correspondence between the theoretical and in vitro results. While the pattern of change is the same for both types of analyses, the magnitudes of relative change are considerably lower in the in vitro study. However, an increase in bending stiffness of between 240% and 530% on addition of the secondary palate may still be considered substantial. The relation of theoretical to experimental results is similar to that of Frankel and Burstein (1965), who compared the properties of whole and partly split human tibiae.

The results above all deal with changes in stiffness. To assess structural strength, the skull must be loaded to failure, so tests with and without the palate cannot be performed on the same skull. We matched a pair of skulls for length and width, split the palate in one and loaded both in bending, via the canines, to failure. The skull with the split palate failed at 245 N; one maxilla broke away along the naso-maxillary suture. The whole skull failed at 484 N, breaking through the braincase, not the rostrum. Thus, splitting the palate does weaken the rostrum by at least 50%.

The changes in stiffness and strength of the rostrum of *Didelphis,* whether assessed theoretically or in vitro, support the hypothesis that mechanical factors may have been important in the evolutionary development of the secondary palate in the ancestors of mammals.

The Mechanical Function of the Nasal Septum and Vomer. The nasal septum is shaped and positioned to brace the rostrum against dorso-ventral bending (Preuschoft et al. 1986). The vomer attaches the secondary palate to the neurocranial base, and would appear to have a similar function. In the theoretical analysis of the didelphid rostrum, it was logistically impossible to account for the effect of these elements on rostral stiffness and strength because of the difficulties in accurately digitizing them. However, their mechanical effect could be investigated in the in vitro stiffness experiment simply by removing them in sequence (stages b and c). The results are a little difficult to interpret because of the variability and low magnitude of the change in deflection following removal of these elements, and the apparent small increase in stiffness in some cases. However, the picture that emerges is that the nasal septum and vomer appear to make only minor contributions to the structural properties of the adult rostrum, despite the importance of the former in the ontogeny of facial form.

The Way of the Future: Finite-Element Analysis

A new and different approach to cranial form lies within the field of finite-element analysis, a technique now widely used in engineering for problems in structural mechanics (Moss 1985). Finite-element analysis relies on the determination of nodal coordinates of two- or three-dimensional objects and was initially developed as an engineering technique for the behavioral analysis of solids and fluids responding to external forces. In such analyses the structure is divided into an assembly of elements of finite proportions. These are then assumed to be connected at their peripheral nodal points. The coordinate positions of each nodal point are accurately determined in order to be able to describe the geometrical shape of the structure in mathematical terms. For mechanical analyses the material properties of the structure and appropriate loading data must be evaluated. The stiffness of the elements and the loading criteria are computed and assembled into an overall system stiffness matrix and load vector. The system matrix, a large array of algebraic simultaneous equations, is solved by evaluating the unknown nodal displacements. Stresses and bending moments may then be calculated from the displacements, and from these, principal stresses and bending moments in other directions can be determined.

Although in biological terms it was initially applied to aspects of growth (Moss et al. 1981), finite-element analysis has the potential to be a powerful tool in mechanical analysis. The details of finite-element analysis for studying change of form through time were outlined by Moss (1985) and Richtsmeier and Cheverud (1986).

The advantage within the finite-element method of being able to identify homologous points, and to see how they relate to areas of deformation, has been the impetus for adapting finite-element analysis for mechanical studies. So far such analysis has been attempted only for an avian example, the shoebill (see below), but it has great potential for application to the mechanical analysis of the mammalian head skeleton.

Guillet et al. (1985) attempted a three-dimensional numerical stress analysis of the skull of the shoebill. Nodal coordinates were determined for the shoebill skull by stereophotogrammetric methods, and finite elements were delimited by these nodes. Although Guillet et al. (1985) emphasized that material properties and loading data must be specified, they failed to provide such data in their analysis. Thus, although the finite-element method has considerable potential for mechanical analysis of the head skeleton, a great deal of information that is not readily available must be accumulated. Strain-gauge data can be recorded from a limited number of sites and only from the surface, while finite-element analysis offers a much broader scope. Unfortunately, real data are not yet sufficiently available to be able to employ effectively the finite-element method in the analysis of cranial mechanics. However, if the logistical difficulties in obtaining sufficient data on material properties and structural form for the head skeleton can be overcome, the finite-element method will come into its own. At that time the analysis of cranial mechanics will advance rapidly from first approximations to the level of interpretation of individual, rather than gross, differences in form.

REFERENCES

Alberius, P., and P.-E. Isberg. 1987. Relationships between growth [sic] at the sutures of the rabbit calvarium. American Journal of Physical Anthropology 72: 431–435.

Alberius, P., and G. Selvik. 1986. Long-term analysis of calvarial growth in rabbits. Anatomischer Anzeiger 162: 153–170.

Alberius, P., G. Selvik, and M. T. E. Fahlman. 1986. Postnatal sutural growth of the calvarium: A survey with special reference to the rabbit. Gegenbaurs morphologisches Jahrbuch 132: 519–534.

Allin, E. F. 1975. Evolution of the mammalian middle ear. Journal of Morphology 147: 403–438.

Ashman, R. B., G. Rosinia, S. C. Cowin, and M. G. Fontenot. 1985. The bone tissue of the canine mandible is elastically isotropic. Journal of Biomechanics 18: 717–721.

Becht, G. 1953. Comparative biologic-anatomical researches on mastication in some mammals. I and II. Verhandelingen der Koninklijke Nederlandse Akademie van Wetenschappen, Amsterdam 56: 508–527.

de Beer, G. R. 1985. The Development of the Vertebrate Skull. With a new foreword by Brian K. Hall and James Hanken. Chicago: University of Chicago Press.

Behrend, D. A. 1978. Patterns of tooth displacement in simulated chewing cycles in man. Archives of Oral Biology 23: 1089–1093.

Behrents, R. G., D. S. Carlson, and T. Abdelnour. 1978. In vivo analysis of bone strain about the sagittal suture in Macaca mulatta during masticatory movements. Journal of Dental Research 57: 904–908.

Bouvier, M. 1986. Biomechanical scaling of mandibular dimensions in New World monkeys. Journal of Primatology 7: 551–567.

Bouvier, M., and W. L. Hylander. 1981. Effect of bone strain on cortical bone structure in macaques (Macaca mulatta). Journal of Morphology 167: 1–12.

Bramble, D. M., and D. B. Wake. 1985. Feeding mechanisms of lower tetrapods. In Functional Vertebrate Morphology, M. Hildebrand, D. M. Bramble, K. F. Liem, and D. B. Wake, eds. Cambridge, Mass.: Belknap Press, pp. 230–261.

Brehnan, K., R. L. Boyd, J. Laskin, C. H. Gibbs, and P. Mahan. 1981. Direct measurement of loads at the temporomandibular joint in Macaca arctoides. Journal of Dental Research 60: 1820–1824.

Buckland-Wright, J. C. 1978. Bone structure and the patterns of force transmission in the cat skull (Felis catus). Journal of Morphology 155: 35–62.

Chierici, G. 1977. Experiments on the influence of oriented stress on bone formation replacing bone grafts. Cleft Palate Journal 14: 114–123.

Condon, K. 1987. A kinematic analysis of mesokinesis in the Nile monitor (Varanus niloticus). Experimental Biology 47: 73–87.

Conroy, G. C., and M. W. Vannier. 1984. Noninvasive three dimensional computer imaging of matrix-filled fossils by high-resolution computed tomography. Science 226: 456–458.

Crompton, A. W. 1955. A possible explanation for the origin of the mammalian brain and skull. South African Journal of Science 52: 130–133.

Crompton, A. W., and P. Parker. 1978. Evolution of the mammalian masticatory apparatus. American Scientist 66: 192–201.

Currey, J. E. 1984. The mechanical adaptations of bones. Princeton: Princeton University Press.

Dahl, E., S. Krieborg, B. L. Jensen, and P. Fogh-Andersen. 1982. Comparison of craniofacial morphology in infants with incomplete cleft lip and infants with isolated cleft palate. Cleft Palate Journal 19: 258–266.

Dechow, P. C., and D. S. Carlson. 1983. A method of bite force measurement in primates. Journal of Biomechanics 16: 797–802.

De Lussanet de la Sablonière, R. M., and P. F. Van Der Stelt. 1985. CT-scanning in palatoschizis. Acta morphologica neerlando-scandinavica 23: 289–296.

Demes, B. 1982. The resistance of primate skulls against mechanical stresses. Journal of Human Evolution 11: 687–691.

———. 1984. Mechanical stresses at the primate skull base caused by the temporomandibular joint force. In *Food Acquisition and Processing in Primates*, D. J. Chivers, B. A. Wood, and A. Bilsborough, eds. New York: Plenum Press, pp. 407–413.

Dullemeijer, P. 1985. The significance of Van Limborgh's approach to craniofacial biology. Acta morphologica neerlando-scandinavica 23: 317–324.

Endo, B. 1965. Distribution of stress and strain produced in the human facial skeleton by the masticatory force. Journal of the Anthropological Society, Nippon 73: 123–136.

Faulkner, M. G., D. C. Hatcher, and A. Hay. 1987. A three-dimensional investigation of temporomandibular joint loading. Journal of Biomechanics 20: 997–1002.

Flint, O. P., and D. A. Ede. 1978. Facial development in the mouse: A comparison between normal and mutant (amputated) mouse embryos. Journal of Embryology and Experimental Morphology 48: 249–267.

Frankel, V. H., and A. H. Burstein. 1965. Load capacity of tubular bone. In *Biomechanics and Related Engineering Topics*, R. M. Kenedi, ed. Oxford: Pergamon Press, pp. 381–396.

Freeman, P. W. 1979. Specialized insectivory: Beetle-eating and moth-eating molossid bats. Journal of Mammalogy 60: 467–479.

Gans, C., and G. Northcutt. 1983. Neural crest and the origin of vertebrates: A new head. Science 220: 268–274.

Gingerich, P. D. 1979. The human mandible: Lever, link, or both? American Journal of Physical Anthropology 51: 135–138.

Greaves, W. S. 1985. The mammalian post-orbital bar as a torsion-resisting helical strut. Journal of Zoology, London 207: 125–136.

———. 1988. The maximum average bite force for a given jaw length. Journal of Zoology, London 214: 295–306.

Griffioen, F. M. M., and J. H. Smit-Vis. 1985. The skull: Mould or cast? Acta morphologica neerlando-scandinavica 23: 325–335.

Guillet, A., W. S. Doyle, and H. Rüther. 1985. The combination of photogrammetry and finite elements for a fine grained functional analysis of anatomical structures. Zoomorphology 105: 51–59.

Haraldson, T., G. E. Carlsson, L. Dahlström, and T. Jansson. 1985. Relationship between myoelectric activity in masticatory muscles and bite force. Scandinavian Journal of Dental Research 93: 539–545.

Herring, S. W. 1985. The ontogeny of mammalian mastication. American Zoologist 25: 339–349.

Hiiemae, K. M., and A. W. Crompton. 1985. Mastication, food transport, and swallowing. In *Functional Vertebrate Morphology*, M. Hildebrand, D. M. Bramble, K. F. Liem, and D. B. Wake, eds. Cambridge, Mass.: Belknap Press, pp. 262–290.

Hinton, R. J. 1981. Form and function in the temporomandibular joint. In *Craniofacial Biology,* D. S. Carlson ed. Monograph no. 10, Craniofacial Growth Series. Ann Arbor, Mich.: Center for Human Growth and Development, pp. 37–60.

Hotton, N., III, P. D. MacLean, J. J. Roth, and E. C. Roth, eds. 1986. *The Ecology and Biology of the Mammal-like Reptiles.* Washington, D.C.: Smithsonian Institution Press.

Huiskes, R., and E. S. Y. Chao. 1983. A survey of finite-element analysis in orthopedic biomechanics: The first decade. Journal of Biomechanics 16: 385–409.

Hylander, W. L. 1979. Mandibular function in *Galago crassicaudatus* and *Macaca fascicularis:* An *in vivo* approach to stress analysis of the mandible. Journal of Morphology 159: 253–296.

———. 1981. Patterns of stress and strain in the macaque mandible. In *Craniofacial Biology,* D. S. Carlson, ed. Monograph no. 10, Craniofacial Growth Series. Ann Arbor, Mich.: Center for Human Growth and Development, pp. 1–35.

———. 1986. *In vivo* bone strain as an indicator of masticatory bite force in *Macaca fascicularis.* Archives of Oral Biology 31: 149–157.

Hylander, W. L., and A. W. Crompton. 1986. Jaw movements and patterns of mandibular bone strain during mastication in the monkey *Macaca fascicularis.* Archives of Oral Biology 31: 841–848.

Hylander, W. L., K. R. Johnson, and A. W. Crompton. 1987. Loading patterns and jaw movements during mastication in *Macaca fascicularis:* A bone-strain, electromyographic, and cineradiographic analysis. American Journal of Physical Anthropology 72: 287–314.

Kemp, T. S. 1972. Whaitsiid therocephalia and the origin of cynodonts. Philosophical Transactions of the Royal Society of London, ser. B, 264: 1–54.

———. 1982. *Mammal-like Reptiles and the Origin of Mammals.* New York: Academic Press.

Klaauw, C. J. van der. 1963. Projections, deepenings, and undulations of the surface of the skull in relation to the attachment of muscles. Verhandelingen der Koninklijke Nederlandse Akademie van Wetenschappen, Afdeling Natuurkunde, Tweede Reeks 55: 1–247, 26 plates.

Krogman, W. M., R. B. Jain, and S. W. Oka. 1982. Craniofacial growth in different cleft types from one month to ten years. Cleft Palate Journal 19: 206–211.

Lanyon, L. E. 1987. Functional strain in bone tissue as an objective, and controlling stimulus for adaptive bone remodelling. Journal of Biomechanics 20: 1083–1093.

Lanyon, L. E., and S. Bourne. 1979. The influences of mechanical function on the development and remodelling of the tibia. Journal of Bone and Joint Surgery 61A: 539–546.

Lauder, G. V. 1985. Aquatic feeding in lower vertebrates. In *Functional Vertebrate Morphology,* M. Hildebrand, D. M. Bramble, K. F. Liem, and D. B. Wake, eds. Cambridge, Mass.: Belknap Press, pp. 210–229.

Lauder, G. V., and L. Lanyon. 1980. Functional anatomy of feeding in the bluegill sunfish *Lepomis macrochirus: In vivo* measurement of bone strain. Journal of Experimental Biology 84: 33–55.

Linderholm, H., and A. Wennström. 1970. Isometric bite force and its relation to general muscle force and body build. Acta odontologica scandinavica 28: 679–689.

Long, C. A. 1985. Intricate sutures as fractal curves. Journal of Morphology 185: 285–295.

Lucas, P. W., R. R. K. Ow, G. M. Ritchie, C. L. Chew, and S. B. Keng. 1986. Relationship between jaw movement and food breakdown in human mastication. Journal of Dental Research 65: 400–404.

Moore, W. J. 1965. Masticatory function and skull growth. Journal of Zoology, London 146: 123–131.

———. 1980. *The Mammalian Skull*. Cambridge: Cambridge University Press.

Moss, J. L., and W. C. Feliciano. 1977. A functional analysis of the fenestrated maxillary bone of the rabbit (*Oryctolagus cuniculus*). Zentralblatt für Veterinärmedizin, Reihe C, Anatomia, Histologia, Embryologia 6: 167–187.

Moss, J. L., H. Vilmann, G. Dasgupta, and R. Skalak. 1981. Craniofacial growth in space-time. In *Craniofacial Biology*, D. S. Carlson, ed. Monograph no. 10, Craniofacial Growth Series. Ann Arbor, Mich.: Center for Human Growth and Development, pp. 61–81.

Moss, M. L. 1985. The application of the finite element method to the analysis of craniofacial growth and form. Acta morphologica neerlando-scandinavica 23: 337–356.

Moss, M. L.,and R. W. Young. 1960. A functional approach to craniology. American Journal of Physical Anthropology 18: 281–292.

Nanda, R., and W. Hickory. 1984. Zygomatico-maxillary suture adaptations incident to anteriorly-directed forces in rhesus monkeys. Angle Orthodontist 54: 199–210.

Park, A. W., and B. J. A. Nowosielski-Slepowron. 1983. Postnatal somatometry of the rat facial skeleton. Acta morphologica neerlando-scandinavica 21: 1–33.

Phillips, P. C.,and R. H. Kaplan. 1987. A personal computer–microscope interface for the analysis of size and shape. Herpetologica 43: 384–385.

Picq, P. G., J. M. Plavcan, and W. L. Hylander. 1987. Nonlever action of the mandible: The return of the Hydra. American Journal of Physical Anthropology 74: 305–307.

Preuschoft, H., B. Demes, M. Meier, and H. F. Bär. 1985. Die biomechanischen Prinzipien im Oberkiefer von langschnauzigen Wirbeltieren. Zeitschrift für morphologisches Anthropologie 76: 1–24.

———. 1986. The biomechanical principles realized in the upper jaw of long-snouted primates. In *Primate Evolution*, vol. 1, J. G. Else and P. C. Lee, eds. Cambridge: Cambridge University Press, pp. 249–264.

Proffit, W. R., and H. W. Fields. 1983. Occlusal forces in normal- and long-face children. Journal of Dental Research 62: 571–574.

Proffit, W. R., H. W. Fields, and W. L. Nixon. 1983. Occlusal forces in normal- and long-face adults. Journal of Dental Research 62: 566–571.

Pruim, G. J., H. J. de Jongh, and J. J. ten Bosch. 1980. Forces acting on the mandible during bilateral static bite at different bite force levels. Journal of Biomechanics 13: 755–763.

Radinsky, L. B. 1970. A new approach to mammalian cranial analysis, illustrated by examples of prosimian primates. Journal of Morphology 124: 167–180.

Richtsmeier, J. T., and J. M. Cheverud. 1986. Finite element scaling analysis of human craniofacial growth. Journal of Craniofacial Genetics and Developmental Biology 6: 289–323.

Ringqvist, M. 1973. Isometric bite force and its relation to dimensions of the facial skeleton. Acta odontologica scandinavica 31: 35–42.

Roark, R. J., and W. C. Young. 1975. *Formulas for Stress and Strain,* 5th ed. New York: McGraw-Hill.

Sarnat, B. G. 1971. Clinical and experimental considerations in facial bone biology: Growth, remodeling, and repair. Journal of the American Dental Association 82: 876–889.

Schoof, S., J. Fanghänel, H. G. Mildschlag, F. Kannmann, and G. H. Schumacher. 1986. Schädeldeformitäten als Folge unilateraler mandibulärer Dysbalance. 2. Quantitative Erfassung der Sekundärveränderungen. Anatomischer Anzeiger 161: 209–214.

Schumacher, G.-H., S. Schoof, J. Fanghänel, G. Mildschlag, and F. Kannmann. 1986. Schädeldeformitäten als Folge unilateraler mandibulärer Dysbalance. 1. Allgemeine Übersichtüber die Sekundärveränderungen. Anatomischer Anzeiger 161: 105–111.

Shipman, P., A. Walker, and D. Bichell. 1985. *The Human Skeleton.* Cambridge: Harvard University Press.

Sinclair, A. G., and R. McN. Alexander. 1987. Estimates of forces exerted by the jaw muscles of some reptiles. Journal of Zoology, London 213: 107–115.

Smiley, G. R., J. C. Hart, and A. D. Dixon. 1971. Growth of the craniofacial complex during formation of the secondary palate. Journal of Dental Research 50 (suppl. to no. 6): 1506–1507.

Smith, D. M., K. R. McLachlan, and W. D. McCall, Jr. 1986. A numerical model of temporomandibular joint loading. Journal of Dental Research 65: 1046–1052.

Smith, J. M., and R. J. G. Savage. 1959. The mechanics of mammalian jaws. School Science Review 40: 289–301.

Smith, K. K., and W. L. Hylander. 1985. Strain gauge measurement of mesokinetic movement in the lizard *Varanus exanthematicus.* Journal of Experimental Biology 114: 53–70.

Thomason, J. J., and A. P. Russell. 1986. Mechanical factors in the evolution of the mammalian secondary palate: A theoretical analysis. Journal of Morphology 189: 199–213.

Thomason, J. J., A. P. Russell, and M. Morgeli. 1990. Forces of biting, body size, and masticatory muscle tension in the opossum *Didelphis virginiana.* Canadian Journal of Zoology 68: 318–324.

Throckmorton, G. S. 1985. Quantitative calculations of temporomandibular joint reaction forces. II. The importance of the direction of the jaw muscle forces. Journal of Biomechanics 18: 453–461.

Tucker, R. 1954a. Studies in functional and analytical craniology. I. The elements of analysis. Australian Journal of Zoology 2: 381–390.

———. 1954b. Studies in functional and analytical craniology. II. The functional classification of mammalian skulls. Australian Journal of Zoology 2: 391–398.

———. 1954c. Studies in functional and analytical craniology. III. The breviarcuate skull and its analysis. Australian Journal of Zoology 2: 399–411.

———. 1954d. Studies in functional and analytical craniology. IV. More extreme forms of the breviarcuate skull. Australian Journal of Zoology 2: 412–418.

———. 1954e. Studies in functional and analytical craniology. VI. Strains and the direction of certain vectors in the breviarcuate skull. Australian Journal of Zoology 2: 427–430.

———. 1955a. Studies in functional and analytical craniology. VII. The longoarcuate skull. Australian Journal of Zoology 3: 513–522.

———. 1955b. Studies in functional and analytical craniology. VIII. The planoarcuate skull. Australian Journal of Zoology 3: 523–529.

———. 1955c. Studies in functional and analytical craniology. IX. The comparative evolutional outlook. Australian Journal of Zoology 3: 530–540.

———. 1955d. Studies in functional and analytical craniology. X. The density of the bony tissue in nodes and tracts. Australian Journal of Zoology 3: 541–546.

Turnbull, W. D. 1970. Mammalian masticatory apparatus. Fieldiana: Geology 18: 149–356.

Urbanus, N. A. M. 1985. The significance of skull growth studies for the treatment of cleft palate patients. Acta morphologica neerlando-scandinavica 23: 369–382.

Van Valkenburgh, B., and C. B. Ruff. 1987. Canine tooth strength and killing behaviour in large carnivores. Journal of Zoology, London 212: 379–397.

Wayne, R. K. 1986. Cranial morphology of domestic and wild canids: The influence of development on morphological change. Evolution 40: 243–261.

Weijs, W. A., P. Brugman, and E. M. Klok. 1987. The growth of the skull and jaw muscles and its functional consequences in the New Zealand rabbit (*Oryctolagus cuniculus*). Journal of Morphology 194: 143–161.

Weijs, W. A., and B. Hillen. 1985. Cross-sectional areas and estimated intrinsic strength of the human jaw muscles. Acta morphologica neerlando-scandinavica 23: 267–274.

Wolff, J. 1892. Das Gestz der Transformation der Knochen. Berlin: A. Hirschwald.

Wragg, L. E. 1971. Facial growth and secondary palate formation. Journal of Dental Research (suppl. to no. 6) 50: 1508–1509.

9

Scaling, Allometry, and Skull Design

SHARON B. EMERSON AND DENNIS M. BRAMBLE

ALL VERTEBRATES INCREASE IN SIZE during development: some such as alligators and bears may grow as much as three orders of magnitude from newborn to adult. Similarly, within the major vertebrate classes, adults of even closely related species often vary widely in body size. ("Body size" refers to mass unless otherwise indicated.) The consequences of such changes of size for morphological shape and function of the skull have long been of interest to biologists.

The vertebrate skull is an extremely complex structure (see, e.g., Moore 1981) involved in a multitude of biological roles from brain protection to food acquisition and processing. The skull can be divided into two functional components, the cerebral skull composed of the braincase and major sensory capsules (eyes and ears), and a facial skull consisting of the jaw apparatus and associated muscle scaffolding (van der Klaauw 1946; Radinsky 1981). Using a simple model of geometric similarity, it is possible to predict how aspects of these components of the vertebrate skull might scale with changes in body size as well as some possible functional consequences of the maintenance of shape. For this chapter a model of geometric similarity will often be used as the null hypothesis against which we compare empirically determined coefficients of scaling within and across species of vertebrates. We chose this model because it is based on the rules and predictions of Euclidean geometry and entails no a priori biological assumptions. Consequently, significant deviations from geometric scaling may be biologically meaningful (or at least potentially so) and can be studied in the context of possible adaptation and constraint.

The cerebral and facial components of the vertebrate skull can be evaluated against a variety of standards—basicranial axis length, skull length, and body size—depending on the particular question under study (Radinsky 1984a). The relationship of any cranial variable to skull length gives an indirect estimation of the effect of size on that cranial variable (because skull length is usually highly correlated with body size), and a direct measure of scale effects on skull shape. (Body weights are rarely known for fossil species; it is therefore common to use skull length as an indirect indicator of size in paleontological studies.) However, some aspects of the facial skull such as jaw length or tooth row length usually comprise a large portion of the skull length. For these components it is advisable to take another independent standard (Radinsky 1981 and references therein). Basicranial axis length has sometimes been used in such situations (e.g., Shea 1985) because it is generally conservative, changing little when other parts of the skull change (Radinsky 1984a). Other skull variables such as brain and sensory capsule size and muscle insertion size are probably determined by overall body size rather than skull length (Radinsky 1981) and so in those cases body size is often a more appropriate standard.

The geometric similarity model predicts that as an object scales up so that its linear dimensions are increased by n, area dimensions will be multiplied by n^2 and volume (or mass) by n^3. These relationships define isometry or maintenance of shape with increases in size. Allometry, or changes in shape with size, occurs when the scaling exponent is greater (= positive allometry) or less (= negative allometry) than that predicted on the basis of geometric similarity. The scaling expectations for some skull variables when maintaining geometric similarity are as follows: orbit area and tooth row surface area will scale as $(mass)^{2/3}$ while brain and bullae volume should scale as $(mass)^{1.0}$. Muscle force, which is a function of the cross-sectional area of a muscle, should scale as $(mass)^{2/3}$, while linear measurements such as jaw length, jaw muscle moment arm length, and tooth row length should all scale as $(mass)^{1/3}$.

The predicted geometric relationships indicate that there can be important functional consequences to maintaining shape with increasing or decreasing size. For example, larger animals have relatively less muscle force, relatively smaller eyes, and relatively less tooth surface area. Deviations from geometric similarity can, on the other hand, produce marked differences in skull shape. For example, empirical work indicates that cranial volume does not scale isometrically with body size but rather with a strong negative allometry (see, e.g., Radinsky 1981). Negative allometry of the cerebral skull with respect to body size results in very differently shaped skulls in large and small animals even among very closely related taxa (fig. 9.1).

The importance of scaling in the evolution of the vertebrate skull can be approached from many perspectives, but we have emphasized the relationship between scaling and constraint, that is, that changes in size can result in a relative loss of function unless there are compensatory adjustments in shape. We will assess this proposition in three sections, which examine: (1) the scaling of the facial skull as a trophic apparatus; (2) the scaling of the cerebral skull through comparison of relative brain and

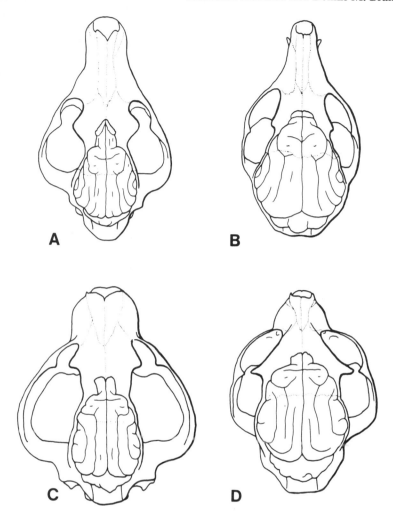

Fig. 9.1. Skulls and brains of large and small canids and felids, to show the effects of changes in shape with size. A. Wolf. B. Desert fox. C. Tiger. D. Domestic cat. All drawn to same length.

braincase size; and (3) ontogenetic scaling of the skull and its implications for phylogenetic change, mechanical performance, and life history patterns.

SCALING OF THE FACIAL SKULL AS THE TROPHIC APPARATUS

The scaling of morphological features of the skull with increasing body size is often suggested to play an important role in determining prey type and size. But this idea has rarely been tested by comparing actual performance via direct comparisons of relative prey size and the slope of prey size/predator size curves with predictions based on the scaling of relevant morphological features (but see Hespenheide 1971; Schoener 1974; Toft 1980). Instead, what little work that has been done has concentrated on the relationship between skull shape and prey type.

The importance of morphological scaling in relation to prey type has probably been explored most thoroughly in mammals. Here the skull shapes of some herbivores and carnivores appear to parallel, in part, those of large and small animals. Herbivorous ungulate mammals have long facial components with large angular processes and a large moment arm for the masseter muscle, while the temporal fossa and coronoid process are reduced relative to most carnivores. Appropriate out-group comparisons indicate that the carnivore morphology represents the primitive condition of mammalian skull and jaw proportions (Radinsky 1985b). Ungulates generally have larger body sizes than most carnivorers. The question then arises as to whether scaling factors related to differences in body size alone can account for the contrasting skull designs of ungulates and carnivores.

A comparison of slopes for the various morphological features of the skull reveals that the moment arm of the masseter and size of the angular process scale isometrically to cheek tooth resistance arm in both carnivores and ungulates (Radinsky 1985b). However, in most modern ungulates temporal fossa length and coronoid process height are negatively allometric with respect to cheek tooth resistance arm, while in carnivores the relationships are generally isometric. This suggests that for most modern ungulates these features will be relatively smaller in larger species. Facial skull length scales with positive allometry on basicranial axis length in both ungulates and carnivores. These data indicate that some of the distinctions in skull shape between smaller carnivores and larger herbivorous ungulates (i.e., temporal fossa length, coronoid process height, facial skull length) do indeed appear to be a consequence of simple allometric scaling. Nonetheless, the enlarged angular process, which has evolved independently at least 12 times in herbivorous mammals (Radinsky 1985b), cannot be explained in this way. Rather, this feature has arisen through transpositional shifts (changes in y-intercept without corresponding adjustments in slope) that are unrelated to body size (Radinsky 1985a).

Two Southeast Asian frogs, *Rana ingeri* and *Rana ibanorum,* offer an interesting example of how the intraspecific scaling of skull morphology can influence feeding behavior. In both species there is marked sexual dimorphism in the size of the jaw-closing musculature and dimensions of the skull. Relative to females, males have broader, longer skulls and a more robust jaw musculature as a result of a positive growth allometry in these features (Smith 1922; Inger 1966). A survey of the stomach contents shows

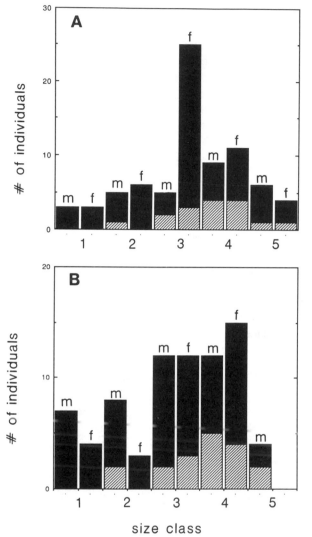

Fig. 9.2. A. Stomach contents of *Rana ingeri*. Size classes are indicated by numbers 1 to 5. Size class 1 includes males (m) and females (f) less than 70 mm in snout vent length. Size class 2 shows animals 70 to 80 mm. Animals in size class 3 are 80 to 90 mm and in size class 4, 90 to 100 mm. Size class 5 animals are over 100 mm snout vent length. Shaded area represents the number of stomachs containing crabs. Black area shows the total number of stomachs examined. B. Stomach contents of *Rana ibanorum*. Symbols are the same as in (A).

that crabs make up a small but significant portion of the diet for both species (Inger 1969). An analysis of crab eating as a function of body size reveals that the stomachs of juvenile frogs (< 70 mm) never contain crabs (fig. 9.2). Presumably this is because either the juvenile frogs cannot generate the absolute muscle force necessary to crack the crab, or the mouth of the juvenile frog is too small to accommodate the size of the crabs available. For frogs between 70 and 80 mm in body length only males have crabs in their diet. At body sizes exceeding 80 mm, crabs are found in the stomachs of both males and females. Owing to differential allometries for some features of the skull, males are able to incorporate a new food type into their diet at a smaller size than are females.

For most vertebrates, prey size increases with predator size. The use of predictive models of prey size to predator size to link skull morphology to prey choice has so far been restricted largely to those cases where prey size is actually limited by bite force (e.g., Kiltie 1982; Wainwright 1987). It is, however, possible to make precise quantitative predictions about the expected slope of the relationship between prey size and predator size for any pertinent morphological variable. To do so requires, however, that the biomechanics of feeding be understood for the particular food type.

In the general case,

$$S \ \alpha \ K_1 M^{x_1},$$

where S = skull variable involved in prey capture or processing; K_1 = constant, M = predator size; x_1 = allometric coefficient, and

$$P \ \alpha \ K_2 S^{x_2},$$

where P = prey size, K_2 = constant, x_2 = allometric coefficient by substitution,

$$P \ \alpha \ K_2 \ (K_1 M^{x_1})^{x_2}$$

and

$$P \ \alpha \ constant \ (M)^{x_1 \cdot x_2}$$

Prey size should scale to predator size as the product of the allometric coefficients of predator skull morphology to predator size and prey size to that particular aspect of skull morphology (fig. 9.3).

Most previous studies which have attempted to relate aspects of skull morphology to prey size have relied on measures of correlation (e.g., Grant et al. 1976; Toft 1980). Generally, most features of the body are correlated with overall body size and their effects on prey size are similarly correlated (Wainwright 1987). Through a comparison of the slopes of the relationship between (1) prey size and predator size, (2) feeding morphology and prey size, and (3) feeding morphology and predator size, one can test hypotheses of causality linking prey size to aspects of skull morphology. If there is no congruence in slope between that predicted on the basis of the scaling of a specific skull variable and actual prey/predator size relationship, the hypothesis that a particular aspect of the skull limits prey size is not supported, at least over the known size range of the animals. (It is possible that a particular feature of the skull could be limiting at a specific size, but not over the entire intra- or interspecific size range under study.) In those cases where there is no match between slopes it may be that other mor-

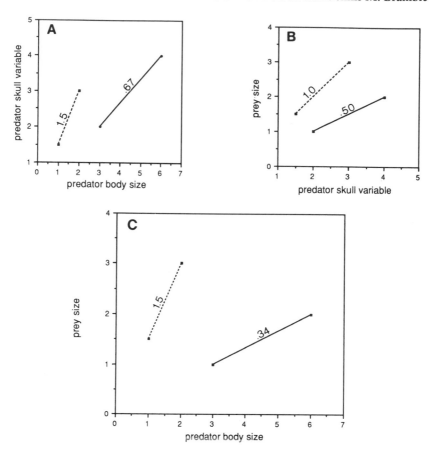

Fig. 9.3. Two hypothetical examples illustrating the multiplicative effect of the scaling relationship of (A) predator skull variable to predator body size and (B) prey size to the same predator skull variable on (C) the slope of the prey/predator size curve. The dotted line represents a predator with a positive allometry in skull trophic morphology and the solid line a predator with a negative allometry in the same variable. Notice the differing effect of these allometries on the prey/predator slopes of the two predators. (See text for further explanation.)

phological features of the skull, prey availability, or competition from other species in the community are influencing the slope of the prey/predator size curve. A test for similarity of slopes can be used to examine the first of these possibilities. Nonequality of slopes for a series of morphological variables certainly suggests consideration of nonmechanical factors.

By testing for similarity of slopes between an actual prey/predator curve and that predicted on the basis of the scaling of a particular morphological feature of the skull to predator and prey size, the scaling approach can be extended beyond features which are absolutely limiting (e.g., bite force) to include aspects of the trophic apparatus which only indirectly determine prey size. Morphological aspects of the skull can impose a scaling constraint on the prey/predator size relationship even if they are not absolutely limiting. For example, differences in head size between fossorial and nonfossorial lizards result in a different scaling relationship between relative prey size and time to swallow and chew prey (Andrews et al. 1987). Fossorial lizards can eat food the same size as nonfossorial lizards up to a prey/predator mass ratio of .068, but the costs associated with eating increase with a much steeper slope in the fossorial lizards. The steepness of the cost of total time to chew and swallow prey effectively "limits" fossorial lizards to smaller prey even though they could physically take much larger items. In this case head size is scaling with prey size but is not imposing an absolute mechanical limit in contrast to those examples involving bite force (e.g., Kiltie 1982; Wainwright 1987). Instead, the scaling of head shape appears to be mediating the prey/predator size relationship in fossorial lizards through scaling differences in prey handling costs.

Given a predicted slope for the relationship between prey size and predator size, it is possible to ask the degree to which scale effects impose a constraint on relative prey size for the system as well as whether identified biomechanical aspects of the skull morphology determine prey capture and/or processing ability.

The model as presented shows a multiplicative effect of the scaling of skull morphology to predator size and to prey size (fig. 9.3). Any morphological variable scaling with a negative allometry to either predator size or prey size will strongly depress the prey/predator curve (fig. 9.3). A skull variable scaling with a positive allometry will greatly increase relative prey size (fig. 9.3). Clades that show a strong positive allometry in skull variables relative to body size might be expected to have their biggest members eat relatively larger prey than clades that lack positive allometry. Conversely, those big animals eating relatively large prey might be predicted to belong most frequently to clades exhibiting a strong positive allometry for trophic components of the skull. This particular association has rarely been examined by quantifying prey/predator sizes across the same taxa for which morphological data on the skull have been gathered, but it has sometimes been examined in a more qualitative fashion (e.g., Toft 1980; Emerson 1985).

Four genera of frogs which eat relatively large prey, *Ceratophrys, Lepidobatrachus, Pyxicephalus,* and *Megophrys,* are among the largest members of their respective families (Emerson 1985). Biomechanical models predict that in frogs a wide skull and long jaws will be important determinants of prey size (Toft 1980; Emerson 1985). Skull width scales with positive allometry in two of the three families to which these genera belong. Jaw length scales isometrically with body length in all three families.

Varanus komodoensis, the Komodo dragon, is a giant among lizards, reaching a body size in excess of 50 kg (Auffenberg 1981). Members of this species commonly feed on prey equal to or larger than themselves (Auffenberg 1981). Most smaller species of *Varanus* eat relatively smaller prey and even the occasional large item in their diet is only a fraction of their size (Greene 1986; Losos and Greene 1988). Komodo dragons do not swallow their large prey whole but divide it into sections for swallow-

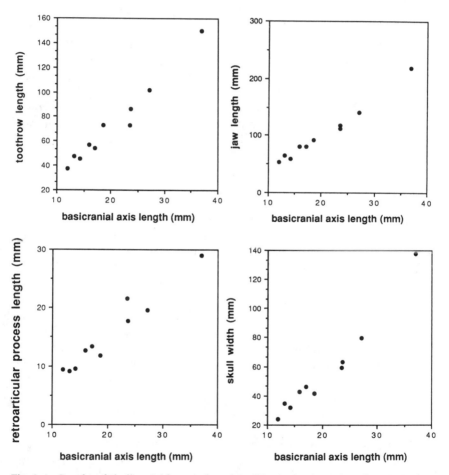

Fig. 9.4. Graphs of skull variables as a function of basicranial axis length (BCAL) for nine species of varanid lizards. *Varanus komodoensis* has the longest basicranial axis length in all graphs. See table 9.1 for regression equations.

TABLE 9.1   Interspecific scaling of skull variables in varanid lizards (N = 9)

Variable	Least-squares slope (b)	Intercept (a)	Correlation coefficient (r)
Tooth row length (TRL)	1.11	.400	.97
Skull width (SW)	1.26[a]	.069	.96
Temporal fossa width (TFW)	1.30[a]	−.373	.90
Retroarticular process length (RAL)	1.09	−.236	.94
Jaw length (JL)	1.18[a]	.467	.99

Notes: All values based on equation: log y = b log (BCAL) + a. Key to measurements and their functional/biological significance: BCAL, basicranial axis length measured from occipital condyle to tip of dorsum sellae. JL, measured from center of articulation for quadrate to tip of symphysis. Measures moment arm of resistance when biting at front of mouth. RAL, measured from center of glenoid on mandible to tip of process. Estimates moment arm of the depressor mandibulae. SW, measured across outer edges of quadrates. TFW, width of the upper temporal fenestra, measured across longest diameter, estimates size of the adductor mandibulae externus medialis and pseudotemporalis. TRL, measured from base of most posterior tooth present in jaw to base of most anterior tooth.
[a] Indicates significant positive allometry (slopes > 1.00).

ing. Nonetheless, *V. komodoensis* is characterized as an extremely fast feeder who swallows very large pieces of prey at one time (Auffenberg 1981).

Simple biomechanical models (e.g., Radinsky 1981; Emerson 1985) extrapolated to the reptile skull suggest that skull width, tooth row length, size of the adductor musculature, jaw length, and length of the retroarticular process are important morphological variables in relation to the rapid eating of large food items. These variables were measured in nine species of *Varanus* and regressed against basicranial axis length (total size was unavailable for most specimens). Figure 9.4 shows that *V. komodoensis* has a typical skull (in terms of measured variables) for a monitor lizard of that size. Table 9.1 indicates that most of the measured morphological variables of the skull scale with positive allometry is varanids. The retroarticular process or moment arm of the jaw depressor muscle, however, does not show positive allometry. This finding is consistent with predictions from biomechanical models that indicate an inverse relationship between length of the retroarticular process and speed of jaw opening (Emerson 1985). The Komodo dragon may be one example where strong phylogenetic allometry has resulted in a dramatic shift in relative prey size in descendant species of large body size.

RELATIVE BRAIN SIZE AND SCALING OF THE CEREBRAL SKULL

For many vertebrates the brain completely fills the cranial cavity and differences in brain size reflect variation in braincase shape. While the literature has focused on relative brain size, the same data also reflect the scaling of the braincase component of the cerebral skull. In fact, measurements of brain size constitute the largest available data set on intra- and interspecific scaling of the vertebrate skull. These data show a clear, repetitive pattern across vertebrates. Both intra- and interspecifically, braincase size scales with a negative allometry to body size.

This scaling relationship may have interesting biomechanical ramifications for other aspects of skull morphology and function. For example, as shown in the previous section, the scaling exponent of the trophic apparatus to body size has a multiplicative effect on the scaling relationship of prey size to predator size. If geometric similarity is maintained in the relationship of jaw muscle cross-sectional area to body size, the masticatory muscles of larger animals will generate relatively less force than those of smaller animals. This, in turn, will markedly depress the slope of the prey/predator size relationship. However, the negative allometry of the braincase results in larger animals having a relatively as well as absolutely wider space between the braincase and zygomatic arch (fig. 9.1). Since this space accommodates part of the jaw musculature, its relative increase with size could provide an avenue for larger animals to maintain trophic function (i.e., prey/predator size relationships) through a positive allometry in jaw muscle size.

Unfortunately, analyses such as that suggested by the preceding example (i.e., the biomechanical consequences of the scaling relationship between braincase and body size) have not been explored for any group of vertebrates. Rather, workers have concentrated on differences in relative brain size. A review of this literature is presented below in order to exemplify some of the limitations that may arise in allometric studies when causation is implied from correlation. It also provides an opportunity to evaluate recent quantitative genetic approaches toward an understanding of the mechanisms responsible for allometric scaling patterns.

The usefulness of models such as that of geometric similarity depends on some a priori knowledge of the functional significance of a skull variable when generating predictions of its scaling relationship to body size. Where insufficient information is available and a posteriori interpretations of slope are attempted, insights appear to be more limited. Perhaps the best example of this problem can be found in the literature on brain size/body size relationships. Numerous studies across vertebrates initially documented differences in relative brain size and the scaling relationships between brain and body size. Closely related species or adults of a single species often show an allometric coefficient of 0.2 to 0.4 (but see Martin and Harvey 1985). Across higher taxonomic levels the relationship shifts to 0.50 to 0.77. Subsequent work on relative brain size has concentrated on trying to explain these divergent scaling coefficients as well as their biological meaning.

A slope of 0.67 among distantly related taxa has suggested to some workers (e.g., Jerison 1973) that brain size is actually correlated with body surface. This argument presumes that surface effectors and receptors determine, in large measure, brain size (Brandt 1867). This relationship requires, in turn, that surface area of the body scale with a slope of 0.67 on body mass and that the density of surface effectors and receptors remain constant and size independent (Armstrong 1985). Empirical data show that while surface area generally does scale as the 0.67 power of body mass, the density of effectors and receptors is variable (Armstrong 1985).

The slope of 0.75 has led others to link relative brain size to metabolism. It has been argued that brain size might scale as a metabolic variable for two reasons: (1) the development of the embryonic brain depends on maternal metabolic turnover (Martin 1981) and (2) the size of the brain is constrained by the amount of available oxygen and energy, and metabolic rate estimates such availability (Armstrong 1983). Whatever the reason for the particular scaling relationship among distantly related taxa, it is important to keep in mind that the slope depends, in part, on which taxa are included in the calculations (Armstrong 1985; Martin and Harvey 1985). Therefore the fact that a particular exponent is correlated with one biological process or another is not a strong argument for causality.

One possible explanation for the discrepancy of slope between taxonomic levels is that brain and body size are genetically correlated and that selection during differentiation of closely related species works primarily on body size. But the steeper slope at higher taxonomic levels is thought to reflect selection acting (in parallel in various lineages) directly on brain size (Lande 1979 and references therein). Evidence supporting this hypothesis comes from artificial selection experiments in mice which show a genetic correlation between brain and body size and that selection on body size alone yields an allometric slope of 0.36 while selection for brain size alone yields a slope of 0.77 (Lande 1979).

More recently, another group of workers (Atchley et al. 1984) has suggested that differences in slope at various taxonomic levels are again the result of a genetic correlation between brain and body size, but with selection working directly on body size in both cases. They postulate that selection operating on body size at early stages of development produces the slope of 0.67 seen among distantly related taxa while selection on body size at later ontogenetic stages produces the lower slope of 0.2 to 0.4 seen among closely related species (Riska and Atchley 1985). As evidence, they offer the results of an ontogenetic study on mice which show that the genetic correlation between brain and body size varies during development, being higher during the early stages of ontogeny. Furthermore, early growth is generally characterized by an increase in cell number, while later growth is largely hypertrophic, occurring through an increase in cell size. Distantly related taxa of different sizes are primarily characterized by differences in cell number. This observation is offered as supportive evidence that a major divergence in body size results from selection on the earlier stages of growth.

Both of these explanations, while plausible, rest on assumptions for which there are no, few, or contradictory data. Both hypotheses assume that the genetic correlations found in mice are ubiquitous among mammals (in fact all vertebrates) and are also constant through evolutionary time (Turelli 1988). Recent work has shown, however, that variance-covariance matrices are not necessarily similar even among closely related species (e.g., Loftsvold 1986). Moreover, in house mice indirect genetic effects have now been found to play a significant role in the evolution of brain size (Leamy 1988). Additionally, a study on Japanese quail revealed no indirect response of brain size to direct selection on body size at four weeks of age, again suggesting that there was no genetic correlation between brain and body size in this species (Ricklefs and Marks 1984). Both explanations also assume that selection has worked primarily on body size with brain size changes reflecting an indirect response due to pleiotropy. There is no reason to suppose, however, that selection could not work on both traits or even on some other character to which both brain and body size are linked. Also, while both hypotheses provide plausible mechanisms for producing the differences in slope at various taxonomic levels, neither explicitly suggests an explanation for why the same scaling coefficients occur repeatedly across vertebrates.

Most recently it has been suggested that the discrepancy in slopes across taxonomic levels might be, in part, statistical artifact (Pagel and Harvey 1988). Simulations show that unequal variances of x and y variables can result in slope shifts between levels of comparison similar to those observed for brain-body size relationships in mammals. While we may be closer to understanding the mechanisms which might produce varying slopes or scaling relationships of brain size (and braincase) to body size, we still have little insight into the biological significance of specific, recurrent allometric coefficients in vertebrates.

ONTOGENETIC SCALING

Perhaps more explicitly than any other, the concept of ontogenetic scaling embodies Haeckel's classic notion of a causal linkage between development and phylogeny. In the sense used here (sensu Shea 1985), ontogenetic scaling implies that size-correlated proportional differences between populations or species are the same as those produced within a single population by the extension of a common growth trajectory. Thus, the shape of larger (or older) individuals may depart significantly from that of smaller individuals only because the former have progressed farther along a growth curve that is strongly allometric. The general topic of ontogenetic scaling has been the subject of several thoughtful discussions (Cock 1966; Gould 1966; Shea 1983b, c, 1985).

That phylogenetic alterations in form and function might arise easily and perhaps rapidly via simple extension or truncation of an ancestral developmental pattern is intrinsically appealing and, indeed, has often been invoked as a causal explanation for observed evolutionary change (Huxley 1932; Hersch 1934; Rensch 1959; Robb 1935a; Gould 1966; Reeve 1941; Giles 1956; Shea 1983a, 1985; Strauss 1984). The appeal of ontogenetic scaling as a vehicle for evolutionary change has no doubt been heightened by renewed interest in "simple" developmental mechanisms as a plausible basis for rapid, macroevolutionary change (Gould 1977; Alberch et al. 1979; Alberch 1980). Recently, however, workers in quantitative genetics have pointed out serious problems with inferring mechanisms of evolutionary change from these "simple" patterns of phenotypic allometry (Lande 1979, 1985; Cheverud 1982; Atchley and Rutledge 1980; Atchley 1983). At the least such an inference assumes that phenotypic and genotypic covariance patterns are similar. Yet, in the few species of vertebrates for which information has become available, phenotypic relationships do not necessarily mirror genetic relationships (e.g., Atchley 1983; Emerson et al. 1988; but see Cheverud 1988). Therefore, patterns of phenotypic allometry do not, by themselves, constitute an adequate test for the hypothesis that evolutionary changes in shape with size are the result of a simple process—i.e., sliding up or down an ancestral ontogenetic trajectory. They can, however, provide important data on the maintenance of structural integrity and shifts in functional capability associated with changes in size. This issue is the primary focus of the following discussion. Classic terms from the literature on heterochrony (see, e.g., Alberch et al. 1979) will be used to describe patterns of change in shape with size, but should not be taken to imply mechanism.

By way of introduction, we have tabulated some characteristic patterns of morphologic change that accompany postnatal cranial growth in tetrapod vertebrates (table 9.2). Empirical observations indicate that in nearly all cases accelerated differentiation of the CNS and sensory capsules yields embryos and neonates having large braincases, eyes, and auditory regions relative to the trophic components of the craniomandibular complex (fig. 9.5A). Consequently, relative reduction of the braincase and primary sensory structures coupled with proportional enlargement of the facial/rostral region are inherent features of normal postnatal skull development (figs. 9.5B, C). These changes are, of course, invariably associated with absolute size increase.

TABLE 9.2 Expected cranial allometries in tetrapod postnatal development

Feature	Isometry	Positive allometry	Negative allometry
Sensory capsules[1]			+
Braincase			+
Foramen magnum			+
Rostral (jaw) length	+	+	
Tooth area		+	
Muscle mass[2]		+	
Skeletal mass		+	

Note: All comparisons are intracranial using basal length as the standard of skull size.
[1] Applies only to auditory and optic capsules.
[2] Applies to chief adductor muscles.

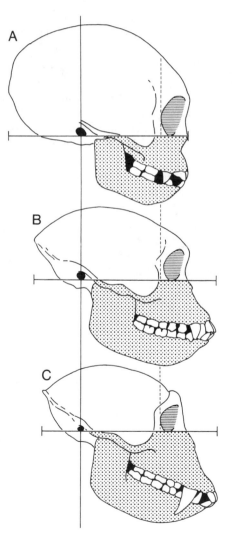

Fig. 9.5. Ontogenetic allometry in the rhesus monkey, *Macaca mulatta,* illustrating influence of age, size, and sex on cranial morphology. Specimens are an infant (A) and female (B) and male (C) adults. All skulls have been drawn to the same maximum skull length (= incisors to occipital prominence). Skulls are oriented to the same horizontal plane and aligned on a vertical axis passing through the external auditory meatus. The figure reveals strong negative allometry of the braincase (unshaded) and orbits (hatched) as well as pronounced positive allometry of the primary trophic complex (stippled). Notice that the relative reduction of the postotic braincase is much greater than the preotic braincase. Also note that the relative distance between the otic and orbital regions remains nearly constant despite substantial allometric distortion in the surrounding areas of the skull. (Modified from Cochard 1985.)

Thus, simple evolutionary extensions of the ancestral growth curve (i.e., hypermorphosis) will necessarily involve size increase and relative reduction of optic and auditory (but not olfactory) components together with an increase in the ratio of facial to braincase size. Exactly the opposite trend will apply to those phylogenetic transformations showing a pattern of simple ontogenetic truncation (i.e., progenesis). It must be emphasized, however, that these are the anticipated consequences of pure ontogenetic scaling. Not only are such cases likely to be rare in nature (see below), but there also exist more complex situations in which, for example, adjustments in the rate of growth can alter the relationship between absolute size and shape (Alberch et al. 1979; Shea 1983a, b, 1985).

On the intraspecific level there are a number of instances in which sexually dimorphic cranial traits may be traced to ontogenetic scaling (fig. 9.5). Recent studies of macaques (Cochard 1985) and gorillas (Shea 1983c, 1985) have shown that most of the major shape differences that serve to distinguish the crania of adult males from those of females are not the expression of sexual differences in ontogenetic growth allometries. Instead, they reflect only the fact that males, which are considerably larger than females, are routed further along a mutual growth trajectory which incorporates significant allometry (figs. 9.6A, B). It is worth noting, however, that in these examples and most others not all sexually dimorphic features can be explained on this basis. In macaques, for instance, the ontogenetic scaling of most dental traits differs strongly between the sexes (Cochard 1985). Hence the dramatically larger canines of adult males are not simply a consequence of growth to larger body size, but are attributable to the much higher allometric coefficient for canine length in males ($b = 1.91$ versus 0.94 for females, where isometry is 1.0) throughout ontogeny (fig. 9.6D). The apparent uncoupling of dental from skeletal allometry also occurs in gorillas (Shea 1983c).

Strong parallels between intraspecific ontogenetic allometry and interspecific scaling relationships have been documented in a number of tetrapod groups. Included are animals as phylogenetically diverse as cichlid fishes (Strauss 1984), plethodontid salamanders (Alberch and Alberch 1981), iguanid lizards (Dodson 1975b), anteaters (Reeve 1941), dogs (Lumer 1940; Wayne 1986), and great apes (Shea 1983a, b, c, 1985). In the latter case, quantitative data now seem to support Giles's (1956) earlier hypothesis that the exaggerated cranial morphology of the gorilla (especially adult males) is more or less what would be expected had this very large ape evolved from a much smaller chimplike ancestor via simple hypermorphosis. Most basic cranial dimensions, exclusive of the dentition, are in fact closely predicted by simple extension of the chimp growth curve (Shea 1983c, 1985).

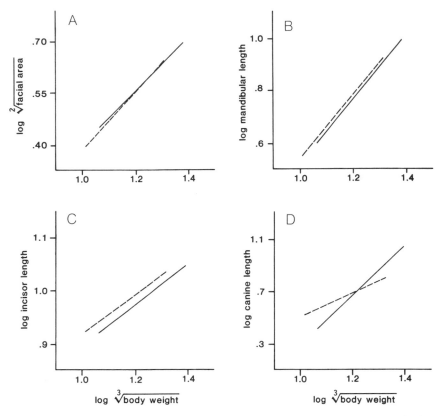

Fig. 9.6. Ontogenetic allometries for selected skull parameters regressed against body weight in growth series of male (solid lines) and female (broken lines) *Macaca mulatta.* Facial area (A) and mandibular length (B) are examples of ontogenetic scaling. Relative incisor length (C) is significantly larger in females than in males and is an example of an allometric transposition. The relatively larger canines (D) of adult males result from a much higher allometric growth coefficient than in females. See text. (Modified from Cochard 1985.)

In another presumably simple and well-publicized example of onto-genetic scaling, the actual situation has proven to be much more complex. Robb's (1935a, b) original study seemed to suggest that the historical transformation of the equid cranium from Eocene *Hyracotherium* to modern *Equus* could be understood largely in terms of simple ontogenetic scaling. In particular, it was asserted that the relative elongation of the muzzle as recorded in Tertiary horse evolution was more or less exactly mirrored in the allometric growth trajectory of modern *Equus*. However, Reeve and Murray's (1942) subsequent analysis revealed that equid cranial phylogeny did not repeat *Equus* ontogeny. They instead argued that the horse skull had undergone significant structural reorganization during its evolution. This was particularly true of the facial region, presumably in response to the appearance (in the mid-Tertiary) of large, high-crowned cheek teeth.

Using more sophisticated quantitative approaches, Radinsky (1983, 1984b) has since demonstrated that evolution of the equid skull is a complex amalgam of both ontogenetic scaling and morphologic reorganization. He found, for example, that total tooth row length (a close measure of rostral length) does scale with strong positive interspecific allometry in fossil equids, but the scaling coefficient (b = ~1.24) is not meaningfully different in lineages possessing low- or high-crowned cheek teeth. This relationship alone predicts that relative elongation of the muzzle will accompany phylogenetic size increase during horse evolution. However, the postnatal ontogenetic trajectory for this parameter (= total tooth row length) in domestic horses scales very differently and, in fact, shows strong negative allometry (b = 0.803). The same scaling relationship holds for static intraspecific comparisons among a size-graded series of adult horses. Nonetheless, another functionally relevant parameter of the equid cranium, the moment arm of the masseter muscle, scales with essentially the same positively allometric exponent (b = ~1.31) in the postnatal ontogeny of domestic horses and phylogenetic series of low-crowned equids (Radinsky 1984a, b).

Devillers et al. (1984) have also reexamined equid cranial evolution in light of growth patterns. Their data indicate that in equids generally, postnatal growth of the muzzle (= preorbital region) scales isometrically with the braincase (= postorbital region). Throughout much of prenatal development, however, a different relationship obtains. In utero the scaling coefficient for muzzle length relative to braincase length declines from approximately 1.58 early in development to roughly 1.02 at the time of birth. Both the median and mean scaling values provided by Devillers et al. (1984) suggest that the average prenatal scaling factor for relative muzzle length is about 1.30. This is much closer to the overall phylogenetic exponent (~1.24) calculated by Radinsky (1984b) than is his value for postnatal growth (i.e., ~0.80). Unfortunately, Radinsky (1984b) and Devillers et al. (1984) use different measures of muzzle and braincase length and, hence, their results cannot be compared directly. Given that modern horses are highly precocial, with extended prenatal development, it is possible that in utero scaling relationships may be more relevant to a complete assessment of ontogenetic and phylogenetic scaling than would otherwise be expected.

Evolutionary Potential of Ontogenetic Scaling Patterns

That developmental processes can be a major reservoir of raw material for evolutionary morphologic change is so widely acknowledged as to require no additional comment. That any given ontogenetic trajectory could simply be extended and thus serve as the basis for phylogenetic transformation is, however, a much more explicit and debatable proposal. Still, to the extent that such curves may be extended, they might legitimately be viewed as mechanisms of preadaptation whose evolutionary promise is expressed chiefly through the "power of extrapolation" (Frazzetta 1975; Shea 1985).

Any suggestion that ontogenies are evolutionarily preadaptive via extrapolation assumes that such a process will not be precluded by intrinsic constraints. To our knowledge there are few quantitative data bearing either on the developmental limitations or on the functional consequences of ontogenetic extension within or between species. Certainly within normal development, serious limitations are imposed by differential growth (Huxley 1932; Gould 1966). Many structures which experienced very rapid size increase early in development (e.g., brain and sensory capsules) must later shift to isometric or negative allometric growth if undesirable distortions of the adult cranium are to be avoided.

Growth trajectories that incorporate strong allometries necessarily mean that substantial shape change will accompany size increase. In theory this may serve to maintain function that would otherwise be sacrificed were growth to proceed geometrically. But in most cases, significant ontogenetic alteration in size, shape, and proportion almost certainly yields functional change as well. Here growth is viewed properly as a continuum of size- (and age-) correlated shifts in function wherein the cessation of growth may well be required in order to hold morphological form within functionally acceptable limits.

For these reasons, we suspect that many ontogenetic trajectories may not be extrapolatable to any great extent without functional compromise. The more pronounced the allometries involved, the more likely that this is true. Whereas selection for significantly larger body size was made functionally permissible by the ontogenetic trajectory of the chimplike ancestor of gorillas (Shea 1983c, 1985), it is not at all certain that the much more exaggerated craniofacial allometries inherent in baboon growth could be extended to a comparable degree. Within a much more restricted range of size, however, the fairly pronounced differences in skull proportions among species or races of *Papio* do seem to reflect ontogenetic scaling (Freedman 1962).

Black-tailed jackrabbits (*Lepus californicus*) provide one possible example wherein intrinsic growth trajectories limit the potential for ontogenetic extrapolation. During growth the cranium of these hares becomes relatively lighter, such that overall skull mass scales with significant negative allometry on skull length (fig. 9.7) (Bramble 1989). Lightening of the cranium is accomplished in two ways: (1) progressive fenestration of the lat-

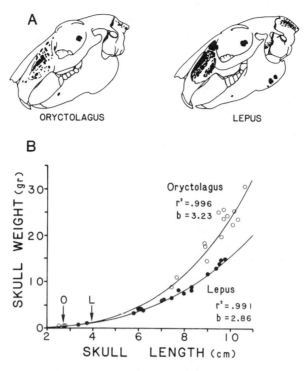

Fig. 9.7. Allometric growth in cranial fenestration and its influence on skull weight in the leporid lagomorphs, *Oryctolagus cuniculus* and *Lepus californicus*. A. Adult crania showing more extensive fenestration (especially rostral) of *Lepus*. B. Allometric growth relationships between skull weight and length in the two species. *Oryctolagus* exhibits positive allometry and *Lepus* negative allometry. Both curves differ significantly from isometry (b = 3.00). Arrows indicate approximate sizes of crania at birth (from Bramble 1989).

eral rostrum and the occipital regions; (2) relative expansion of the large incisive foramina and choanal passages. The latter tends to reduce the size of the osseous palate. As a consequence of these growth processes, the adult skull of *L. californicus* is remarkably lightweight, having only about half the mass of a rabbit (i.e., *Oryctolagus*) cranium of equal size. The light skull of *Lepus* is thought to be one of several strategies for reducing overall head weight which, in turn, may facilitate the maintenance of head stability in these highly cursorial leporids (Bramble 1989).

But these same, presumably adaptive, growth processes would also appear to limit developmental and evolutionary extrapolation in *Lepus*. The scaling of skull mass indicates that if extended to significantly larger size, the cranium would become increasingly fragile and, in fact, would be expected to have little bone remaining in those areas that are heavily fenestrated. At some point this would presumably lead to structural compromise or failure. Secondly, the scaling of palatal length as compared to the length of the incisive foramina predicts that the latter will approach and then exceed the former in specimens having a basicranial length roughly four times larger than a modern adult *L. californicus* (Bramble, unpublished data). Because the incisive foramina are large, unossified vacuities within the palate, it is probable that the structural integrity and load-bearing capacity of the rostrum would become limiting well before the incisive foramina actually expanded to the full length of the palate.

In theory, ontogenetic scaling as a vehicle of morphologic change in evolution should exhibit a directional bias. That is, simple extensions of growth trajectories (= hypermorphosis) are necessarily made into uncharted territory as regards functional capacity and structural integration. (An exception would be those species earlier evolved through progenesis.) Conversely, evolutionary truncation of development, as in progenesis, amounts to a retreat into morphological space that is known to be viable. From this perspective we expect that phylogenetic size reduction might frequently be accompanied by ontogenetic scaling of shape variables without meaningful departure from ancestral growth curves. This should not be true, however, of phylogenetic size increase involving extension of growth trajectories. The latter should more often be characterized by developmental reorganization as required to circumvent structural/functional limitations. Such reorganizational patterns include those that permit an uncoupling of size and shape (e.g., allometric transposition) or a change in the allometric coefficient (as in neoteny).

In this general context ontogenetic scaling, like geometric scaling, can constitute a null hypothesis when it is employed as "a criterion of subtraction" (Pilbeam and Gould 1974; Gould 1975; Shea 1985). That is, the extension (or truncation) of a known growth trajectory gives a quantitative prediction of morphological organization in possible descendant species. Adults of closely related species of varying body size can then be compared to this standard in order to determine whether and in what way(s) they deviate from it. In this manner expected size-correlated shape changes can be factored out or "subtracted" from the actual morphology of the species under examination. Significant residuals (i.e., following subtraction) signal departure from the null hypothesis (= simple ontolgenetic scaling). These signals may be used to identify morphological parameters which possibly required alteration of the ancestral growth pattern during phylogenetic transformation either to maintain function at differing body size (i.e., biomechanical scaling; Shea 1985) or as adaptive responses to shifts in function, behavior, or ecology.

The criterion of subtraction is itself a test of the hypothesis of an ontogenetic scaling pattern. Though qualified data sets are relatively few, the incidence of discordant scaling in ontogenetic versus interspecific series does suggest that simple extrapolation of ancestral growth allometries is infrequently the basis of phylogenetic transformation. Even in examples which largely conform to the expectations of ontogenetic scaling, close examination reveals an appreciable suite of growth parameters that do not fit this model. Thus, although most measures of overall skull shape indicate ontogenetic scaling in the pygmy chimp–common chimp–gorilla series studied by Shea (1983c), many detailed aspects of cranial morphology do not. Much the same situation exists for the scaling of skull form in lizards (Dodson 1975b), dogs (Wayne 1986), and also for some aspects of sexual dimorphism in macaque crania (fig. 9.6) (Cochard 1985).

Species-specific differences in allometric scaling exponents are to be expected if one accepts the view that strong growth allometries may set an upper limit on adult body size (Gould 1966, 1971; Dodson 1975b). More specifically, there should exist an inverse relationship between body size and the strength of the allometric coefficient for the growth of homologous structures among closely related species. Dodson (1975b) found support for this prediction in the skull growth and allometry of the lizard *Sceloporus*. Progressive reduction of the scaling exponent for the area of the temporal fossa is also found among a size-graded series of great apes (Shea 1983c). In this case the functional result is that the area occupied by the muscle mass is appreciably less in adult gorillas than would be expected on the basis of extrapolation of the growth curves of chimpanzees.

Allometric transpositions, or changes in the scaling constant without adjustments in the scaling coefficient, are commonly encountered in inter- and sometimes intraspecific comparisons of growth trajectories (fig. 9.6C) as well as in static intraspecific allometries (Walton and Hammond 1938; Kurten 1954, 1955; Meunier 1959; Bohlken 1964; Jerison 1961; Gould 1966, 1971; White and Gould 1965). Mechanistically, transpositions may arise from simple shifts in the timing of development, such as the onset of growth in one feature relative to another without a corresponding change in the specific growth rate of either feature (Gould 1971). It has been suggested that allometric transposition allows for an uncoupling of size and shape and that this may then permit the extension of ancestral body proportions to larger size (i.e., the maintenance of geometric similarity) in descendant species (Gould 1971). This should be particularly important for cases in which the ancestral growth trajectory is strongly allometric and consequently size-limiting. Transpositional allometry may also facilitate rapid phylogenetic size increase, particularly when its genetic basis is simple (Gould 1971). In contradiction to this, however, Shea (1983c) shows that allometric transpositions in great apes frequently act not to preserve geometric similarity over an extended range of body size, but instead actually introduce substantial cranial allometry.

Ontogenetic Scaling and Maintenance of Function

Implicit in much of the foregoing discussion is that growth-induced allometric size and shape changes effect measurable differences in function and therefore in the performance of important biological tasks. Where developmental pathways contain profound discontinuities (e.g., metamorphosis in anurans), the attendant functional shifts are quite obvious. But what of the more gradual continuum that typifies the ontogeny of most vertebrates? Here again there have been almost no detailed, quantitative assessments of the relationships among growth stage, morphological differentiation, and performance.

Significant ontogenetic change in relative mass, line of action, and even fiber type and architecture have now been recorded for the adductor muscles in several species of mammals (e.g., goats, pigs, rats; see reviews by Herring 1985; Gorniak 1988). But the functional consequences of these changes are far less clear. In sheep (Zey 1940) and pigs (Herring 1977; Herring and Wineski 1986), for example, certain ontogenetic changes in oral function can be related to changes in the geometry of the masticatory apparatus. However, in hamsters, the ontogenetic appearance of large-scale jaw movements and associated muscle activity seems to be more clearly related to the maturation of the neural circuitry than to that of the musculo-skeletal complex (Lakars and Herring 1980).

In a particularly fine study, Otten (1982) has traced the effects of allometric growth on the mouth-opening mechanism in a generalized cichlid, *Haplochromis elegans* (fig. 9.8). In early larval stages the geniohyoideus muscle provides the only means of mouth opening. Subsequently, however, rapid growth of the suspensorium causes the quadrate jaw articulation to be displaced relative to the traction line of the genioglossus, whose function is then suddenly switched from mandibular depression to mandibular adduction (when the mouth is at low gape angles). However, growth is closely coordinated and an alternative depressor mechanism, involving the opercular complex, is substituted for the geniohyoideus at almost exactly this time (fig. 9.9). Important alterations in the kinematic profiles of the mandible and hyoid complex during normal respiratory function accompany this abrupt, and developmentally mandated, shift in jaw mechanics. In *Salmo gairdneri*, in which the jaw articulation experiences relatively little relocation during larval growth, the geniohyoideus continues to operate as the mouth opener and the opercular mechanism develops very late compared to that in *H. elegans* (fig. 9.9).

Other aspects of the growth trajectory of *H. elegans* illustrate the manner in which closely coordinated, preprogrammed developmental change can act to maintain functional continuity (Otten 1983). The geometry of

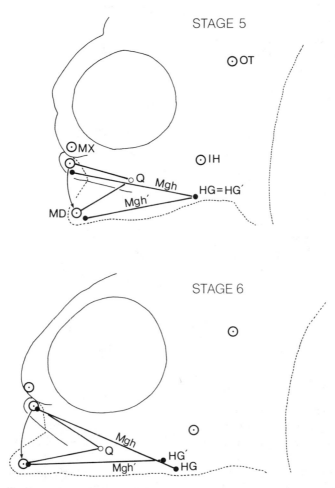

Fig. 9.8. Functional consequences of growth allometry during larval development in the cichlid fish *Haplochromis elegans*. With mouth closed (= solid outlines), line of action of the geniohyoideus muscle (Mgh) passes ventral to the quadratal jaw joint (Q) in the earlier growth stage. Owing to shifts in jaw joint position, the traction line of this muscle comes to lie dorsal to the joint in the later stage. The function of the geniohyoideus therefore changes from a depressor (stage 5) to an elevator (stage 6) of the mandible. When the mouth is widely open (= broken outlines), the muscle acts as a depressor in both ontogenetic stages. Other abbreviations: HG, hyoid-m. geniohyoideus connection with mouth closed; HG′, same with mouth open; IH, interhyal-hyoid joint; MD, mandibular symphysis marker; MX, maxillary marker; Mgh′, traction line of geniohyoideus with mouth open; OT, otolith marker. (Modified from Otten 1982.)

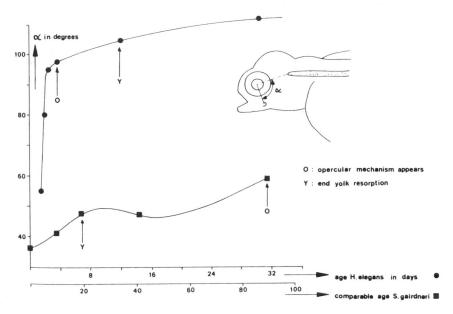

Fig. 9.9. Angular displacement (α) of the lower jaw articulation during growth in *Haplochromis elegans* and *Salmo gairdneri* in relation to the timing of the development of the opercular mouth-opening mechanism. (From Otten 1982.)

the mandibular skeletal complex (e.g., lever relationships) in young fish is mechanically superior to that of adults with respect to the production of bite force. However, the bite forces generated by juveniles are not significantly different from those produced by adults. The explanation rests with the fact that the alignment of the adductor mandibulae musculature in the young fish is suboptimal. This alignment is apparently related to spatial constraints imposed by a relatively large eye at this stage of growth. Negative growth allometry produces a less restrictive eye size in adult *H. elegans* and, therefore, a more favorable orientation of the jaw-closing muscles as well as a relatively larger muscle mass. But the same growth interval alters the geometry of the mandibular complex, and thereby reduces its mechanical advantage. The net consequence of these opposing changes is that force production stays roughly constant during ontogeny.

So far the only detailed quantitative evaluation of the mechanical consequences of skull growth in mammals is that of Weijs et al. (1987). These workers found that despite large allometric changes in craniomandibular shape together with relative muscle mass and orientation, the direction of the resultant force produced by the adductor muscles and its mechanical advantage remained essentially unchanged between young and adult rabbits. In this sense the developmental program of *Orcytolagus* also apparently preserves certain aspects of function over much of the growth curve. At the same time, ontogenetic changes in morphological organization result in adult rabbits being able to produce slightly larger maximum bite forces than juveniles but over a more restricted range of gape (fig. 9.10).

In fact, the ontogenetic shifts in mechanical performance reported by Weijs et al. (1987) are very likely to be conservative estimates, since their younger growth stage represented animals that were already postweaning and their oldest specimens were young adults. A more complete indication of the full range of ontogenetic shape change in *Oryctolagus* and its influ-

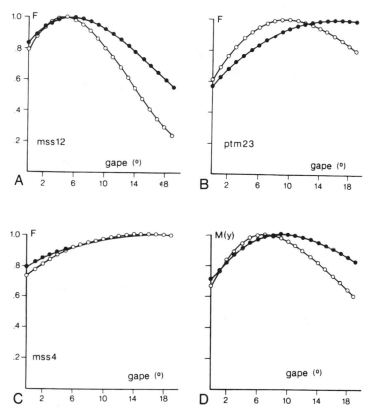

Fig. 9.10. Growth-related changes in the functional properties of the masticatory muscles of the rabbit, *Oryctolagus cuniculus*. A–C illustrate modeled shifts in force-gape curves for the superficial masseter (A), medial pterygoid (B), and posterior portion of the superficial masseter (C). Closed-circle curves are for a young rabbit; open-circle curves represent a young adult. D. Composite curve for total jaw-closing force (= moment). Note that large bite forces are restricted to a narrower range of gape in the adult. In all cases, force is expressed as a fraction of that available at an optimum gape. (Modified from Weijs et al. 1987.)

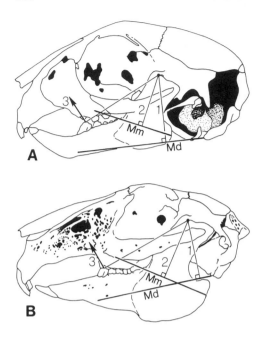

Fig. 9.11. Comparison of cranial proportions and their effect on the lever relationships of major adductor and depressor muscles in *Oryctolagus cuniculus*. In the newborn (A) cranial configuration favors the mechanics of mandibular depression and is reflected in the relatively greater moment arm (1) of the digastric muscle (Md). The moment arm (2) of the superficial masseter (Mm) is absolutely less than that of the digastric. In the adult (B) the lever relationships have reversed. The relatively greater area of attachment of masseter muscle is indicated by the enlarged masseteric fossa of the adult. Despite these changes, the vector direction of the bite force (3) remains approximately constant throughout growth. The mechanical demand of feeding (= suckling) favors early ossification of the jaws in neonates as compared to other regions of the skull (e.g., lateral braincase posterior to jaw joint) with no such mechanical requirement.

ence on organization of the masticatory musculature is provided in figure 9.11. Some of these shape changes are probably adaptive and related to the dietary differences between neonates and older individuals (see below). Because Weijs et al. (1987) sampled only two growth stages, it is not possible to determine the true scaling relationships for either morphological or biomechanical parameters from their data.

Phenotypic Plasticity in Ontogenetic Scaling

Rather striking structural and functional adjustments are associated with skull growth in certain species of aquatic turtles (e.g., some *Trionyx, Graptemys, Sternotherus, Emydura*). In these chelonians some or most older individuals of one sex (females in *Graptemys,* males of *Sternotherus*) or both sexes (*Trionyx, Emydura*) develop oversized heads in which the jaws are expanded to form broad crushing plates and the adductor muscles (and associated bony attachments) are greatly hypertrophied. Available information suggests that such "megacephalic" individuals tend to become increasingly durophagous in their feeding habits, often including large quantities of shellfish (Carr 1952; Berry 1975).

Intraspecific cranial allometries and some of their mechanical consequences have been most extensively examined in *Trionyx* (Dalrymple 1977). In this taxon both males and females show similar allometric trends in cranial modification with increasing body size. The most extreme examples of trophic hypertrophy are found in very large females. Nonetheless, individual variation among both sexes is pronounced and analyses of gut contents often do not confirm a close correspondence with skull configuration. Moreover, allometric hypertrophy of one component of the feeding mechanism is not always associated with a corresponding enlargement of other components. The data for *Trionyx*, then, indicate that although allometric growth trends can effect substantial modification in trophic form and function, the pattern itself is complex and extremely variable in its expression both among individuals and populations. Dalrymple interprets the evidence from *Trionyx* as indicative of a trophic apparatus that is loosely integrated and highly plastic, with the corresponding capacity to respond to the homeostatic needs of individuals. The high degree of variation witnessed in *Trionyx* and some other turtles (e.g., some species of *Emydura*; Legler 1981, 1989) in allometric skull development hints that an underlying genetic propensity for cranial hypertrophy is to a considerable extent modulated by individual feeding behavior/history. If so, much of the relative enlargement of trophic morphology in these turtles may reflect a physiological response to increased mechanical stress (Dalrymple 1977).

A more concrete, experimentally determined example of ontogenetic phenotypic plasticity is Meyer's (1987) study of the influence of diet and feeding mode on cranial form in a New World cichlid, *Cichlasoma managuense*. Full sib hatchlings were divided into two groups and each was raised on a different diet. After 8.5 months the two groups differed significantly in nearly all measures of cranial size and shape. The morphometric analysis demonstrated that one group had retained a rounded, blunt skull similar to those normally observed in hatchlings of this species, while the other developed a relatively more elongate cranium, similar to those of wild cichlid species that emphasize a suction mode of prey capture. When, subsequently, some blunt-headed fish were transferred to the other diet (= brine shrimp nauplii) they responded by developing the elongate skull and were ultimately indistinguishable from the original members of that dietary class.

These data not only document considerable phenotypic plasticity in cranial form and function in this cichlid, but also indicate that differences in diet (or correlated modes of feeding) can strongly influence developmental morphology. Although the proximate mechanism(s) by which food or feeding mode help to canalize growth along a specific trajectory are not known (again, bone response to differing levels of mechanical stress is a distinct possibility), the blunt-headed fish appear to be paedomorphs in which somatic development has been retarded. Conversely, some of these same fish exhibited an accelerated rate of shape change following a dietary shift.

Finally, data from humans (Corruccini and Lee 1984; Corruccini et al. 1985), rats (Beecher and Corruccini 1981a), macaques (Beecher and Corruccini 1981b), and squirrel monkeys (Corruccini and Beecher 1982) indicate that growth of the mammalian skull is also influenced by diet. Furthermore, like the situation in *Trionyx*, there is differential plasticity among phenotypic features of the skull. Thus, while mandibular growth in humans is affected by diet, tooth size is not.

Scaling Relationships and Life History Patterns

It should be clear that many scaling trends, both intra- and interspecific, have been selected in relation to specific life history requirements. Among the most obvious and well known of these are a variety of sexually dimorphic cranial specializations reflective of sexual selection. Most secondary cranial structures such as horns and antlers are of this type. All horns result from positive allometric growth during an animal's lifetime and interspecific comparisons reveal pronounced relative enlargement of these structures with increasing body size in numerous lineages of mammals and some dinosaurs (Gould 1974; Dodson 1975c).

One aspect of life history strategy that seems very likely to influence patterns of cranial growth and allometry is that of parental care. The topic appears to have been little studied. If there is no parental investment in the postnatal development of the young, then it must be expected that the trophic apparatus will be appropriately configured at birth for self-sufficiency. This need not be true of evolutionarily derived species in which parental care involves direct feeding of the young. On the other hand, provisioning of this sort may demand its own set of structural specializations. In this sense parental care can constitute a new and additional feeding dimension for which developmental and functional adjustments of the neonatal trophic apparatus are required. Therian mammals offer a possible illustration.

From birth until weaning therians derive all or most of their nourishment from a liquid diet produced by the mother's mammary glands. The mechanics of suckling have been investigated in only a few species (Ardran and Kemp 1959; Gordon and Herring 1987), but it appears probable that in virtually all cases active suction is required either to extract milk from the mammary gland or to transport it to the pharynx or both. Suction is generated chiefly by active displacements of the posterior region of the tongue and the floor of the buccal chamber. The associated kinematics and muscle activity patterns are generally similar to those seen in the jaw-opening movements of adult mammals when chewing. The mechanical demands of suckling may well account for the observation that the relative development and geometry of the mandible in neonatal mammals is biased in favor of the mechanics of jaw opening (Herring 1985). Subsequent growth progressively emphasizes those musculoskeletal features related to jaw-closing mechanisms (and, hence, effective biting and chewing). This pattern is well illustrated by cranial shape in neonatal versus adult *Oryctolagus* (fig. 9.11). In the former (fig. 9.11A) the mechanical advantage of the digastric actually exceeds that of the masseter. Moreover, not only is the leverage of this mandibular depressor favored by neonatal skull proportions, but the relative size of this muscle is also enhanced in suckling individuals. Thus, whereas the digastric constitutes about 5.6% of the total jaw musculature in adult *Oryctolagus,* it is approximately 15.5% in individuals one week of age (Langenbach and Weijs, unpublished data).

It is also likely that the special trophic requirements of newborn mammals select for earlier structural competency in the mandible and rostrum/palate relative to other regions of the cranial complex. In *Oryctolagus,* for example, which has altricial young, both the rostrum and mandible are well ossified at birth, whereas the posterior braincase contains a conspicuous, unossified hiatus (fig. 9.11A). A recent report indicates that rostral/mandibular ossification is also accelerated relative to other parts of the head skeleton in the extremely altricial neonates of some marsupials (Clark 1987).

Another developmental imperative seemingly imposed by the suckling habit of young mammals is that of rostral length. Compared with other tetrapods, most mammals are born with proportionally very short faces. We suggest that this is reflective of a basic functional requirement of suction feeding. If, as seems likely, mechanical efficiency depends on the suction forces being produced in close proximity to the tip of the nipple, then short muzzles and restricted labial openings will be favored. As postnatal growth proceeds, both relative and absolute lengthening of the rostrum will take place. Eventually this will tend to place a mechanical limitation on effective suckling unless there are compensatory changes in mammary structure (e.g., facultative nipple elongation). It might be anticipated that the switch from liquid to solid food would be correlated with the relative growth of some aspects of the facial region in mammals. For those species in which the inherent growth curve permits the retention of a short rostrum (e.g., many primates; felids) there is at least the mechanical potential for prolonged postnatal suckling. This will not be the case in species characterized by fairly rapid development (i.e., strong positive allometry) of an elongated muzzle (e.g., wild canids). Many precocial grazing ungulates (e.g., horses) initiate life with a well-developed rostrum. In these same mammals, however, an elongate and specialized teat has replaced the shorter and more primitive nipple as the milk-delivering structure.

CONCLUDING REMARKS

There has been much renewed interest in the role of scaling and allometry as either determinants or predictors of biological organization and function. Much of this reawakening may be traced to the influential papers of Gould (1966, 1971, 1977), Cock (1966) and others beginning in the mid-1960s. Within the past few years alone, several major volumes on these topics have appeared (e.g., Peters 1983; Schmidt-Nielsen 1984; Calder 1984). The major focus of these works, however, is the physiological and ecological consequences of scaling. Those aspects concerned with the morphological and functional implications of allometry have dealt primarily with issues of body support and locomotion. There have been no comparable treatments of cranial allometry and its significance for the evolution of the vertebrate skull.

Detailed quantitative analyses of ontogenetic growth of the vertebrate skull are few and mostly for domestic mammals. Much additional descriptive information of this type is needed for two primary reasons. First, only these data can provide empirical documentation of the pattern and sequence of growth processes that establish normal adult cranial form and function. Secondly, adequate quantitative descriptions of growth- and size-correlated shape change are prerequisite to meaningful tests of the hypothesis of ontogenetic scaling and related ideas that seek to clarify the connections between species-specific developmental processes and those witnessed in phylogenetic transformation. In this context the extraordinary developmental and phenotypic plasticity observed in some taxa serves as a cautionary warning that growth trajectories obtained from a few individuals or even a restricted sampling of populations will not always permit adequate description of ontogenetic change or of its evolutionary potential. In order to better understand how such flexibility is achieved and maintained, genetical studies of the type that exist for captive species (e.g., Atchley 1983) should be applied to naturally occurring forms that display an exceptional degree of developmental phenotypic plasticity.

Two recurring themes in evolutionary considerations of scaling are those related to "constraint" and "opportunity." We believe this general area of inquiry deserves much more emphasis. In many respects, the vertebrate skull may be more amenable to the examination of size-shape and growth-related constraints on function than is the postcranial locomotor complex, if only because its full range of functions (i.e., mechanical) is more limited. Hylander's (1985) recent study of allometric constraints and the design of the mandible in macaques stands as an excellent but unfortunately isolated example. It nicely demonstrates how experimentally based functional morphology can be joined with scaling and engineering theory to achieve a quantitative, predictive model of morphological and evolutionary constraint. Hylander shows that intrinsic allometric patterns of mandibular length and width combined with the scaling of adductor muscle mass in cercopithecine monkeys will necessarily result in disproportionately large mechanical stresses at the symphyseal region during normal feeding. Therefore, relative enlargement and enhanced buttressing of the mandibular symphysis in larger species of this lineage appears to be required in order to maintain functional equivalence.

The preceding example is one of functional limits set by interspecific scaling. But, as we have emphasized, the size-shape changes associated with ontogeny are nearly always vastly greater than those occurring in either adult static or interspecific allometries. Though there is little reason to expect that simple extension of ontogenetic growth curves will very often characterize interspecific evolutionary transformations, this does not mean that the general thesis embodied in the phrase "the power of extrapolation" is without merit. Indeed, it is clear that there must be continuity between ancestral and descendant growth processes. One approach to evaluating the question of "extrapolatability" would be to apply a historical approach to the study of ontogenetic trajectories (sensu Lauder 1981). Comparisons could then be made within clades where speciation has involved major changes in body size to seek matching patterns of ontogenetic scaling coefficients within sister groups that have undergone similar, but independent, size changes. In this way it might be possible to identify certain growth trajectories as more amenable to extrapolation, at least in a functional sense.

Clearly, much work is left to be done on the relationship between scaling and evolution of the vertebrate skull.

ACKNOWLEDGMENTS

We thank Bob Zanon for data on varanid lizards. Eric Charnov and Jon Seger provided insights into the allometry of prey/predator relationships. Brian Shea, Wim Weijs, Harry Greene, and Peter Dodson provided helpful comments on an earlier draft of the manuscript. Over the years, both of us had many hours of

stimulating discussion on the vertebrate skull with Leonard Radinsky. It is a plea-
sure to acknowledge his contribution to the ideas presented in this paper.

REFERENCES

Alberch, P. 1980. Ontogenesis and morphological diversification. American Zoologist 20: 653–667.

Alberch, P., and J. Alberch. 1981. Heterochronic mechanisms of morphological
diversification and evolutionary change in the Neotropical salamander, *Bolitoglossa occidentalis* (Amphibia: Plethodontidae). Journal of Morphology
167: 249–264.

Alberch, P., S. J. Gould, G. F. Oster, and D. B. Wake. 1979. Size and shape in
ontogeny and phylogeny. Paleobiology 5: 296–317.

Andrews, R., F. Pough, A. Collazo, and A. deQuciroz. 1987. The ecological cost
of morphological specialization: Feeding by a fossorial lizard. Oecologia 73:
139–145.

Ardran, G. M., and F. H. Kemp.1959. A correlation between suckling pressures
and movements of the tongue. Acta paediatrica 48: 261–271.

Armstrong, E. 1983. Relative brain size and metabolism in mammals. Science 220:
1302–1304.

———. 1985. Allometric considerations of the adult mammalian brain, with special emphasis on primates. In *Size and Scaling in Primate Biology,* W. L. Jungers, ed. New York, Plenum Press, pp. 115–146.

Atchley, W. 1983. Some genetic aspects of morphometric variation. In *Numerical
Taxonomy,* J. Felsenstein, Berlin, Springer-Verlag, pp. 346–363.

Atchley, W., B. Riska, L. Kohn, A. Plummer, and J. Rutledge. 1984. A quantitative
genetic analysis of brain and body size associations, their origin and ontogeny:
Data from mice. Evolution 38: 1165–1179.

Atchley, W., and J. Rutledge. 1980. Genetic components of size and shape. I. Dynamics of components of phenotypic variability and covariability during ontogeny in the laboratory rat. Evolution 34: 1161–1173.

Auffenberg, W. 1981. *The Behavioral Ecology of the Komodo Monitor.* Gaines-
ville: University Presses of Florida.

Beecher, R. M., and R. S. Corruccini. 1981a. Effects of dietary consistency on craniofacial and occlusal development in the rat. Angle Orthodontist 51: 61–69.

———. 1981b. Effects of dietary consistency on maxillary arch breadth in macaques. Journal of Dental Research 60: 68.

Berry, J. F. 1975. The population effects of ecological sympatry on the musk turtles
in northern Florida. Copeia: 692–701.

Bohlken, H. 1964. Vergleichende Untersuchungenan den Schädeln wilder und do-
mestizeiter Rinder. Zeitschrift für Wissenschaftliche Zoologie 170: 324–418.

Bramble, D. M. 1989. Cranial specialization and locomotor habit in the Lagomor-
pha. American Zoologist 29: 303–317.

Brandt, A. 1867. Sur le rapport du poids du cerveau à celui du corps chez diffé-
rents animaux. Société Impériale des Naturalistes de Moscou, Bulletin 40:
525–543.

Calder, W. A., III. 1984. *Size, Function, and Life History.* Cambridge: Harvard University Press.

Capel-Williams, G., and D. Pratten. 1978. The diet of adult and juvenile *Agama bibroni* (Reptilia: Lacertae) and a study of the jaw mechanisms in the two age groups. Journal of Zoology, London 185: 309–318.

Carr, A. F. 1952. *Handbook of Turtles.* Ithaca, N.Y.: Comstock Publishing Associates.

Cheverud, J. 1982. Relationships among ontogenetic, static, and evolutionary allometry. American Journal of Physical Anthropology 59: 139–149.

———. 1988. A comparison of genetic and phenotypic correlations. Evolution 42: 958–968.

Clark, C. 1987. Craniofacial osteogenesis in a marsupial. American Zoologist 34A (Abstract).

Cochard, L. R. 1985. Ontogenetic allometry of the skull and dentition of the rhesus monkey (*Macaca mulatta*). In *Size and Scaling in Primate Biology,* W. L. Jungers, ed. New York: Plenum Press, pp. 231–255.

Cock, A. 1966. Genetical aspects of metrical growth and form in animals. Quarterly Review of Biology 41: 131–190.

Corruccini, R. S., and R. M. Beecher. 1982. Occlusal variation related to soft diet in a nonhuman primate. Science 218: 74–76.

Corruccini, R. S., and G. T. R. Lee. 1984. Occlusal variation in Chinese immigrants to the United Kingdom and their offspring. Archives of Oral Biology 29: 779–782.

Corruccini, R. S., L. D. Whitley, S. S. Kaul, L. B. Flander, and C. A. Morrow. 1985. Facial height and breadth relative to dietary consistency and oral breathing in two populations (North India and U.S.). Human Biology 57: 151–161.

Dalrymple, G. H. 1977. Intraspecific variation in the cranial feeding mechanism of turtles of the genus *Trionyx* (Reptilia, Testudines, Trionychidae). Journal of Herpetology 11: 255–285.

Devillers, Ch., J. Mahe, D. Ambroise, R. Bauchot, and E. Chatelain. 1984. Allometric studies on the skull of living and fossil Equidae (Mammalia: Perissodactyla). Journal of Vertebrate Paleontology 4: 471–480.

Dodson, P. 1975a. Functional and ecological significance of relative growth in *Alligator.* Journal of Zoology, London 175: 315–355.

———. 1975b. Relative growth in two sympatric species of *Sceloporus.* American Midland Naturalist 94: 421–450.

———. 1975c. Taxonomic implications of relative growth in lambeosaurine hadrosaurs. Systematic Zoology 24: 37–54.

Emerson, S. 1985. Skull shape in frogs: Correlations with diet. Herpetologica 41: 177–188.

Emerson, S., J. Travis, and M. Blouin. 1988. Evaluating a hypothesis about heterochrony: Larval life-history traits and juvenile hindlimb morphology in *Hyla crucifer.* Evolution 42: 68–78.

Frazzetta, T. H. 1975. *Complex Adaptations in Evolving Populations.* Sunderland, Mass.: Sinauer.

Freedman, L. 1962. Growth of muzzle length relative to calvaria length in *Papio.* Growth 26: 117–128.

Giles, E. 1956. Cranial allometry in the great apes. Human Biology 28: 43–58.

Gordon, K. R., and S. W. Herring. 1987. Activity patterns within the genioglossus during suckling in domestic dogs and pigs: Interspecific and intraspecific plasticity. Brain, Behavior, and Evolution 30: 249–262.

Gorniak, G. C. 1988. Morphological and functional questions on the growth and plasticity of mammalian and avian jaw muscles. American Zoologist 28: 247–255.

Gould, S. J. 1966. Allometry and size in ontogeny and phylogeny. Biological Reviews 41: 587–640.

———. 1971. Geometric scaling in allometric growth: A contribution to the problem of scaling in the evolution of size. American Naturalist 105: 113–136.

———. 1974. The evolutionary significance of "bizarre" structures: Antler size and skull size in the "Irish Elk," Megaloceros giganteus. Evolution 28: 191–220.

———. 1975. Allometry in primates, with emphasis on scaling and the evolution of the brain. Contributions to Primatology 5: 244–292.

———. 1977. Ontogeny and Phylogeny. Cambridge: Harvard University Press.

Grant, P., B. Grant, J. Smith, I. Abbott, and L. Abbott. 1976. Darwin's finches: Population variation and natural selection. Proceedings of the National Academy of Science 73: 257–261.

Greene, H. 1986. Diet and arboreality in the emerald monitor, Varanus prasinus, with comments on the study of adaptation. Fieldiana: Zoology, n.s., 31: 1–12.

Herring, S. W. 1977. Mastication and maturity: A longitudinal study in pigs. Journal of Dental Research 56: 1377–1382.

———. 1985. The ontogeny of mammalian mastication. American Zoologist 25: 339–349.

Herring, S. W., and L. E. Wineski. 1986. Development of the masseter muscle and oral behavior in the pig. Journal of Experimental Zoology 237: 191–207.

Hersch, A. H. 1934. Evolutionary relative growth in titanotheres. American Naturalist 168: 537–561.

Hespenheide, H. 1971. Food preference and the extent of overlap in some insectivorous birds, with special reference to the Tyrannidae. Ibis 113: 59–72.

Huxley, J. S. 1932. Problems of Relative Growth. London: MacVeagh.

Hylander, W. L. 1985. Mandibular function and biomechanical stress and scaling. American Zoologist 25: 315–330.

Inger, R. 1966. The systematics and zoogeography of the Amphibia of Borneo. Fieldiana: Zoology 52: 1–402.

———. 1969. Organization of communities of frogs along small rain forest streams in Sarawak. Journal of Animal Ecology 38: 123–148.

Jerison, H. 1961. Quantitative analysis of evolution of the brain in mammals. Science 133: 1012–1014.

———. 1973. Evolution of Brain Size and Intelligence. New York: Academic Press.

Kiltie, R. 1982. Bite force as a basis for niche differentiation between rain forest peccaries (Tayassu tajacu and T. pecari). Biotropica 14: 188–195.

Kurtén, B. 1954. Observations on allometry in mammalian dentitions: Its interpretation and evolutionary significance. Acta zoologica fennica 85: 1–13.

———. 1955. Contribution to the history of a mutation during 1,000,000 years. Evolution 9: 107–118.

Lakars, T. C., and S. W. Herring. 1980. Ontogeny of oral function in hamsters (*Mesocricetus auratus*). Journal of Morphology 165: 237–254.

Lande, R. 1979. Quantitative genetic analysis of multivariate evolution, applied to brain:body size allometry. Evolution 33: 402–416.

———. 1985. Genetic and evolutionary aspects of allometry. In *Size and Scaling in Primate Biology,* W. L. Jungers, ed. New York: Plenum Press, pp. 21–32.

Lauder, G. 1981. Form and function: Structural analysis in evolutionary morphology. Paleobiology 7: 430–442.

Leamy, L. 1988. Genetic and maternal influences on brain and body size in randombred house mice. Evolution 42: 42–53.

Legler, J. M. 1981. The taxonomy, distribution, and ecology of Australian turtles (Testudines: Pleurodira: Chelidae). National Geographic Society Research Reports 13: 391–404.

———. 1989. Diet and head size in Australian chelid turtles, genus *Emydura.* Annales de la Société royale Zoologique de Belgique 119: 10.

Loftsvold, D. 1986. Quantitative genetics of morphological differentiation in *Peromyscus.* I. Tests of the homogeneity of genetic covariance structure among species and subspecies. Evolution 40: 559–573.

Losos, J., and H. W. Greene. 1988. Ecological and evolutionary implications of diet in monitor lizards. Biological Journal of the Linnean Society 35: 379–407.

Lumer, H. 1940. Evolutionary allometry in the skeleton of the domestic dog. American Naturalist 74: 439–467.

Martin, R. 1981. Relative brain size and basal metabolic rate in terrestrial vertebrates. Nature 293: 57–60.

Martin, R., and P. Harvey. 1985. Brain size allometry: Ontogeny and phylogeny. In *Size and Scaling in Primate Biology,* W. L. Jungers, ed. New York: Plenum Press, pp. 147–174.

Meunier, K. 1959. Die Allometrie des Vogelflügels. Zeitschrift für Wissenschaftliche Zoologie 161: 444–482.

Meyer, A. 1987. Phenotypic plasticity and heterochrony in *Cichlasoma managuense* (Pisces, Cichlidae) and their implications for speciation in cichlid fishes. Evolution 41: 1357–1369.

Moore, W. 1981. *The Mammalian Skull.* Cambridge: Cambridge University Press.

Otten, E. 1982. The development of a mouth-opening mechanism in a generalized *Haplochromis* species: *H. elegans* Trewavas 1933 (Pisces, Cichlidae). Netherlands Journal of Zoology 32: 31–48.

———. 1983. The jaw mechanism during growth of a generalized *Haplochromis* species: *H. elegans* Trewavas 1933 (Pisces, Cichlidae). Netherlands Journal of Zoology 33: 55–98.

Pagel, M., and P. Harvey. 1988. The taxon-level problem in the evolution of mammalian brain size: Facts and artifacts. American Naturalist 132: 344–359.

Peters, R. H. 1983. *The Ecological Implications of Body Size.* Cambridge: Cambridge University Press.

Pilbeam, D. R., and S. J. Gould. 1974. Size and scaling in human evolution. Science 186: 892–901.

Radinsky, L. 1981. Evolution of skull shape in carnivores. I. Representative modern carnivores. Biological Journal of the Linnean Society 15: 369–388.

———. 1983. Allometry and reorganization in horse skull proportions. Science 221: 1189–1191.

———. 1984a. Basicranial axis length v. skull length in analysis of carnivore skull shape. Biological Journal of the Linnean Society 22: 31–41.

———. 1984b. Ontogeny and phylogeny in horse skull evolution. Evolution 38: 1–15.

———. 1985a. Approaches in evolutionary morphology: A search for patterns. Annual Review of Ecology and Systematics 16: 1–14.

———. 1985b. Patterns in the evolution of ungulate jaw shape. American Zoologist 25: 303–314.

Reeve, E. C. R. 1941. A statistical analysis of taxonomic differences within the genus *Tamandua* Gray (Xenarthra). Proceedings of the Zoological Society of London 111: 279–302.

Reeve, E. C. R., and P. D. F. Murray. 1942. Evolution in the horse's skull. Nature 150: 402–403.

Reilly, S. M., and G. V. Lauder. 1988. Ontogeny of aquatic feeding performance in the eastern newt, *Notophthalmus viridescens* (Salamandridae). Copeia: 87–91.

Rensch, B. 1959. *Evolution above the Species Level.* New York: Columbia University Press.

Ricklefs, R., and H. Marks. 1984. Insensitivity of brain growth to selection of four-week body mass in Japanese quail. Evolution 38: 1180–1185.

Riska, B., and W. Atchley. 1985. Genetics of growth predict patterns of brain-size evolution. Science 229: 668–671.

Robb, R. C. 1935a. A study of mutations in evolution. I. Evolution of the equine skull. Journal of Genetics 31: 39–46.

———. 1935b. A study of mutations in evolution. II. Ontogeny in the equine skull. Journal of Genetics 31: 47–52.

Schmidt-Nielsen, K. 1984. *Scaling: Why Is Animal Size so Important?* New York: Cambridge University Press.

Schoener, T. 1974. Resource partitioning in ecological communities. Science 185: 27–39.

Shea, B. T. 1983a. Allometry and heterochrony in the African apes. American Journal of Physical Anthropology 62: 275–289.

———. 1983b. Paedomorphosis and neoteny in the pygmy chimpanzee. Science 222: 521–522.

———. 1983c. Size and diet in the evolution of African ape craniodental form. Folia primatologica 40: 32–68.

———. 1985. Ontogenetic allometry and scaling: A discussion based on the growth and form of the skull in African apes. In *Size and Scaling in Primate Biology*, W. L. Jungers, New York: Plenum Press, pp. 175–205.

Smith, M. 1922. The frogs allied to *Rana doriae*. Journal of the Natural History Society of Siam 4: 215–225.

Strauss, R. E. 1984. Allometry and functional morphology in haplochromine cichlids. In *Evolution of Fish Species Flocks*, A. A. Echelle and I. Kornfield, eds. Orono: University of Maine Press, pp. 217–229.

Toft, C. 1980. Feeding ecology of thirteen syntropic species of anurans in a seasonal tropical environment. Oecologia 45: 131–141.

Turelli, M. 1988. Phenotypic evolution, constant covariances, and the maintenance of additive variance. Evolution 42: 1342–1347.

van der Klaauw, C. 1946. Cerebral skull and facial skull: A contribution to the knowledge of skull structure. Archives néerlandaises de zoologie 7: 16–37.

Wainwright, P. 1987. Biomechanical limits to ecological performance: Mollusc crushing by the Caribbean hogfish, *Lachnolaimus maximus*. Journal of Zoology, London 213: 283–297.

Wake, M. 1986. The morphology of *Idiocranium russeli* (Amphibia: Gymnophiona), with comments on miniaturization through heterochrony. Journal of Morphology 189: 1–16.

Walton, A., and J. Hammond. 1938. The maternal effects on growth and conformation in Shire horse–Shetland pony crosses. Proceedings of the Royal Society of London 125: 311–335.

Wayne, R. K. 1986. Cranial morphology of domestic and wild canids: The influence of development on morphological change. Evolution 40: 243–261.

Weijs, W. A., D. Brugman, and E. M. Klok. 1987. The growth of the skull and jaw muscles and its functional consequences in the New Zealand rabbit (*Oryctolagus cuniculus*). Journal of Morphology 194: 143–161.

White, J. F., and S. J. Gould. 1965. Interpretation of the coefficient in the allometric equation. American Naturalist 99: 5–18.

Zey, A. 1940. Funktion des Kauapparates und Schädelgestaltung bei den Wiederkaüern. Diss., University of Frankfurt-am-Main.

10

Ecomorphology of the Teleostean Skull

KAREL F. LIEM

INTRODUCTION

RECENT RESEARCH IN EXPERIMENTAL FUNCTIONAL MORPHOLOGY has revolutionized our understanding of the biomechanics of the vertebrate skull (e.g. Bemis and Lauder 1986; Bramble and Wake 1985; Hiiemae and Crompton 1985; Lauder 1985). Likewise, ecologists have provided key advances in elucidating the mechanisms underlying predator-prey interactions (e.g., Hespenheide 1973), competition (Schoener 1983), resource partitioning (Werner 1977; Werner and Hall 1979; Mittelbach 1984), and prey switching during ecological "bottlenecks" (e.g., Grant et al. 1976; Wiens 1977). In spite of the explosive growth of both ecology and morphology, interdisciplinary studies have lagged behind. As a result only a few influential concepts can be identified from the partnership of morphological and ecological research involving the vertebrate skull. The lack of broad concepts has not been caused by the dearth of empirical data (van der Klaauw 1948; Lederer 1984; Leisler and Winkler 1985; Karr and James 1975). It is partially due to the blind acceptance that an organism's morphology fits manifestly well in its environment and that the apparent optimal matching of the organism's form and function with its environment is molded by natural selection (Bock, 1977a, b; Bock and von Wahlert 1965; Zweers 1979). In the absence of a broad conceptual framework, many ecomorphological studies have either described the ecological role of morphological features without any knowledge of their functions (the "nonfunctional approach"; e.g., DeMartini 1969; Keast and Webb 1966; Emery 1973; De Silva et al. 1980) or measured everything with the hope that some significant correlations would emerge (the "shotgun approach"; e.g. Gatz 1979a, b; Felley 1984). Both approaches accept a priori that natural selection has molded each part of the organism as an adaptive device to a prevailing environmental parameter (Lewontin 1978).

In this chapter, I will discuss ecomorphological aspects of the teleost skull mainly because the functional relationships of teleostean cranial morphology are rooted in a solid experimental foundation (e.g., Aerts et al. 1987; Lauder 1980, 1983a, c; Liem 1978, 1980b; Muller et al. 1982). The ecological principles are supported by a vast empirical data base for teleosts (Bentsen and McPhail 1984; Chao and Musick 1977; Keast and Webb 1966; Smith and Tyler 1973; Witte 1984). Wherever good data on other vertebrates are available, the reader is referred to appropriate key references. The chapter is subdivided into five parts. First the experimental foundation is discussed to provide the necessary background for the subsequent sections on the ecomorphological paradigm, the nature and significance of varying repertoires, and the emerging concepts of ecomorphology.

THE EXPERIMENTAL FOUNDATION

Kinematic analyses have revealed three basic teleostean strategies of prey capture: (a) suction, during which prey is sucked into the buccopharynx by the stationary predator; (b) ram feeding, in which the moving predator overtakes the prey with an open mouth; and (c) biting, in which the teeth of upper and lower oral jaws are applied to the prey or food in various ways (Liem 1990a; Norton 1989).

Functional analysis applying high-speed cinematography, electromyography, and pressure-transducer recordings have revealed that suction feeders generate very large negative pressures in the buccal cavity, while ram feeders produce very small negative pressures (Lauder 1980, 1983c; Brainerd 1985; Muller and Osse 1984; Muller et al. 1982). Biters (e.g., *Astatoreochromis*) do generate negative pressures to transport the collected food toward the esophagus (Liem 1990a).

The prey-capture apparatus of teleosts has been modeled as a truncated cone that can be expanded and compressed in various ways by the action of muscles (Osse and Muller 1980; Brainerd 1985). Coordinated activity of the epaxial, sternohyoideus, levator arcus palatini, and dilatator operculi muscles results in the explosive expansion of the cone-shaped buccopharyngeal cavity. This produces a steep negative pressure in the buccal cavity (fig. 10.1). Compression of the cone is effected by actions of the adductor mandibulae, adductor arcus palatini, and geniohyoideus muscles. Patterns of muscle actions are conserved in many taxa (Wainwright and Lauder 1966; Sanderson 1988), while in others intraspecific variation is pervasive (Liem 1980; Lauder 1981). For many teleosts neuromuscular patterns change in response to the kind and position of prey under attack (Liem 1978, 1979, 1980b; Elshoud-Oldenhave and Osse 1976; Lauder 1980).

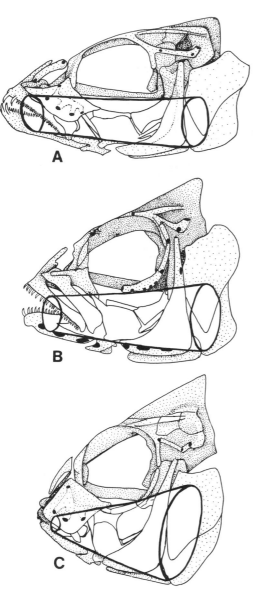

Figure 10.1. Schematic representations of three differently designed cichlid fish skulls. The buccopharyngeal cavities are highlighted with heavy outlines. A. Design of a typical ram feeder as exemplified in *Lamprologus elongatus* with a cylindrically shaped buccopharyngeal cavity. B. The intermediate design of a combined ram and suction feeder as found in *Grammatotria lemairei*. C. The truncated cone design characteristic for suction feeders as found in *Tylochromis microlepis*. (From Liem 1990a)

Many generalized teleosts can combine elements of suction feeding, ram feeding, and biting in response to the functional demands presented by particular prey. A detailed examination of variation in feeding kinematics due to these various demands provides insight into the functional and ecological significance of morphologies found in specialists. The cichlid

Hemitilapia oxyrhynchus exhibits a wide repertoire of modes of prey capture ranging from suction feeding in midwater, suction from the surface and bottom, ram feeding on elusive prey, a combination of ram and suction feeding when capturing various kinds of zooplankton and prey, to biting and scraping. It represents an ideal model to assess how the expanding cone is adjusted in shape and kinematic velocity to maximize prey capture. Thus it exhibits the initial divergence of designs for the various ways in which different types of prey are captured most efficiently.

Suction Feeding

When suction feeding, *H. oxyrhynchus* begins with shaping the buccopharynx as an attenuated cone by early activity of the geniohyoideus muscle (fig. 10.2). This decreases the initial volume of the buccal cavity and is immediately followed by a sudden expansion of the base of the cone by actions of the epaxial and sternohyoideus muscle, a protrusion of the upper jaw brought about by various couplings (Liem 1979; Otten 1983b), and prolonged activity of the levator arcus palatini muscle. Expansion of the base of the cone and jaw protrusion while keeping the gape to a minimum (fig. 10.2) result in a steep drop of the pressure in the buccal cavity (fig. 10.3), leading to effective prey capture by suction. A small gape increases the water flowing by the prey.

Based on the pattern of suction feeding in *H. oxyrhynchus,* it can be predicted that a design to enhance suction would involve a high supraoccipital crest or a wide skull (e.g., cottids) for insertion of a well-developed epaxial muscle mass, a deep suspensory apparatus to accommodate an elongate and highly differentiated levator arcus palatini muscle, a protrusible upper jaw, relatively short mandible, maxilla, and dentigerous arm of the premaxilla, a small gape, and a deep urohyal with large insertion sites for a strongly developed sternohyoideus to expand the base of the cone ventrally.

Ram Feeding

When capturing a relatively large and elusive prey from midwater, *H. oxyrhynchus* overtakes the prey at high velocity, producing a large gape accompanied by jaw protrusion. Early and abbreviated activity of the levator arcus palatini and sternohyoideus muscles seems to result in a large gape. The originally cone-shaped buccopharyngeal cavity is transformed into a cylinder (fig. 10.2) rather than an attenuated cone. The large gape is only slightly smaller in diameter than the base of the cone.

This pattern, so characteristic for body ram feeders, causes only a very small drop in pressure in the buccal cavity, and very little suction is generated (fig. 10.3).

According to the pattern of ram feeding in *H. oxyrhynchus*, a design which would enhance the efficiency of ram feeding would incorporate a long mandible, maxilla, and dentigerous arm of the premaxilla, a shallow suspensory apparatus with a modest levator arcus palatini, an elongate hyoid rami, and an elongate sternohyoideus muscle to displace the hyoid apparatus more posteriorly than ventrally. The supraoccipital crest can remain shallow, since the epaxial muscle mass plays only a minor role. In many jaw ram feeders jaw protrusion shortens the predator-prey distance

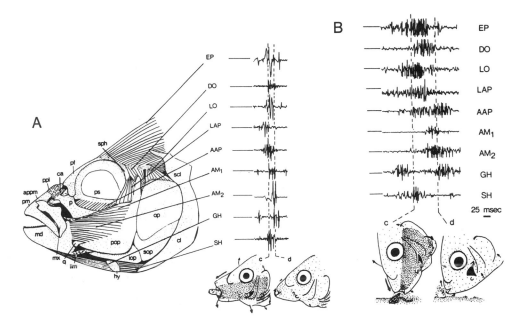

Fig. 10.2. Lateral view of major head muscles of the cichlid *Hemitilapia oxyrhynchus* with accompanying electromyograms and major kinematic events during ram feeding and during suction feeding. When capturing elusive prey from midwater the fish overtakes its prey by forward velocity and large gape, producing a cylindrical buccopharyngeal cavity (outlined with dense stipples). When suction feeding the fish creates a conical buccopharyngeal cavity with a small circular gape. Note the differences in the patterns of electromyograms in respect to duration of activity. (Modified from Liem 1990a.) Abbreviations: AAP, adductor arcus palatini; AM1, A1 portion of adductor mandibulae; AM2, A2 portion of adductor mandibulae; appm, ascending process of premaxilla; ca, rostral cartilage; cl, cleithrum; DO, dilatator operculi; GH, geniohyoideus; hy, hyoid; iop, interoperculum; LAP, levator arcus palatini; lim, interoperculo-mandibular ligament; LO, levator operculi; md, mandible; mx, maxilla; p, palatine; pm, premaxilla; pop, preoperculum; ppl, palatopalatine ligament; ps, parasphenoid; q, quadrate; SH, sternohyoideus; sop, suboperculum; sph, sphenotic.

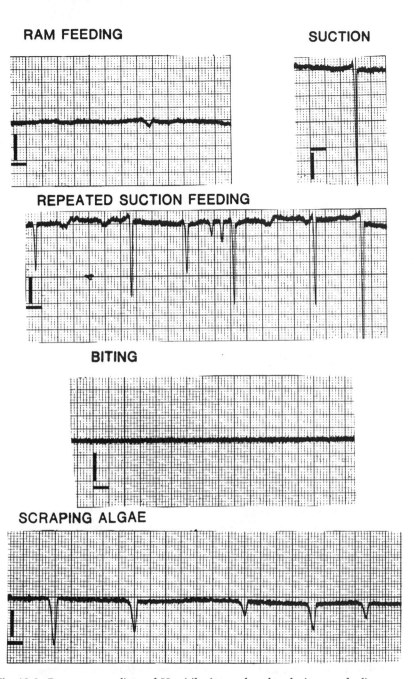

Fig. 10.3. Pressure recordings of *Hemitilapia oxyrhynchus* during ram feeding, suction feeding in a single strike, repeated suction feeding, biting, and scraping. When ram feeding the fish generates only a very slight "negative" pressure (25–40 cm of water). In sharp contrast a very large negative pressure (over 500 cm of water) is produced during suction feeding. Repeated suction feeding is consistently accompanied by large negative pressures. Biting produces no change in pressure within the buccal cavity. Scraping algae is characterized by the generation of moderately negative pressures in a rhythmic pattern to transport the collected algae into the buccopharynx.

(e.g., *Epibulus* [Westneat and Wainwright 1989], *Luciocephalus* [Lauder and Liem 1981], *Chromis* [Coughlin and Strickler 1990]).

Biting

During a "pure" bite *H. oxyrhynchus* does not generate any negative pressure in the buccopharyngeal cavity (fig. 10.3). A large gape is produced by head lifting by action of the epaxial, levator operculi, and sternohyoideus muscles. Pronounced and prolonged activity is found in the adductor mandibulae muscle complex and the geniohyoideus muscle (fig. 10.4). The original cone-shaped buccopharyngeal cavity is transformed into a cylinder. The side walls of the buccal cavity are not abducted by the levator arcus palatini muscle, which remains silent.

Based on the pure biting pattern of *H. oxyrhynchus,* the design that

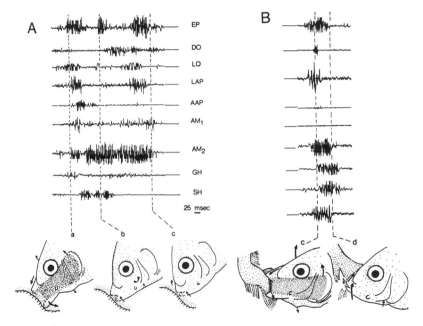

Fig. 10.4. During algae scraping *Hemitilapia oxyrhynchus* (A) produces a large gape and a cylindrical buccopharyngeal cavity. The accompanying electromyograms differ greatly from those during ram and suction feeding. When biting (B), the kinematic events closely resemble those during scraping, but the electromyograms differ in having the levator arcus palatini and adductor arcus palatini silent. For abbreviations see legend of fig. 10.2. (Modified from Liem 1990a)

enhances the bite would maximize the adductor mandibulae muscle in size as well as architecture. Likewise the epaxial muscle mass should be greatly expanded for strong suction. To accommodate a large adductor mandibulae complex with a favorable lever arm, the suspensory apparatus should increase in depth, while increased insertion sites for the epaxial muscle mass can be realized by a high supraoccipital crest. This design is therefore compatible with the design enhancing suction.

Actually, *H. oxyrhynchus* usually combines biting with suction when scraping algae with a large gape. During scraping, the fish seems to create suction at regular intervals to draw the loosened algae into the buccopharyngeal cavity (fig. 10.3). The electromyographic and kinematic pattern exhibited by *H. oxyrhynchus* during scraping (fig. 10.4) does combine the designs that enhance suction and biting, i.e., a high supraoccipital crest, a large adductor mandibulae complex, highly differentiated epaxial and levator arcus palatini muscles, a deep configuration of the suspensory apparatus, and relatively short jaws.

DESIGN AND PERFORMANCE

Very few studies have offered unequivocal evidence for the precise matching of a particular design with improved execution of a biological role (Arnold 1983). Norton (1989), in a series of elegant experiments, has shown that sculpins (Cottidae) with a ram-feeding design exhibit a significantly higher prey-capture success when feeding on elusive prey than do sculpins possessing the design characteristics of suction feeders.

Bentsen and McPhail (1984) discovered two morphologically distinct and sympatric species of the three-spined stickleback (*Gasterosteus*): limnetics and benthics. The feeding performance of the two forms was tested experimentally under both laboratory and field conditions. The limnetic form possesses the design of a ram feeder, a more elongate snout and shallower suspensory apparatus. The benthic form has the design of a suction feeder with a shorter, broader snout and deeper suspensory apparatus. The limnetics were significantly more successful in capturing elusive zooplankton than were the benthics.

During low food abundance, the molariform morph of the polymorphic cichlid species *Cichlasoma minckleyi* with a crushing pharyngeal jaw design was significantly more successful in capturing and processing snail prey than the papilliform morph without such a design (Liem and Kaufman 1984). Hoogerhoud (1986), working on the mollusk-feeding cichlid species *Astatoreochromis alluaudi*, offers experimental evidence that profitability parameters such as handling time and cost of shell ejection, shell crushing, and shell ingestion can be related to the morphology of the prey and of the predator. Wainwright (1987, 1988) has drawn the same conclusions in an elegant experimental study of the mollusk-crushing labrid species *Lachnolaimus maximus*. Finally, Stein et al. (1984) and Mittelbach (1984) correlate differences in handling times of snails and zooplankton to morphological differences in gill rakers and pharyngeal jaw apparatus between the centrarchids *Lepomis macrochirus* and *L. gibbosus*.

Thus, the available evidence supports the notion that the experimentally deduced design matches the relative efficiency of the execution of the biological role in several lineages of teleost fishes. Experimental studies in progress (in the laboratories of Philip Motta, Stephen Norton, and Peter Wainwright) lend support to ecomorphology, which attempts to relate performance with experimentally derived design.

THE ECOMORPHOLOGICAL PARADIGM

Davis and Birdsong (1973), Smith and Tyler (1973), Ebeling and Cailliet (1974), Liem (1980a, b), Barel (1983), Yamaoka (1982, 1983, 1987), Motta (1988), and Clements and Bellwood (1988) have stated the ecomorphological paradigm as currently accepted: morphology of the skull relates to how the animal feeds. Interspecific (or intraspecific) variation in morphology is correlated with observed interspecific differences in diet. The assumption is that such a correlation is caused by differences in feeding efficiency. Thus the ecomorphological paradigm accepts a close fit between feeding morphology and prey capture and processing.

The ecomorphological paradigm can best be illustrated with examples from the Cichlidae of the Great Lakes of Africa, different lineages of coral reef fishes, and the Chaetodontidae (Motta 1988).

Cichlidae

Cichlids are well known both from the perspective of functional morphology and ecology (Fryer and Iles 1972; Greenwood 1978; Liem 1979, 1980a, b; Barel 1983; Barel et al. 1989; Witte 1984; Yamaoka 1982, 1983; McKaye and Marsh 1983; Hoogerhoud 1986; Ribbink et al. 1983). Many of the morphologically specialized cichlids of different lineages exhibit convergence in ecology. Specialized examples of suction feeders, ram feeders, and biters are discussed as centerpieces of the ecomorphological paradigm.

Ram-feeding cichlids demonstrate in an exaggerated form the features predicted from *H. oxyrhynchus* when ram feeding. The buccopharyngeal cavity is cylindrical, and the jaws are elongate, while the suspensory apparatus is shallow, and the gape very large (fig. 10.5B). The hyoid apparatus is positioned in a more dorsal configuration almost reaching the roof of the mouth. The shallow suspensory apparatus accommodates a modest adductor mandibulae complex. The narrow elongate head has an effect on

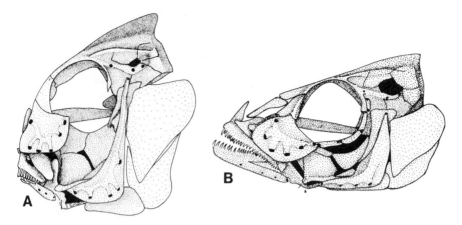

Fig. 10.5. Sharp contrast in skull design between (A) an algae scraper (*Simochromis curvifrons*) and (B) a ram feeder (*Bathybates ferox*). The ram feeder has a large gape, an elongate snout, shallow suspensory apparatus, and relatively slender jaws. The algae scraper ("biter") has an abbreviated snout, small gape, deep suspensory apparatus, and stout jaws (from Liem 1980a)

the angle between the rami of the mandible which ranges only between 15° and 37° (Barel 1983, fig. 8). The muscles responsible for buccal expansion, i.e., levator arcus palatini, epaxial muscles, and sternohyoideus, are only moderate in size. This design is not conducive to the generation of a steep negative pressure within the expanding cylindrical buccopharyngeal cavity (Brainerd 1985). Intraoral pressures confirm this prediction (fig. 10.3). Ram-feeding cichlids rely on high-velocity forward locomotion when overtaking and engulfing the prey with a large gape. All ram-feeding cichlids exhibit striking convergences in design, e.g., *Bathybates* and *Hemibates* of Lake Tanganyika (Liem 1978), *Ramphochromis* (Lake Malawi; personal observation), *Cichla* (neotropical; Brainerd 1985).

Ram feeders are often pursuit-hunting piscivores foraging for midwater prey. There is little doubt that high-velocity ram-feeding design and tactics are highly successful in the capture of large or small elusive prey, not only fish, but also shrimp and some zooplankton. Streamlining of the elongate head and torpedo-shaped body enhances swimming velocity, while the enormous gape allows for the engulfment of large prey. However, ram-feeding design is also conducive for the capture of small midwater prey such as copepods, as exhibited by *Haplotaxodon* (fig. 10.6). Fishes with this typical ram-feeding design are ineffective in capturing prey from near the bottom or in highly structured habitats. Ram feeders are unable to bite and inefficient in capturing prey from in between rocks or crevices.

Suction feeders and biters have very similar designs, the latter exhib-

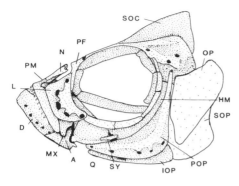

Fig. 10.6. Lateral aspect of the skull of the elusive zooplankton feeder *Haplotaxodon microlepis.* This zooplankton feeder possesses the design of a piscivorous ram feeder: its gape is large, the suspensory apparatus is quite shallow, and the jaws are slender with the oblique gape directed upward. Abbreviations: A, angular; D, dentary; HM, hyomandibula; IOP, interoperculum; L, lachrymal; MX, maxilla; N, nasal; OP, operculum; PF, prefrontal; PM, premaxilla; POP, preoperculum; Q, quadrate; SOC, supraoccipital; SOP, suboperculum; SY, symplectic.

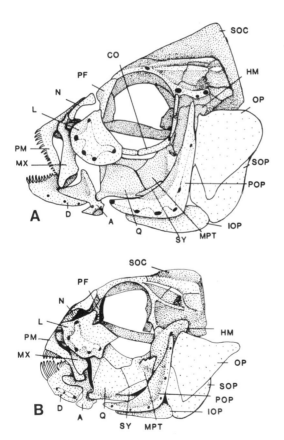

Fig. 10.7. Skull designs of (A) a suction feeder, *Cynotilapia afra,* with a deepened suspensory apparatus, a smaller gape, and shorter mandible; and (B) a biter, *Telmatochromis temporalis,* with a very deep suspensory apparatus, a fossa on the preoperculum for accomodation of the hypertrophied adductor mandibulae complex, and a very short and stout mandible, in which the dentary is greatly enlarged. Abbreviations: A, angular (articular); CO, circumorbital; D, dentary; HM, hyomandibula; IOP, interoperculum; L, lachrymal; MPT, metapterygoid; MX, maxilla; N, nasal; OP, operculum; PF, prefrontal; PM, premaxilla; POP, preoperculum; Q, quadrate; SOC, supraoccipital; SOP, suboperculum; SY, symplectic.

iting exaggerated specializations found in the former. Biters and suction feeders typically have a design already foreshadowed in *H. oxyrhynchus* when it feeds by suction or by scraping and biting (figs. 10.2, 10.4). The buccopharyngeal cavity is shaped as an attenuated truncated cone and the gape is much smaller as a result of the short and stout mandible, premaxilla, and maxilla (fig. 10.7). The suspensory apparatus is deep, creating extensive sites of attachments for the massive adductor mandibulae complex which is expanded medially, invading the lateral surfaces of the preoperculum. The suspensory apparatus has large crests for the insertion of the levator arcus palatini. The articulation between the suspensory apparatus and the hyoid is shifted ventrally while the hyoid becomes positioned obliquely and far ventrally from the buccal roof. The shorter mandibular rami meet at much greater angles, i.e., 38°–87° (Barel 1983), than in ram feeders. The wider angle provides not only a more effective bite, but also space for greatly enlarged geniohyoideus muscles (fig. 10.8). Often the pre-

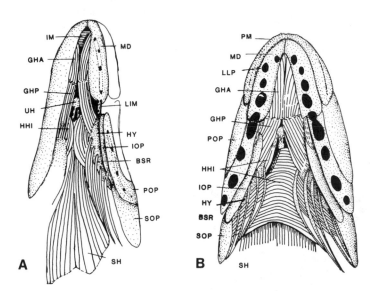

Fig. 10.8. Ventral musculature of the head of a typical ram-feeding design (A. *Lamprologus attenuatus*), and a characteristic suction/biter design (B. *Lamprologus tretocephalus*). In the ram feeder, the angle of the mandibular and hyoid rami is acute and the geniohyoideus muscle is elongate and slender, while the hyohyoideus inferior is only weakly developed. In the suction/biter, the angle between the mandibular and hyoid rami is much less acute, while the geniohyoideus and hyohyoideus inferior muscles are hypertrophied. Abbreviations: BSR, branchiostegal ray; GHA, geniohyoideus anterior; GHP, geniohyoideus posterior; HHI, hyohyoideus inferior; HY, hyoid; IM, intermandibularis; IOP, interoperculum; LIM, interoperculomandibular ligament; LLP, lateral line canal pore; MD, mandible; PM, premaxilla; POP, preoperculum; SH, sternohyoideus; SOP, suboperculum; UH, urohyal.

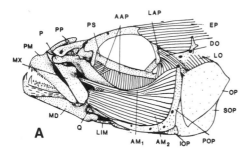

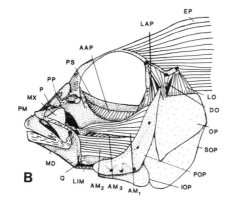

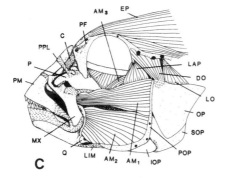

Fig. 10.9. Lateral head musculature of (A) a ram feeder (*Lamprologus attenuatus*), (B) a primarily suction feeder (*Tylochromis polylepsis*), and (C) a biter (*Telmatochromis temporalis*). Abbreviations: AAP, adductor arcus palatini; AM₁, AM₂, AM₃, parts A1, A2, and A3 of the adductor mandibulae complex; C, rostral cartilage; DO, dilatator operculi; EP, epaxial; IOP, interoperculum; LAP, levator arcus palatini; LIM, interoperculomandibular ligament; LO, levator operculi; MD, mandible; MX, maxilla; OP, operculum; P, palatine; PF, prefrontal; POP, preoperculum; PM, premaxilla; PP or PPL, palatopalatine ligament; PS, parasphenoid; Q, quadrate; SOP, suboperculum.

orbital region of the skull is abbreviated while the supraoccipital crest is high, providing the necessary sites for insertions of the epaxial muscle mass (fig. 10.9).

The biter design is basically an exaggeration of the specialized design of suction feeders (fig. 10.9).

Biters are quite effective in grasping prey or algae between the teeth with a great force. Among biters are algae scrapers (e.g., *Petrochromis*,

Yamaoka 1982), scale eaters, and fin biters (e.g., *Genyochromis mento*). Suction feeders are represented by numerous cichlid species, from bottom feeders (*Xenotilapia*) to benthic feeders (e.g., *Haplochromis elegans*) and mollusk feeders (*Tylochromis*, fig. 10.9).

Other Teleosts: Coral Reefs and Ontogenetic Stages

A test of the ecomorphological hypothesis can now be made by searching for similar trends in other teleost lineages. Based on the work by Davis and Birdsong (1973) and Kotrschal and Thomson (1989), a comparison can be made between benthic foragers (suction feeders) and water-column foragers (ram feeders) in coral reef fishes. Among the Lutjanidae, the ram feeder *Lutjanus griseus* exhibits many of the skull design elements that are found in the ram-feeding cichlids (fig. 10.10), while the suction feeder *Emmelichthyops atlanticus* exhibits the same trends found in the cichlid suction-feeding/biter design: shorter mandible, deeper suspensory apparatus. Similar contrasts in ram-feeder versus suction-feeder designs can be found in Serranidae: *Epinephelus cruentatus* versus *Schultzea beta*

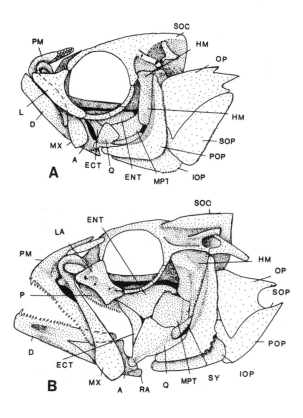

Fig. 10.10. Contrasting skull designs within the lineage Lutjanidae: A, the benthic suction feeder *Emmelichthyops;* B, the midwater ram feeder *Lutjanus griseus.* Abbreviations: A, articular (angular); D, dentary; ECT, ectopterygoid; ENT, entopterygoid; HM, hyomandibula; IOP, interoperculum; L or LA, lachrymal; MPT, metapterygoid; MX, maxilla; OP, operculum; P, palatine; PM, premaxilla; POP, preoperculum; Q, quadrate; RA, retroarticular; SOC, supraoccipital; SOP, suboperculum; SY, symplectic.

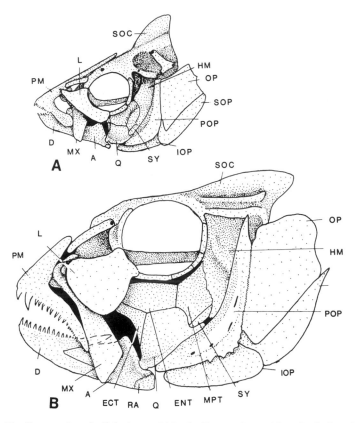

Fig. 10.11. Contrasting skull designs within the lineage Serranidae. A. the benthic suction feeder *Schultzea beta*. B. the ram-feeding *Epinephelus cruentatus* (abbreviations as in fig. 10.10).

(fig. 10.11); in Pomacentridae: *Chromis* versus *Abudefduf* (Emery 1973); in Labridae: *Clepticus parai* versus *Halichoeres poeyi* (Davis and Birdsong 1973); and in Haemulidae: *Haemulon striatus* versus *Haemulon sciurus* (Davis and Birdsong 1973).

The ecomorphological hypothesis also applies to early life history stages of fishes. During the development of the clown fish *Amphiprion frenatus,* the early larva feeds by ram feeding on rotifers. During this stage the skull possesses the typical ram-feeding design with a relatively large gape, shallow suspensory apparatus, and dorsally positioned hyoid, resulting in a cylindrically shaped buccopharyngeal cavity (fig. 10.12). As ontogeny proceeds rapidly, the larva switches from a ram-feeding mode of prey capture to a suction-feeding strategy (Dilling 1989; Coughlin 1991; Liem 1991). It is during this switch that the design of the skull assumes the

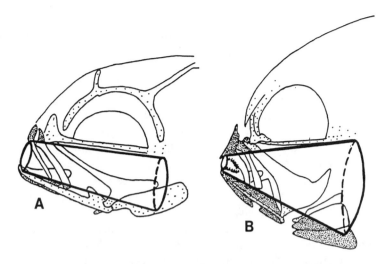

Fig. 10.12. Diagrammatic representation of major components of the jaw apparatus and shape of the buccopharyngeal cavity (outlined with heavy line) in a newly hatched larva (A) and a 21-day-old juvenile of *Amphiprion frenatus* (B). Note the drastic change from the cylindrical ram-feeding design to the truncated cone suction-feeder design (from Dilling 1989).

form of a typical suction feeder with a more ventral disposition of the hyoid, a deeper suspensory apparatus resulting in a conical buccopharyngeal cavity (fig. 10.12; Dilling 1989; Liem 1991). This switch in design coincides with a switch in prey-capture tactics and not in the kind of prey, since in both developmental stages the fish feeds on rotifers. The good fit of skull design with the way the developing fish feeds throughout its ontogeny represents evidence in favor of the ecomorphological hypothesis. Radical ontogenetic changes in skull form accompany the major changes in prey-capture strategy, and each change in design can be interpreted in terms of maximizing the shifting biological roles.

CHALLENGES TO THE ECOMORPHOLOGICAL PARADIGM

The ecomorphological paradigm is firmly rooted in the notion that inclusive fitness is reflected in the net energy gained from environmental resources (Barel et al. 1989). Since the net energy gain equals the energy content of the resource minus the costs of the design in executing its biological role, an optimal gain can be realized if the underlying anatomical and functional systems perform at their highest possible efficiencies (Barel et al. 1989). Thus the common currency is energy. Two major assumptions are made in this reasoning: (1) energy is not only the universal currency, but is also a limited resource for which there is competition; (2) historical factors (e.g., developmental constraints and canalization, the degree of genotypic and phenotypic variation, phylogenetic constraints) are not important.

Historical factors may well play a significant role in molding the skull, producing forms which do not follow the prediction made on ecomorphological arguments. Among chaetodontids (Motta 1988) *Forcipiger longirostris* is a suction feeder on small invertebrates living in crevices and between coral branches, while *F. flavissimus* bites, grabs, and tears pieces of larger, benthic noncoralline invertebrates. Yet they have skulls of strikingly similar design (Motta 1988). The resemblance reflects a close phylogenetic relationship of the two species rather than optimization of suction feeding and biting, respectively.

Most teleost fishes possess skulls that are intermediate between ram-feeder and suction-feeder designs. Such intermediate designs are found in species that combine either suction- and ram-feeding strategies equally or are predominantly suction feeders.

For example, many cichlids with intermediate skull designs are capable of ram feeding, suction feeding, and biting, as exhibited in *Hemitilapia* (figs. 10.2, 10.4), *Petrotilapia* (Liem 1980b), *Limnotilapia* (Liem 1984), *Lobochilotes* (Liem 1980b), and *Cichlasoma* (Liem and Kaufman 1984). In *Petrotilapia* and *Hemitilapia*, the preferred diet consists of zooplankton, shrimp, and insect larva, which are captured by a combination of suction- and ram-feeding strategies (Liem 1980b; McKaye, personal communication). The accompanying electromyograms, kinematics of the expanding cone, and pressure profiles (figs. 10.2, 10.3, 10.4) support the notion that the teleostean skull possesses a plasticity driven by different patterns of neuromuscular outputs. Under laboratory conditions, *Petrotilapia* and *Hemitilapia* prefer insect larvae and zooplankton over algae when food resources are abundant. Only when food resources are in short supply do *Petrotilapia* and *Hemitilapia* switch to scraping algae, for which their skull forms are well designed with a relatively deep suspensory apparatus, short jaws, and high supraoccipital crest. Teleost fishes engage in extensive diet switching in response to variations in prey abundance (Stoner 1980; McKaye and Marsh 1983; Goulding 1980). It seems that fishes with intermediate skull design readily switch from ram feeding to suction feeding and even to biting. Some morphologies (e.g., *Cichlasoma, Petrotilapia, Geospiza* in the Galapagos) appear to be of selective advantage only during ecological bottlenecks. They are bet-hedging strategies. At the same time the generalized morphologies of many species may also represent a bet-hedging strategy against fluctuations in resources. This becomes a fascinating question when we consider the evolutionary longevities of specialist versus generalist species. In embiotocids, Schmitt and

Coyer (1982) found that disparate foraging behaviors resulted in great differences in diets between *Embiotoca lateralis* and *E. jacksoni* with identical skull morphologies. Motta (1988) observed that *Chaetodon miliaris, C. quadrimaculatus,* and *Forcipiger flavissimus* are noticeably opportunistic in their feeding. Although they feed primarily on polychaete worms, the three species can feed exclusively on abundant plankton sources for extended times.

In the polymorphic cichlid species *Cichlasoma minckleyi,* papilliform as well as the molariform morphs prefer to feed on the larvae of Odonata. Only during a simulated ecological bottleneck of low food abundance do the two morphs segregate their diets, the molariform morph feeding preferentially on snails. The specialized morphology of the masticatory apparatus of the molariform morph is adapted for a refugium diet of snails rather than for its otherwise preferred Odonata larvae when food is abundant in the environment (Liem and Kaufman 1984).

In the chaetodontid fishes, *Chaetodon auriga* and *Forcipiger flavissimus* have very different morphologies but strikingly similar diets, while *Forcipiger longirostris* and *F. flavissimus* have similar gross morphologies although the former is a suction feeder and the latter a biter (Motta 1988).

The data of these studies on teleost fishes do not support the notion that skull morphology is a consistently good predictor of the preferred prey type. The data indicate that behavioral parameters often play a greater role than skull design in the exploitation of prey and that there are multiple and diverse and not necessarily optimal solutions to capturing a particular prey type. At best the ecomorphological paradigm involves a fairly close fit between skull design and prey capture and handling. Future research in ecomorphology should focus on the occurrence, nature, and significance of feeding repertoires in relation to skull design.

Ecomorphological research attempts to demonstrate how superior design from an engineer's point of view enhances inclusive fitness, which in turn can be measured indirectly from the net energy gained from environmental resources (Barel et al. 1989). Relative efficiencies of various skull designs in relation to prey capture and processing have been postulated exclusively from anatomy and functional morphology or from search, capture, and prey handling times (Stein et al. 1984; Werner and Hall 1979; Yamaoka 1983, 1987). None of the ecomorphological studies to date have furnished empirical data on the energetics of prey capture and processing in teleost fishes. At best, only approximate estimates of relative efficiencies can be made. For teleosts, hypothetical models state how the relation between the form of the eye and the form of the expanding cone of the teleostean prey-capture apparatus will determine the interaction with various prey types, resulting in different energy gains (Barel et al. 1989). However, without direct measurements of net total energy gain, the assertions that

certain designs are more efficient machines than others will remain speculative. Future research programs in ecomorphology should measure the
functional efficiency or performance of different designs in a common currency that expresses their respective adaptive values (Arnold 1983; Barel
et al. 1989; Wainwright 1988; Norton 1989). However, in selecting the
skull and associated structures as traits optimally designed by natural selection for their biological roles, ecomorphologists may generate flawed
interpretations, since the assumed common currency, food resources (energy), may actually not be the limiting factor in the majority of the teleost
fish communities, which have been analyzed. Actually, energy is the typical
currency, but the usual feature optimized is the net rate of energy intake.
Even if food is abundant, extra time spent foraging may be time not spent
in other important activities (such as breeding) or it may increase exposure
to predators. When part-by-part optimization is not found, the design of
the skull is still interpreted as the best compromise among competing demands on the basis of constructional morphology (e.g., Barel et al. 1989).
Thus, interaction among components is retained completely within the notion of the best possible design for the whole. Within the framework of
constructional morphology of the teleost skull, the immediate utility of the
components is overemphasized and other attributes of the design are un-
deremphasized as multipartite trade-offs or arbitrarily excluded as being
incompatible to the performance of functions (Barel et al. 1989). However,
these very functions are actually being executed by the fishes under both
laboratory (Liem 1980a, b) and field conditions (McKaye and Marsh 1983;
Ribbink et al. 1983).

ECOMORPHOLOGY EMERGING

Gould and Lewontin (1979) stated that "Too often, the adaptationist programme gave us an evolutionary biology of parts and genes, but not of
organisms." They further argued that "the potential rewards of abandoning exclusive focus on the adaptationist programme are very great indeed"
and they "advocated the richness that a pluralistic approach, so akin to
Darwin's spirit, can provide." Ecomorphology may well offer this pluralistic approach by abandoning the exclusive focus on the adaptationist program and by a thorough consideration of the key role of historical
constraints and integrated developmental functional units.

We must recognize that organisms belong to two hierarchies: genealogical or historical, in which genetic information is transferred, and
ecological or economic, in which energy is transferred. Current ecomorphological studies focus exclusively on the economic or ecological interactions in which the transfer of energy reigns supreme. However, the

genealogical side is the source of genetic information and variation and evolution is defined as what happens in the genealogical hierarchy. According to the proposed principle of symecomorphosis, which is defined as the balanced symmetry of the coexisting and mutually interdependent ecological and genealogical hierarchies in nature (Liem 1989), ecomorphological studies must accord equal weighting to both the economic and genealogical factors. To date, the focus has been on the economic (ecological) aspects of skull design in fishes. However, symecomorphosis predicts that the balanced symmetry can be disrupted when there are spontaneous modifications in the transfer of genetic information which would alter the developmental as well as functional design of the participants in the economic arena. Because theory predicts that the informational side of the hierarchy will persist almost indefinitely as long as the economic (ecological) system persists unaltered, many of the studies have indeed confirmed the ecomorphological paradigm: the manifest fit between skull design and feeding ecology (e.g., Davis and Birdsong 1973; Barel 1983; Motta, 1988; Kotrschal 1988; Wainwright 1987, 1988; Yamaoka 1987; Yamaoka et al. 1986). An example of adaptive precision in fish skulls has been functionally and theoretically demonstrated by Otten (1983a, b). By perturbation analysis in computer models he has identified 7 "hot spots" in the heads of fishes. He defines hot spots as anatomical landmarks for which their respective topographies are highly critical in determining the suction and biting forces which play a key role in the economic arena. A transformation from a suction-feeding design to a biting design would involve the following seven changes (as illustrated in cichlids in fig. 10.13):

1. Shortening of the ascending process of the premaxilla (APPM).
2. Steepening of the ascending process of the premaxilla (APPM).
3. The ligament between the maxilla and rostral cartilage moves anteriorly relative to the maxilla (L_2).
4. Lengthening of the maxillary process of the palatine (P).
5. Shortening of the ascending process of the mandible (APA).
6. A dorsal shift of the adductor mandibulae muscle part A1 (AM_1).
7. A caudo-ventral shift of the insertion of the adductor mandibulae A1 tendon on the maxillary head (TAM_1).

It is predicted that such minor shifts of the seven hot spots could result in doubling of the biting force. Comparative ecological and morphological studies have revealed a positive correlation between the topography of these hot spots and the feeding ecology of suckers and biters (Liem, 1991).

In the skulls within the Viperidae the presence of a pit in the maxilla in the pit vipers (Crotalinae) has major constructional consequences for the jaw apparatus (Dullemeijer 1956, 1959; Liem et al. 1971). The presence of the pit, a heat-sensing device, provides a very novel and important

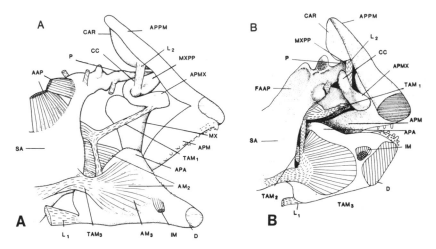

Fig. 10.13. Medial aspect of left jaw apparatus and anterior portion of the suspensory apparatus to show the change in positions of the "hot spots" from (A) a suction feeder *Lobochilotes labiatum* to (B) a biter (*Telmatochromis temporalis*). Abbreviations: AAP, adductor arcus palatini; AM_2, AM_3, portions A2, and A3 of the adductor mandibulae complex; APA, ascending process of the articular (angular); APM, alveolar process of the premaxilla; APMX, articular process of the maxilla; APPM, ascending process of the premaxilla; CAR, rostral cartilage; CC, cranial condyle of the maxilla; D, dentary; FAAP, fossa for the adductor arcus palatini; IM, intermandibularis; L_1, interoperculomandibular ligament; L_2, ligament between rostral cartilage and head of maxilla; MX, maxilla; MXPP, maxillary process of the palatine; P, palatine; SA, suspensory apparatus; TAM_1, tendon of part A1 of the adductor mandibulae; TAM_2, tendon of part A_2 of the adductor mandibulae muscle. TAM_3, tendon of part A3 of the adductor mandibulae.

sensory apparatus greatly affecting the feeding strategies. The pit is housed in a deep base fossa of the maxilla which also carries the fang. Because of the mechanical demands, the maxilla possesses a condyle to articulate with a fossa in the ectopterygoid. In the true vipers devoid of a pit, the fang-bearing maxilla has a fossa instead of a condyle, to receive a condyle of the ectopterygoid. These seemingly slight differences in the maxillary-ectopterygoid joint have important consequences on the axes of movements of the maxilla which underlie the envenomation process (Dullemeijer 1959; Liem et al. 1971; Liem 1990b).

However, not all evolutionary changes in the vertebrate skull can be understood or explained in terms of the manifest fit of skull design with its feeding ecology (e.g. Liem 1980a, b; Goldschmid and Kotrschal 1985, 1989; Kotrschal 1989a, b; Kotrschal 1987; Kotrschal and Lindquist 1986). There are four major reasons that some skull designs are not strictly or directly adaptive:

(1) Many evolutionary changes may be adaptive and yet the resulting differences among taxa in the character may not be adaptive. They may simply represent alternative solutions to the problem because of historical (genealogical) factors. Thus piscivory and capture of large elusive prey may be solved with different skull designs in cichlids, characoids, clupeoids (Liem 1990a), esocoids, and luciocephaloids (Lauder and Liem 1981).

(2) Many design features in the skull evolve as the result of differential growth or allometry (see, e.g., Strauss 1984). The relative growth rates of different parts of the skull of teleosts are different, so that larger fishes do not have all their parts of the skull in the same proportion.

(3) The phenomenon of pleiotropy is well known and documented in many organisms, but because ecomorphologists have been preoccupied working within the conceptual constraints of the ecomorphological (or adaptive) paradigm, pleiotropic effects, which do not relate to the ecological factors in the fish skull, remain to be discovered.

(4) Developmental constraints and early life history stages may hold the decisive rein over possible evolutionary pathways leading to the adult skull designs. It is very likely that early life history stages are often subjected to selection pressures of much higher magnitude than in adult fishes (see, e.g., Balon 1985). Skull design of early life history stages must be critically attuned to the changing biological roles in feeding and respiration throughout the ontogeny of teleost fishes, if the larvae are to survive at all (fig. 10.12; Otten 1983a, b; Drost et al. 1988; Liem 1991). Since early development so strongly restricts later development, the resulting adult skull design may well be a compromise rather than an adaptive optimum. Experimental and field studies have provided ample evidence that adult teleost skulls and associated structures have a built-in functional plasticity conducive to extensive prey switching (Stoner 1980; Liem 1980a, b, 1984; Goulding 1980; Lauder 1981; McKaye and Marsh 1983; Ribbink et al. 1983). Thus, in sharp contrast to the condition in ontogenetic stages, the functional design of the adult teleost head offers generally a greater variety of alternative paths favoring an individual's survival in changing environments with changing food supplies. Such a developmental pattern may produce multiple solutions to the same problems in the feeding apparatus of teleosts belonging to diverse phylogenetic lineages.

However, adaptation is a real phenomenon. Ecomorphology should offer a holistic and pluralistic approach to the study of organismic diversity and adaptation. An exclusive focus on the perfect fit of design with environmental parameters is difficult to test "because simplifying assumptions and ingenious explanations [on compromises in design for constructional reasons] can almost always result in *ad hoc* adaptive explanation" (Lewontin 1978). Thus, ecomorphology should go beyond the exclusive search for adaptive explanations of animal diversity, and include the genealogical factors, which according to the concept of symecomorphosis, are as important as economic factors (Schaefer and Lauder 1986; Liem 1989). Furthermore, in explaining teleost skull diversity, it is essential to understand the developmental pathways of functional units in early life history stages, which may be under strong selection pressures. Ontogeny may hold the decisive reign over possible evolutionary pathways leading to the adult skull. A clear understanding of the nature of polymorphisms and ecomorphological plasticity may shed light on the great variety of alternative paths by which a given skull design may change, so that some of the features will allow selection to act on them without affecting other features adversely (Liem and Kaufman 1984). Allometric relations between various skull components should be analyzed in an ecomorphological framework in order to test the nonadaptive hypothesis as a competing hypothesis of the ecomorphological paradigm (Strauss 1984). Studies (Greenwood 1965; Meyer 1987; Hoogerhoud 1986) have demonstrated how phenotypic plasticity permits some cichlid fishes to mold their skull design to prevailing circumstances of prey items during ontogeny. Such approaches hold considerable promise in future ecomorphological studies. Pluralistic analysis of the biological roles of the functional units should include long-term studies to understand the possible effects of ecological crunches or bottlenecks (Wiens 1977; Liem and Kaufman 1984) during which the adaptive significance of a design feature may suddenly come to light. Some skull designs may not be perfect fits (from economic points of view) for the exploitation of the preferred diet during high food abundance, but appear to be adaptations for secondary refugium prey during ecological bottlenecks or crises.

Boag and Grant (1981) have shown that the design of the bill, jaw apparatus, and musculature in *Geospiza magnirostris* is especially important during periods of intense selection (ecological bottlenecks). Studies on trophic polymorphisms in turtles (John Legler, personal communication), birds (Boag and Grant 1981; Smith 1987) and fishes (Liem and Kaufman 1984; Meyer 1990) provide an important link between functional morphology and ecological tracking of food resources.

Ecomorphological research can become more powerful in elucidating holistic adaptations by developing approaches to measure differential performances emanating from the various neuromuscular outputs intraspecifically and interspecifically. Comparative quantitative assessments of correlations between design, performance, and fitness (e.g., Emerson and Arnold 1989) may become an especially fertile research area for ecomorphologists. Combined comparative field and laboratory studies may then yield the key to a better understanding of adaptation from an ecomorphological perspective, especially if historical factors are included by applying comparative studies within a phylogenetic framework (Lauder and Liem 1989; Jensen 1990).

REFERENCES

Aerts, P., J. W. M. Osse, and W. Verraes. 1987. Model of jaw depression during feeding in *Astatotilapia elegans* (Teleostei: Cichlidae): Mechanisms for energy storage and triggering. Journal of Morphology 194: 85–109.

Arnold, S. J. 1983. Morphology, performance, and fitness. American Zoologist 23: 347–361.

Balon, E. K. 1985. *Early Life Histories of Fishes: New Developmental, Ecological, and Evolutionary Perspectives.* Dordrecht: W. Funk Publishers.

Barel, C. D. N. 1983. Towards a constructional morphology of cichlid fishes (Teleostei: Perciformes). Netherlands Journal of Zoology 33: 357–424.

Barel, C. D. N., G. Ch. Anker, F. Witte, R. J. C. Hoogerhoud, and T. Goldschmidt. 1989. Constructional constraint and its ecomorphological implications. Acta morphologica neerlando-scandinavica 27: 23–109.

Bemis, W. E., and G. V. Lauder. 1986. Morphology and function of the feeding apparatus of the lungfish, *Lepidosiren paradoxa* (Dipnoi). Journal of Morphology 187: 81–108.

Bentsen, P., and J. D. McPhail. 1984. Ecology and evolution of sympatric sticklebacks (*Gasterosteus*): Specialization for alternative trophic niches in the Enos Lake species pair. Canadian Journal of Zoology 62: 2280–2286.

Boag, P. T., and P. R. Grant. 1981. Intense natural selection in a population of Darwin's finches (Geospizinae) in the Galapagos. Science 214: 82–86.

Bock, W. J. 1959. Preadaptation and multiple evolutionary pathways. Evolution 13: 194–211.

———. 1977a. Adaptation and the comparative method. In *Major Patterns in Vertebrate Evolution,* M. K. Hecht, P. C. Goody, and B. M. Hecht, eds. New York: Plenum Press, pp. 57–82.

———. 1977b. Toward an ecological morphology. Die Vogelwarte 29: 127–135.

Bock, W. J., and G. von Wahlert. 1965. Adaptation and the form-function complex. Evolution 19: 269–299.

Bowman, R. I. 1961. Morphological differentiation and adaptation in the Galapagos finches. University of California, Publications in Zoology 58: 1–302.

Brainerd, E. L. 1985. An experimental analysis of prey capture mechanisms in teleost fishes with implications for present hydrodynamical models of suction feeding. Honor's thesis, Harvard University.

Bramble, D., and D. B. Wake. 1985. Feeding mechanisms of lower tetrapods. In *Functional Vertebrate Morphology,* M. Hildebrand, D. M. Bramble, K. F. Liem, and D. Wake, eds. Cambridge: Harvard University Press, pp. 230–261.

Chao, L. N., and J. A. Musick. 1977. Life history, feeding habits, and functional morphology of juvenile sciaenid fishes in the York River estuary, Virginia. Fishery Bulletin, U.S. 75: 657–702.

Clements, K. D., and D. R. Bellwood. 1988. A comparison of the feeding mechanisms of two herbivorous labroid fishes, the temperate *Odax pullus* and the tropical *Scarus rubroviolaceus*. Australian Journal of Marine Freshwater Research 39: 87–107.

Coughlin, D. J. 1991. The ontogeny of feeding behavior during the early life of fishes. Ph.D. diss., Boston University.

Coughlin, D. J., and J. R. Strickler. 1990. Zooplankton capture by a coral reef fish: An adaptive response to evasive prey. Environmental Biology of Fishes 29: 35–42.

Davis, W. P., and R. S. Birdsong. 1973. Coral reef fishes which forage in the water column: A review of their morphology, behavior, ecology, and evolutionary implications. *Helgolander* Wissenschaftliche Meeresuntersuchungen 24: 292–306.

De Martini, E. E. 1969. A correlative study of the ecology and comparative feeding mechanism morphology of the Embiotocidae (surf-fishes) as evidence of the family's adaptive radiation into available ecological niches. *Wasmann* Journal of Biology 27: 177–247.

De Silva, S. S., P. R. T. Cumaranatunga, and C. D. De Silva. 1980. Food, feeding ecology, and morphological features associated with feeding of four co-occuring cyprinids (Pisces: Cyprinide). Netherlands Journal of Zoology 30: 54–73.

Dilling, L. 1989. An ontogenetic study of the jaw morphology and feeding modes in *Amphiprion frenatus* and *A. polymnus*. Honor's thesis, Harvard University.

Drost, M. R., J. W. M. Osse, and M. Muller. 1988. Prey capture by fish larvae, water flow patterns, and the effect of escape movements of prey. Netherlands Journal of Zoology 38: 23–45.

Dullemeijer, P. 1956. The functional morphology of the head of the common viper, *Vipera berus* (L). Archives Néerlandaises de Zoologie 11: 386–497.

———. 1959. A comparative functional anatomical study of the heads of some Viperidae. Morphologische Jahrbuch 99: 881–985.

———. 1972. Explanation in morphology. Acta biotheoretica 21: 260–273.

———. 1974. Concepts and approaches in animal morphology. Assen: Van Gorcum.

———. 1980. Animal ecology and morphology. Netherlands Journal of Zoology 30: 161–178.

Eberling, A. W., and G. M. Cailliet. 1974. Mouth size and predatory strategy of midwater fishes. *Deep-sea Research* 21: 959–968.

Elshoud-Oldenhave, M. J. W., and J. Osse. 1976. Functional morphology of the feeding system of the ruff—*Gymnocephalus cernua* (L. 1758)—Teleostei, Percidae. Journal of Morphology 150: 399–422.

Emerson, S. B., and S. Arnold. 1989. Intra- and interspecific relationships between morphology, performance, and fitness. In *Complex Organismal Functions: Integration and Evolution in Vertebrates,* D. B. Wake and G. Roth, eds. New York: John Wiley, pp. 295–314.

Emery, A. R. 1973. Comparative ecology and functional osteology of fourteen species of damselfish (Pisces: Pomacentridae) at Alligator Reef, Florida Keys. Bulletin of Marine Science 23: 649–770.

Felley, J. D. 1984. Multivariate identification of morphological-environmental relationships within the cyprinidae (Pisces), Copeia: 442–455.

Fryer, G., and T. D. Iles. 1972. *The Cichlid Fishes of the Great Lakes of Africa: Their Biology and Evolution.* Edinburgh: Oliver and Boyd.

Gans, C. 1974. *Biomechanics: An Approach to Vertebrate Biology.* Philadelphia: Lippincott Co.

Gatz, A. J., Jr. 1979a. Community organization in fishes as indicated by morphological features. Ecology 60: 711–718.

———. 1979b. Ecological morphology of freshwater fishes. Tulane Studies in Zoology and Botany 21: 91–124.

Goldschmid, A., and K. Kotrschal. 1985. Morphological and functional adaptations in different feeding types of blennies (Perciformes; Teleostei). Fortschritte der Zoologie 30: 241–244.

Goldschmid, A., and K. Kotrschal. 1989. Ecomorphology: Development and concepts. Fortschritte der Zoologie 35: 501–512.

Gould, S. J., and R. C. Lewontin, 1979. The Spandrels of San Marco and the Panglossian paradigm: A critique of the adaptationist programme. Proceedings of the Royal Society of London B 205: 581–598.

Goulding, M. 1980. *The Fishes and the Forest: Explorations in Amazonian Natural History.* Berkeley: University of California Press.

Grant, P. R. 1986. Ecology and evolution of Darwin's finches. Princeton: Princeton University Press.

Grant, P. R., B. R. Grant, J. N. M. Smith, I. J. Abbott, and L. K. Abbott. 1976. Darwin's finches: Population variation and natural selection. Proceedings of the National Academy of Science 73: 257–261.

Greenwood, P. H. 1965. Environmental effects on the pharyngeal mill of a cichlid fish, *Astatoreochromis alluaudi,* and their taxonomic implications. Proceedings of the Linnean Society, London 176: 1–10.

———. 1978. Cichlid fishes of Lake Victoria, East Africa: The biology and evolution of a species flock. Bulletin of the British Museum of Natural History (Zoology), suppl., 6: 1–134.

Hespenheide, H. A. 1973. Prey characteristics and predator niche width. In *Ecology and Evolution of Communities,* M. L. Cody and J. M. Diamond, eds. Cambridge: Belknap Press, pp. 158–180.

Hiiemae K., and Crompton, A. W. 1985. Mastication, food transport, and swallowing. In *Functional Vertebrate Morphology,* M. Hildebrand, D. M. Bramble, K. F. Liem, and D. Wake, eds. Cambridge: Harvard University Press, pp. 230–261.

Hoogerhoud, R. J. C. 1986. Ecological morphology of some cichlid fishes. Ph.D. diss., University of Leiden, The Netherlands.

Jensen, J. S. 1990. *Plausibility and Testability: Assessing the Consequences of Evolutionary Innovation.* M. Nitecki, ed. Chicago: University of Chicago Press, pp. 171–190.

Karr, J. R., and F. C. James. 1975. Eco-morphological configurations and convergent evolution in species and communities. In *Ecology and Evolution of Communities,* M. L. Cody and J. M. Diamond, eds. Cambridge: Belknap Press, pp. 258–291.

Keast, A., and D. Webb. 1966. Mouth and body form relative to feeding ecology in the fish fauna of a small lake, Lake Opinicon, Ontario. Journal of the Fisheries Research Board of Canada 23: 1845–1874.

Klaauw, C. J. van der. 1948. Ecological studies and reviews. IV. Ecological morphology. *Bibliotheca biotheoretica 4* (2): 27–111.

Kotrschal, K. 1987. Evolutionary patterns in tropical marine reef fishes. Zeitschrift für Zoologisches Systematik und Evolutionsforschung 26: 51–64.

———. 1988. A catalogue of skulls and jaws of eastern tropical Pacific blennioid fishes (Blennioidei: Teleostei): A proposed evolutionary sequence of morphological change. Zeitschrift der Zoologisches Systematik und Evolutionsforschung 26: 442–466.

———. 1989a. On the biological role of form: Evolutionary trophic ecomorphology in 34 Gulf of California blennioid fishes. Fortschritte der Zoologie 35: 517–518.

———. 1989b. Trophic ecomorphology in Eastern Pacific blennioid fishes: Character transformation and associated change of their biological roles. Environmental Biology of Fishes 24: 199–218.

Kotrschal, K., and A. Goldschmid. 1983. Food preferences, morphology, and arrangement of teeth in 14 species of Adriatic blennies. Thalassia jugoslavica 19: 217–219.

Kotrschal, K., and D. G. Lindquist. 1986. The feeding apparatus in four Pacific tube blennies (Teleostei: Chaenopsidae): Lack of ecomorphological divergence in synoptic species. Marine Ecology 7: 241–254.

Kotrschal, K., and D. A. Thomson. 1989. From suckers towards pickers and biters: Evolutionary patterns in trophic ecomorphology of tropical marine reef fishes. Fortschritte der Zoologie 36: 564–568.

Lauder, G. V. 1980. Hydrodynamics of prey capture in teleost fishes. In *Biofluid Mechanics,* vol. 2, D. Schenck, ed. New York: Plenum Press, pp. 661–181.

———. 1981. Intraspecific functional repertoires in the feeding mechanism of the characoid fishes *Lebiasina, Hoplias,* and *Chalceus.* Copeia: 154–168.

———. 1982. Historical biology and the problems of design. Journal of Theoretical Biology 97: 57–67.

———. 1983a. Functional and morphological bases of trophic specialization in sunfishes (Teleostei: Centrarchidae). Journal of Morphology 178: 1–21.

———. 1983b. Neuromuscular patterns and the origin of trophic specialization in fishes. Science 219: 1235–1237.

———. 1983c. Prey capture hydrodynamics in fishes: Experimental tests of two models. Journal of Experimental Biology 104: 1–13.

———. 1985. Aquatic feeding in lower vertebrates. In *Functional Vertebrate Morphology,* M. Hildebrand, D. M. Bramble, K. F. Liem, and D. Wake, eds. Cambridge: Harvard University Press, pp. 210–229.

Lauder, G. V., and K. F. Liem. 1981. Prey capture by *Luciocephalus pulcher:* Implications for models of jaw protrusion in teleost fishes. Environmental Biology of Fishes 6: 257–268.

———. 1989. The role of historical factors in the evolution of complex organismal functions. Dahlem Workshop Reports, W. Berlin: 63–78.

Lederer, H. F. 1984. A review of avian ecomorphological hypotheses. Ökologie der Vögel 6: 119–126.

Leisler, B., and H. Winkler. 1985. Ecomorphology. In *Current Ornithology*, vol. 2, R. F. Johnston, ed. New York: Plenum Publishing, pp. 155–186.

Lewontin, R. C. 1978. Adaptation. Scientific American 157–169.

Liem, K. F. 1974. Evolutionary strategies and morphological innovations: Cichlid pharyngeal jaw. Systematic Zoology 22: 425–441.

———. 1978. Modulatory multiplicity in the functional repertoire of the feeding mechanism in cichlid fishes. I. Piscivores. Journal of Morphology 158: 323–360.

———. 1979. Modulatory multiplicity in the feeding mechanism of cichlid fishes, as exemplified by the invertebrate pickers of Lake Tanganyika. Journal of Zoology, London 189: 93–125.

———. 1980a. Acquisition of energy by teleosts: Adaptive mechanisms and evolutionary patterns. In *Environmental Physiology of Fishes*, M. A. Ali, ed. New York: Plenum Press, pp. 299–334.

———. 1980b. Adaptive significance of intra- and interspecific differences in the feeding repertoires of cichlid fishes. American Zoologist 20: 295–314.

———. 1984. Functional versatility, speciation, and niche overlap: Are fishes different? In *Trophic Interactions within Aquatic Ecosystems*, D. G. Meyers and J. R. Strickler, eds. AAAS Selected Symposium 85. Boulder, Colo.: Westview Press, pp. 269–305.

———. 1989. Functional morphology and phylogenetic testing within the framework of symecomorphosis. Acta morphologica neerlando-scandinavica 27: 119–131.

———. 1990a. Aquatic versus terrestrial feeding modes: Possible impacts on the trophic ecology of vertebrates. American Zoologist 30: 209–221.

———. 1990b. Key evolutionary innovations, differential diversity, and symecomorphosis. In *Evolutionary Innovations*, M. Nitecki ed. Chicago: University of Chicago Press, pp. 147–170.

———. 1991. A functional approach to the development of the head of teleosts: implications on constructional morphology and constraints. In *Constructional Morphology and Evolution*, N. Schmidt-Kittler and K. Vogel, eds. Berlin: Springer-Verlag, pp. 231–249.

Liem, K. F., and L. S. Kaufman. 1984. Intraspecific macroevolution: Functional biology of the polymorphic cichlid species *Cichlasoma minckleyi*. In *Evolution of Fish Species Flocks*, A. A. Echelle and I. Kornfield, eds. Orono: University of Maine at Orono Press, pp. 203–215.

Liem, K. F., H. Marx, and G. B. Rabb. 1971. The viperid snake *Azemiops:* Its comparative cephalic anatomy and phylogenetic position in relation to Viperinae and Crotalinae. Fieldiana: Zoology 59: 67–126.

Liem, K. F., and D. J. Stewart. 1976. Evolution of the scale-eating cichlid fishes of Lake Tanganyika: A generic revision with a description of a new species. Bulletin of the Museum of Comparative Zoology 147: 319–350.

Lombard, R. E., and D. B. Wake. 1976. Tongue evolution in lungless salamanders, family Plethodontidae. I. Introduction, theory, and general model of dynamics. Journal of Morphology 148: 265–286.

————. 1977. Tongue evolution in lungless salamanders, family Plethodontidae. II. Function and evolutionary diversity. Journal of Morphology 153: 39–80.

McKaye, K. R., and A. Marsh. 1983. Food switching by two specialized algae-scraping cichlid fishes in Lake Malawi, Africa. Oecologia, Berlin 56: 245–248.

Meyer, A. 1987. Phenotypic plasticity and heterochrony in *Cichlasoma managuense* (Pisces, Cichlidae) and their implications for speciation in cichlid fishes. Evolution 41: 1357–1369.

————. 1990. Ecological and evolutionary consequences of the trophic polymorphism in *Cichlasoma citrinellum* (Pisces: Cichlidae). Biological Journal of the Linnean Society 39: 279–299.

Mittelbach, G. G. 1984. Predation and resource partitioning in two sunfishes (Centrarchidae). Ecology 65: 499–513.

Motta, P. J. 1988. Functional morphology of the feeding apparatus of ten species of Pacific butterflyfishes (Perciformes: Chaetodontidae): An eco-morphological approach. Environmental Biology of Fishes 22: 39–67.

Moyle, P. P., and F. R. Senanayake. 1984. Resource partitioning among the fishes of rainforest streams in Sri Lanka. Journal of Zoology, London 202: 195–223.

Muller, M., and J. W. M. Osse. 1984. Hydrodynamics of suction feeding in fish. Transactions of the Zoological Society of London 37: 1–136.

Muller, M., J. W. M. Osse, and J. H. G. Verhagen. 1982. A quantitative hydrodynamical model of suction feeding in fish. Journal of Theoretical Biology 95: 49–79.

Norton, S. F. 1989. Constraints on the foraging ecology of subtidal cottid fishes. Ph.D. diss., University of California at Santa Barbara.

Oijen, M. J. P. van. 1982. Ecological differentiation among the haplochromine piscivorous species of Lake Victoria. Netherlands Journal of Zoology 32: 336–363.

Osse, J. W. M., and M. Muller. 1980. A model of suction feeding in teleostean fishes with some implications for ventilation. In *Environmental Physiology of Fishes*, M. A. Ali, ed. New York: Plenum, pp. 335–351.

————. 1985. Jaw protrusion, an optimization of the feeding apparatus of teleosts. *Acta biotheoretica* 34: 219–232.

Otten, E. 1982. The development of a mouth-opening mechanism in a generalized *Haplochromis* species: *H. elegans* Trewavas 1933 (Pisces; Cichlidae). *Netherlands Journal of Zoology* 32: 31–48.

————. 1983a. The jaw mechanism during growth of a generalized *Haplochromis* species: *H. elegans* Trewavas, 1933 (Pisces: Cichlidae). Netherlands Journal of Zoology 33: 55–98.

————. 1983b. Vision and jaw mechanism during growth of the cichlid fish *Haplochromis elegans:* Changes and functional implications. Ph.D. diss., University of Leiden, The Netherlands.

Ribbink, A. J., B. A. Marsh, A. C. Marsh, A. C. Ribbink, and B. J. Sharp. 1983. A preliminary survey of the cichlid fishes of rocky habitats in Lake Malawi. African Journal of Zoology 18: 149–310.

Sanderson, S. L. 1988. Variation in neuromuscular activity during prey capture by trophic specialists and generalists (Pisces: Labridae). Behavior and Evolution 32: 257–268.

Schaefer, S. A., and G. V. Lauder. 1986. Historical transformation of functional design: Evolutionary morphology of the feeding mechanism in loricarioid catfishes. Systematic Zoology 35: 489–508.

Schmitt, R., and A. J. Coyer 1982. The foraging ecology of sympatric marine fish in the genus *Embiotoca* (Embiotocidae): Importance of foraging behavior in prey size selection. Oecologia 55: 369–378.

Schoener, T. W. 1983. Field experiments on intraspecific competition. American Naturalist 122: 240–285.

Smith, C. L., and J. C. Tyler. 1973. Direct observations of resource sharing in coral reef fish. Helgolander wissenschaftliche Meeresuntersuchungen 24: 264–275.

Smith, T. B. 1987. Bill size polymorphism and niche utilization in an African finch. *Nature* 329: 717–719.

Stein, R. A., C. G. Goodman, and E. A. Marshall. 1984. Using time and energetic measures of cost in estimating prey value for fish predators. Ecology 65: 702–715.

Stoner, A. W. 1980. Feeding ecology of *Lagodon rhomboides* (Pisces, Sparidae): Variation and functional responses. Fishery Bulletin, U.S. 78: 337–352.

Strauss, R. E. 1984. Allometry and functional feeding morphology in haplochromine cichlids. In *Evolution of Fish Species Flocks*, A. Echelle and I. Kornfield, eds. Orono: University of Maine.

Wainwright, P. C. 1987. Biomechanical limits to ecological performance: Mollusc-crushing by the Caribbean hogfish, *Lachnolaimus maximus* (Labridae). Journal of Zoology, London 213: 283–297.

———. 1988. Morphology and ecology: Functional basis of feeding constraints in Caribbean labrid fishes. Ecology 69: 635–645.

Wainwright, P. C., and G. V. Lauder. 1986. Feeding biology of sunfishes: Patterns of variation in prey capture. Zoological Journal of the Linnean Society, London 88: 217–288.

Werner, E. E. 1977. Species packing and niche complementarity in three sunfishes. American Naturalist 111: 553–577.

Werner, E. E., and D. J. Hall. 1979. Foraging efficiency and habitat switching in competing sunfishes. Ecology 60: 256–264.

Westneat, M. W., and P. C. Wainwright. 1989. Feeding mechanism of *Epibulus insidiator* (Labridae: Teleostei): Evolution of a novel functional system. Journal of Morphology 202: 129–150.

Wiens, J. A. 1977. On competition and variable environments. American Scientist 65: 590–597.

Witte, F. 1984. Ecological differentiation in Lake Victoria haplochromines: Comparison of cichlid species flocks in African lakes. In *Evolution of Fish Species Flocks,* A. A. Echelle and I. Kornfield, eds. Orono: University of Maine at Orono Press, pp. 155–167.

Yamaoka, K. 1982. Morphology and feeding behavior of five species of genus *Petrochromis* (Teleostei: Cichlidae). Physiological Ecology of Japan 19: 57–75.

————. 1983. Feeding behaviour and dental morphology of algae-scraping cichlids (Pisces: Teleostei) in Lake Tanganyika. African Study Monographs 4: 77–89.

————. 1987. Comparative osteology of the jaw of algal feeding cichlids (Pisces, Teleostei) from Lake Tanganyika. Reports, USA Marine Biological Institute 9: 87–137.

Yamaoka, K., M. Hori, and S. Kuratani. 1986. Ecomorphology of feeding in "Goby-like" cichlid fishes in Lake Tanganyika. Physiological Ecology of Japan 23: 17–29.

Zweers, G. A. 1979. Explanation of structure by optimization and systematization. Netherlands Journal of Zoology 29: 418–440.

LIST OF CONTRIBUTORS

Dennis M. Bramble
Department of Biology
University of Utah
Salt Lake City, Utah 84112
U.S.A.

Sharon B. Emerson
Department of Biology
University of Utah
Salt Lake City, Utah 84112
U.S.A.

Brian K. Hall
Department of Biology
Dalhousie University
Halifax, Nova Scotia B3H 4J1
Canada

James Hanken
Department of Environmental,
    Population, and Organismic Biology
University of Colorado
Boulder, Colorado 80309-0334
U.S.A.

Thomas E. Hetherington
Department of Zoology
Ohio State University
1735 Neil Avenue
Columbus, Ohio 43210-1293
U.S.A.

George V. Lauder
School of Biological Sciences
University of California, Irvine
Irvine, California 92717
U.S.A.

Karel F. Liem
Museum of Comparative Zoology
Harvard University
Cambridge, Massachusetts 02138
U.S.A.

R. Eric Lombard
Department of Organismic Biology
    and Anatomy
University of Chicago
Chicago, Illinois 60637
U.S.A.

Anthony P. Russell
Department of Biological Sciences
University of Calgary
2500 University Drive, N.W.
Calgary, Alberta T2N 1N4
Canada

S. Laurie Sanderson
Department of Biology
College of William and Mary
P.O. Box 8795
Williamsburg, Virginia 23185-8795
U.S.A.

H. Bradley Shaffer
Department of Zoology
University of California, Davis
Davis, California 95616
U.S.A.

Kathleen K. Smith
Department of Biological
   Anthropology and Anatomy
Duke University Medical Center
Durham, North Carolina 27710
U.S.A.

Jeffrey J. Thomason
Basic Sciences
College of Osteopathic Medicine
Ohio University
Athens, Ohio 45701-2979
U.S.A.

Marvalee H. Wake
Department of Integrative Biology and Museu
   of Vertebrate Zoology
University of California, Berkeley
Berkeley, California 94720
U.S.A.

Richard Wassersug
Department of Anatomy
Dalhouse University
Halifax, Nova Scotia B3H 4H7
Canada

David B. Weishampel
Department of Cell Biology
   and Anatomy
School of Medicine
Johns Hopkins University
Baltimore, Maryland 21205
U.S.A.

INDEX